Medical Radiology

Diagnostic Imaging

Series Editors

Hans-Ulrich Kauczor
Paul M. Parizel
Wilfred C. G. Peh

For further volumes:
http://www.springer.com/series/4354

Lluís Donoso-Bach • Giles W. L. Boland
Editors

Quality and Safety in Imaging

Springer

Editors
Lluís Donoso-Bach
Department of Diagnostic Imaging,
Hospital Clinic of Barcelona,
University of Barcelona,
Barcelona
Spain

Giles W. L. Boland
Department of Radiology,
Brigham and Women's Hospital,
Harvard Medical School,
Boston, MA
USA

ISSN 0942-5373 ISSN 2197-4187 (electronic)
Medical Radiology
ISBN 978-3-030-13254-5 ISBN 978-3-319-42578-8 (eBook)
https://doi.org/10.1007/978-3-319-42578-8

This Springer imprint is published by the registered company Springer Nature Switzerland AG
The registered company address is: Gewerbestrasse 11, 6330 Cham, Switzerland

Contents

Contributors

Jane Adam Department of Radiology, St. George's Hospital, London, UK

Angel Alberich-Bayarri Biomedical Imaging Research Group (GIBI230), La Fe Health Research Institute, La Fe Polytechnics and University Hospital, Valencia, Spain

Quantitative Imaging Biomarkers in Medicine (QUIBIM SL), Valencia, Spain

Tarik K. Alkasab Harvard Medical School, Boston, MA, USA

Department of Radiology, Massachusetts General Hospital, Boston, MA, USA

H. Benjamin Harvey Harvard Medical School, Boston, MA, USA

Department of Radiology, Massachusetts General Hospital, Boston, MA, USA

Institute for Technology Assessment, Massachusetts General Hospital, Boston, MA, USA

Lincoln L. Berland Department of Radiology, University of Alabama at Birmingham, Birmingham, AL, USA

Michael Bettmann Wake Forest University School of Medicine, Winston-Salem, NC, USA

American College of Radiology, Reston, VA, USA

Bernardo C. Bizzo Harvard Medical School, Boston, MA, USA

Department of Radiology, Massachusetts General Hospital, Boston, MA, USA

Giles W. L. Boland Department of Radiology, Brigham and Women's Hospital, Boston, MA, USA

Harvard Medical School, Boston, MA, USA

Jan M. L. Bosmans Ghent University Hospital, Ghent, Flanders, Belgium

Ghent University, Ghent, Flanders, Belgium

University of Antwerp, Antwerp, Flanders, Belgium

Brian E. Chapman Department of Radiology and Imaging Sciences, University of Utah School of Medicine, Salt Lake City, UT, USA

Laila Cochon Department of Radiology, Center for Evidence-Based Imaging, Brigham and Women's Hospital, Harvard Medical School, Boston, MA, USA

Justin Cramer Department of Radiology, University of Nebraska Medical Center, Omaha, NE, USA

Jaap Deinum Department for Health Evidence, Health Technology Assessment Group, Radboud Institute for Health Sciences, Radboud University Medical Center, Nijmegen, The Netherlands

Ronald Eisenberg Department of Radiology, Beth Israel Deaconess Medical Center, Harvard Medical School, Boston, MA, USA

Donald P. Frush Pediatric Radiology, Duke Medical Center, Durham, NC, USA

Marta E. Heilbrun Department of Radiology and Imaging Sciences, Emory University School of Medicine, Atlanta, GA, USA

Myriam Hunink Erasmus University Medical Center, Rotterdam, The Netherlands

Harvard T.H. Chan School of Public Health, Boston, MA, USA

Netherlands Institute for Health Sciences (NIHES), Rotterdam, The Netherlands

Mannudeep K. Kalra Divisions of Thoracic and CardioVascular Imaging, Department of Radiology, Webster Center for Quality and Safety, Massachusetts General Hospital, Boston, MA, USA

Ramin Khorasani Department of Radiology, Center for Evidence-Based Imaging, Brigham and Women's Hospital, Harvard Medical School, Boston, MA, USA

Jonathan Kruskal Department of Radiology, Beth Israel Deaconess Medical Center, Harvard Medical School, Boston, MA, USA

Romeo Laroya II Department of Radiology, Center for Evidence-Based Imaging, Brigham and Women's Hospital, Harvard Medical School, Boston, MA, USA

Peter Makai Department for Health Evidence, Health Technology Assessment Group, Radboud Institute for Health Sciences, Radboud University Medical Center, Nijmegen, The Netherlands

Peter Mildenberger Department of Radiology, University Medical Center Mainz, Mainz, Germany

Erik R. Ranschaert EUSOMII, H. Hartziekenhuis, Flanders, Belgium

Gabriela Restovic Health Technology Assessment Unit, Research and Innovation Directorate, Hospital Clínic, University of Barcelona, Barcelona, Spain

Laura Sampietro-Colom Health Technology Assessment Unit, Research and Innovation Directorate, Hospital Clínic, University of Barcelona, Barcelona, Spain

Gert Jan van der Wilt Department for Health Evidence, Health Technology Assessment Group, Radboud Institute for Health Sciences, Radboud University Medical Center, Nijmegen, The Netherlands

Jessica G. Zarzour Department of Radiology, University of Alabama at Birmingham, Birmingham, AL, USA

Part I

Introduction

Framing the Issues

Giles W.L. Boland

Quality and safety is increasingly ascendant in medicine as systems are focused on delivering better value and outcomes to patients and payers. However, even with the many checks and balances being introduced into clinical workflows, medical systems are still challenged to deliver consistent, evidenced-based best practices at the point of care. In the United States, the Institute of Medicine believes that close to 100,000 deaths/annum are created by medical error and some opinions believe that number to be closer to 400,000 lives. There is no known worldwide statistic but it almost certainly runs into the millions. While radiological procedures may usually seem non-life threatening, there is still considerable risk, real or perceived. Certainly, invasive interventional procedures do carry significant risk, even death (i.e., angiography or percutaneous biopsy). Other procedures have theoretical risk such as the effects of radiation dose exposure (even at lower doses) mainly from Computed Tomography, discussed elsewhere in this book. Furthermore, there is widespread variation in the use of appropriate examinations (imaging tests) for a particular condition, sometimes referred to as appropriateness (see other chapters in this book). In fact, despite much evidence on the use of appropriate best practices for radiological procedures (usually promulgated by national radiological societies), variation in the practice of radiology abounds, usually with no two departments alike delivering similar practices and operating procedures. What might seem appropriate in one department is often not seen in another—for instance, what is viewed as an acceptable radiation dose varies across regions, towns, and sometimes even within the same health organization. Given this widespread variation, legislative, payer, and professional bodies are now finding this scenario unacceptable and are introducing legislation or pay-for-performance measures to drive organizations to deliver more consistent and better care with outcomes that meet certain predetermined standards. Furthermore, patients themselves are now demanding better outcomes and less variation, particularly as it has become more evident from the press that outcomes can significantly vary from one organization to another. This has come at a time when demand for imaging services is busier than ever as referrers continue to see imaging as a key tool to reach a diagnosis earlier, monitor therapy more closely, and/or cure and palliate patients through innovative interventional therapies. This significant increase in radiological volume has sometimes come at the cost of quality (and even safety) as radiologists and departments are busier than ever trying to keep up with demand of simply

G.W.L. Boland, M.D.
Department of Radiology, Brigham and Women's Hospital, Francis Street, Boston, MA, USA

Harvard Medical School, Boston, MA, USA
e-mail: Boland.Giles@BWH.HARVARD.EDU

Med Radiol Diagn Imaging (2018)
DOI 10.1007/174_2017_145, © Springer International Publishing AG
Published Online 08 February 2018

performing and interpreting the procedures. Often departments are just too inundated with the workload to take a step back to rethink fundamentally how quality and safety initiatives can be reorganized in a meaningful and systematic way to drive the delivery of care towards better practices and outcomes. Quality and safety measures, which are often difficult to measure, let alone deemed as meaningful in the first place, are then sometimes seen as an afterthought. Even experts often struggle to define standards and then agree upon them. Furthermore, measures put in place to monitor quality and safety are frequently imposed from afar, often by payers (i.e., large bureaucracies such as the Center for Medicare and Medicare Service or the National Health Service) and therefore deemed onerous and unnecessarily imposing by front-line providers. This can result in frustration and ambivalence towards the quality and safety agenda. The approach of many radiologists to many of the quality and safety measures is to simply "check the box" so they can either meet their mandatory compliance standards or, in increasing circumstances, actually get paid. There is a common belief that many of the quality and safety standards are either only tangentially relevant or sometimes not meaningful at all. Added to this frustration, the practice of medicine and radiology keeps changing and even experts find it difficult to keep up with new technologies, treatments, and new care pathways such that creating meaningful, up-to-date, and relevant metrics inevitably lags the innovation. Finally, although pay-for-performance measures are now tying part of payments to performance (sometimes quality and safety), much of what can be achieved through quality and safety initiatives is not reimbursed. Considering the numerous other non-remunerated regulatory and compliance measures required from radiologists, quality and safety initiatives are often viewed as overly burdensome and are relegated to the domain of just "doing the right thing" for the patient rather than a compelling reason to do so.

Despite these challenges and the increasing nonclinical workload that radiologists are facing, it is imperative that all caregivers and departments develop, implement, and monitor a robust quality and safety program to remove unnecessary variation, deliver best practices at the point of care, and ultimately deliver better outcomes for their patients. Achieving this requires a cultural shift within the organization, sometimes referred to as the "culture of safety." This starts with leadership whose role is to impart a compelling reason to their staff as to why quality and safety is integral to every aspect of the workflow, why measurement is important, and why change is mandatory when standards do not meet best practices. In other words, the work needed is not optional and the programs and people put in place need to be held accountable to the mission and goal at hand. As with all leadership, effective translation of the vision will require choosing the right teams to develop meaningful strategies, tactics, and tools to deliver better quality and that these teams need to work with the wider department to ensure consistent delivery of the solutions. Constant monitoring, feedback, and sharing of the data will be necessary to iterate and improve as well as benchmarking departmental and individual performance. This cultural pivot often takes years to implement and requires constant vigilance to ensure that teams and individuals do not lose sight of the primary goal of the processes—the delivery of better outcomes for patients. Otherwise commitment can quickly unravel and quality and safety will again be viewed as a burdensome and relatively unnecessary part of their workload. Performance monitoring and measurement is critical to driving cultural change and offers managers the opportunity to transform their departments towards better practices. Fortunately, while still challenging, measurement is becoming more seamless through electronic health records and data capture and display, which is more presentable and understandable and importantly, up to date. Departments are developing scorecards and dashboards to help providers understand their performance either instantly as in the use of dashboards (i.e., how many patients have been cleared for MRI safety checks on a given day) or over several weeks or months as in scorecards that look at trends in performance over a period of time. Both are meaningful tools with which to benchmark quality and safety practices from which teams can then determine if further improvement and change is needed.

It cannot be understated how important a pivot to a "culture of safety" must be sustained, because it changes the mindset of a department to gear all aspects of the operations with quality and safety in mind. Rather than quality and safety being seen as some arbitrary and unnecessary imposition, it fully embraces the Hippocratic oath of "first do no harm," a foundational medical doctrine that goes as far back as, well… Hippocrates. While this oath is rarely formally taken by physicians nowadays, it surely is in the hearts and minds of all providers as they strive to do the best they can for patients. Yet, doing one's best is often not sufficient, it is better to know what to do and then do one's best (attributed to Edwards Demings). In other words, while caregivers honestly strive to do their best for patients, in reality it may fall well short of current best practices either because of lack of knowledge or systems that are not in place to aid providers to deliver care of the highest quality and safety. Leaders have the challenging task of placing quality and safety at the core of their operations which can then drive all departmental practices accordingly and in a manner that all staff can embrace and support. Only when every member of the overall team believes that working together in a data-driven, supportive, non-punitive, and transparent framework will departments approach the culture of safety.

Once leadership provides the vision for the quality and safety agenda, it is advantageous to frame the approach by considering the operations in totality rather than piecemeal, where individual activities are not viewed as connected or integrated into a larger framework. For instance, a quality and safety agenda may do sterling work on reducing radiation dose for specific CT procedures and the department may be led to believe that they are excelling in this particular arena. While reduction of CT dose is unquestionably appropriate and necessary, the quality efforts to achieve this can quickly be undermined or even rendered useless depending on patient circumstances. For instance, no matter how much work has been invested into reducing dose and no matter how low a CT dose has been achieved, it is meaningless to those patients who underwent a CT, which was not indicated in the first place. In other words, the efforts to reduce CT dose have not been tied to the necessary efforts to reduce imaging inappropriateness. Similarly, efforts by radiologists to become more subspecialized towards precision reporting will be undermined if the report they are generating for an examination was for a test that was inappropriate or non-indicated. In that sense, all unnecessary activities can be viewed as waste and ultimately error, the antithesis of quality and safety. Similarly, variation in performance can also be considered as waste and error as best practice standards are not being consistently met at the point of care. Increasingly waste and variation are being viewed as a cost to the overall system, a major driver for inefficiency in health care (not just one of morbidity and mortality). The Institute of Medicine in the United States believes that medical inefficiencies (waste) contribute up to 33% of medical costs (over $1 trillion in annual waste) so quality and safety measures are now considered a critical component of reducing waste and costs in the system. Furthermore, cost can be understood as not just financial. Redundant and inappropriate care can lead to unnecessary anxiety for patients and inappropriate use of their time and other resources.

So quality and safety measures are now a central and major focus of policy makers, payers, hospital leaders, patient advocates, and in turn care providers as they strive not just to reduce morbidity and mortality for patients but a whole host of other cost issues. Radiology services must in turn address these forces and acknowledge that the efforts ought to be comprehensive and overarching—and address every aspect of the radiology operations. To achieve this, leaders and managers must recognize that all radiology activities and operations are ultimately interlinked. Business leaders have recognized this for decades and some have used a value chain as a metaphor to help understand and frame their operations to improve performance, quality, and even safety.

They teach that each component of an operation or workflow contributes to the overall performance of that operation, whether it be a service or a product. This metaphor is just as apt for radiology and it could be helpful to view the radiology operations as an imaging value chain and the delivery of best practices is only as strong as the weakest link in that chain. Therefore improving quality and safety in one domain (or link) does not necessarily translate into overall effectiveness if other up or downstream efforts have not been similarly addressed.

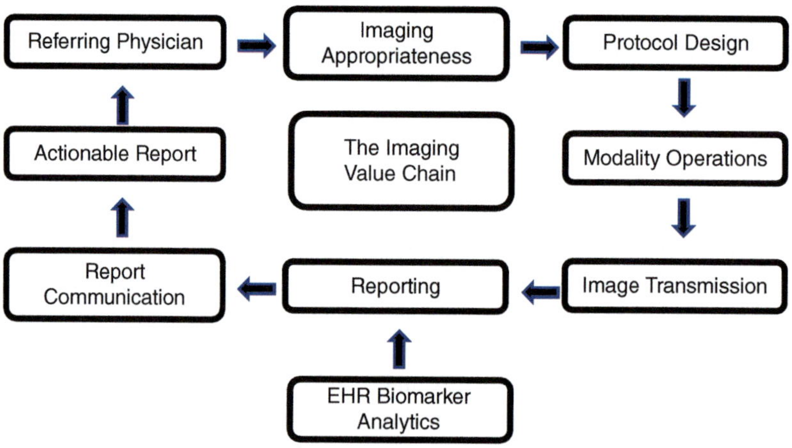

The imaging value chain can be simplistically imagined as the workflow from when a referrer orders an imaging test to when he or she receives a report, hopefully one that is actionable (see graphic). Hopefully the referring physician is familiar with the right test to order for the patient (image appropriateness) but not infrequently they do not know precisely the best test to order at that time for that patient with their current presenting complaint. This can be termed imaging inappropriateness, with some believing this could account for up to 30% of all imaging requests. Once the test is ordered it then needs to be scheduled and protocoled. Then the patient arrives at the imaging suite and the procedure is performed (could be either diagnostic or interventional). The images are acquired and transmitted (and stored) at which point the radiologist interprets the images (with increasing access to collateral biomarker data residing in electronic health record databases). The reports are then communicated to the referring physician, ideally actionable (meaning they are succinct, structured, precise, unambiguous, directional)—in other words a report that the referrer can then use to determine the next best course of action without unnecessary additional tests or actions which might only lead to additional waste and cost in the system.

Using the imaging value chain metaphor, it helps departments to view the operations as a whole and approach quality and safety initiatives as a systems approach so benefits in one part of the system can effectively be translated through to other parts. As discussed, too often managers do not envisage their operations holistically when devising quality and safety measures, rather efforts are fragmented and uncoordinated. For imaging appropriateness, tests should only be ordered when they are deemed absolutely necessary. Given the complexity and pace of modern medicine, this can only realistically be achieved through computerized decision support systems that guide referrers to order the right test for any given clinical scenario. This then sets the stage for the delivery of an actionable report downstream (as an inappropriate test is, by definition, non-actionable). Once the test is chosen, it behooves the operations to perform the test as quickly as possible (otherwise why would the test be necessary). This means scheduling the test expeditiously, ideally through sophisticated electronic order entry systems that allow referrers and patients to choose an imaging location of their choice and convenient time. This may not seem a quality measure but from a customer's point of view (referrer or patient) it very much is a quality metric on overall performance of the operation. Once the time and place of the examination has been chosen (assuming the right test has been chosen in the first place) then the correct, precise protocol should be selected for the indication at hand. For instance, imaging unnecessary body parts only adds to additional radiation (CT) or scan time (MRI). Use of IV contrast may be appropriate for malignant disease but inappropriate for other clinical indications. Increasingly precision protocoling needs to be tailored to the individual patient, their condition, and the question being asked by the referring physician. Protocol appropriateness is a particular problem for many departments as most departments use their own idiosyncratic protocols and there is pervasive variation across institutions and even within departments (some radiologists prefer different protocols for the same clinical indication compared to their colleagues). It is well known, for instance, that radiation dose for the same indication can vary by as much as tenfold depending on the institution, frequently three- to fourfold. Almost no two academic medical centers have similar protocols for the same indications, some with 20, 30, or 45 min MRI protocols for the same indication, for instance.

Similarly modality operations vary considerably from one institution to another. What is seen as an efficient use of assets in one organization is seen as inefficient in another. For instance, one organization may view their 8 a.m.–5 p.m. operation as very busy and productive yet another will operate their scanner from 6 a.m. to 11 p.m. Others will operate their scanners with multiple resources to help expedite patients in and out of the scanner while other organizations will use a single technologist to maneuver the patient on and off the CT table, operate the scanner, send the images to PACS, and go to the waiting room to collect the next patient (a markedly inefficient manner with which to operate an expensive asset). These differences reflect the quality of services as an inefficient operation leads to reduced patient access to scanning (prolonging time to diagnosis) and delays once at the imaging suite (an inconvenience to patients). Once images are generated, radiologists will need the comprehensive set of prior images necessary to determine any new or chronic findings. This has become particularly challenging as organizations consolidate (an increasing trend in the USA) whereby images reside on different and disparate PACS systems which are often poorly connected, if at all. This undermines precision reporting and ability to avoid unnecessary additional imaging tests downstream.

Reporting variation is also widespread both between and within institutions. Even within academic medical centers there is considerable variation of imaging interpretation and analysis of the findings. The reasons are numerous, but imaging has become too complex and sophisticated for any single radiologist (even subspecialty radiologists) to be familiar with the appearances of each disease from each modality with a given protocol. Furthermore, the style and language used by radiologists varies markedly. It is not uncommon for radiologists to offer a range of differential diagnoses without any particular weighting to the chance of one diagnosis being more likely than another. Even the terms to infer degree of risk for a disorder vary from one radiologist to another—one radiologist may believe "consistent with" confers 100% likelihood of disease, another less so (other terms such as likely, suspicious for, concerning for, also have different connotations from one radiologist to another). There is also widespread evidence that the recommendations made by radiologists for additional tests (especially further imaging) vary considerably in both frequency and type. One radiologist's certainty for a particular imaging finding may be sufficient for them to recommend no further tests; another may believe a confirmatory and clarification test is required. For instance, some radiologists who diagnose a hepatic hemangioma by ultrasound may stop there; others might recommend a confirmatory additional test such as a three-phase contrast enhanced CT, while others may recommend an MRI. Yet others will recommend further tests immediately; others at a later date. Some might leave the recommendation vague with terms such as "consider" follow-up MRI (or CT) for example or, even worse, use the term "clinical correlation" required. In short, this variation reduces the radiologist's ability to deliver an actionable report and further undermines the rest of any quality improvements implemented in workflow upstream (as indicated by the imaging value chain). Needless to say, referrers and increasingly patients (who often have ready access to their reports) are frustrated by ambiguous and vague narratives and the sometimes frivolous use of further imaging recommendations. These unwarranted variations in practices serve to undermine all other quality and safety efforts.

Once a report has been generated, the referring physician (and patient) expects to receive that report (hopefully actionable) as soon as possible, ideally electronically (so as to be available to as many caregivers as needed). Yet communication standards vary widely too, with some radiologists calling referrers immediately on some reports but not on others, some for routine findings, and some only for critical findings. One might imagine that critical finding alerts (those reports which must be delivered to appropriate caregivers immediately to prevent serious patient harm) should be consistent between institutions (given they are potentially lifesaving in the immediate short term). Yet most departments have critical finding report communication protocols that differ (albeit slightly) from one department to another. Certainly national recommendations exist. Nonetheless, widespread and uniform implementation of the national guidelines has not been achieved.

In summary quality and safety should not just be framed, as it frequently is, around events that lead to obvious immediate harm (i.e., contrast reactions or interventional complications)—rather they should be framed around the myriad of unique activities that constitute the overall radiology workflow. Many of these activities may, in themselves, seem trivial as to their contribution to risk and adversity (such as the recommendation for an unwarranted test, or minor variations in MRI protocol design) but in aggregate these variations can lead to considerable costs and even harm. Until radiologists recognize that it is the responsibility of the overall team to evaluate every operational activity to determine if it meets best practice standards, quality and safety efforts will be undermined and sometimes ineffective. It is the role of leadership to frame the issues to their departments, then build the teams to create, deliver, and manage solutions using data-driven management techniques and the necessary tools and resources to perpetually drive towards better practices and outcomes.

The chapters in this book help address the quality and safety agenda in a systematic and logical order around the concept of the imaging value chain. Subsequent chapters begin with imaging appropriateness (and the use of clinical decision support tools to establish adherence to national guidelines). Chapter III will address protocol optimization with the informed use of medical radiation in diagnostic imaging and further discuss guidelines and standards for managing radiation dose. Chapters will then address modality operations and use of clinical guidelines, image interpretation, structured reporting, and decision support tools for radiologist reporting. Report communication standards will be addressed. Measurement tools and appropriate use of data that have practical and meaningful implications for management of departmental quality and safety will be addressed. Furthermore peer learning and peer review strategies will be outlined that encourage the development of the "culture of safety." Finally the emerging field of big data and data analytics to manage the quality and safety agenda will highlight the increasing use of IT systems to drive performance in radiology.

Part II

Imaging Appropriateness

Guideline Development

Michael Bettmann and Myriam Hunink

Contents

Abstract

The reason to develop and use Clinical Imaging Guidelines (CIG) is, simply, to improve patient care. CIG development and use are based on the principle that imaging use is not always optimal; reasons for this include lack of expertise (with either the clinical concern or the available imaging modality), nonmedical reasons for requesting the study (medicolegal concerns, possible financial gain), lack of available resources, and expediency. The use of CIG potentially helps in all of these areas, by providing guidance based on high-quality literature and supplemented by expert opinion. CIG answer the question: which, if any, imaging study would be most helpful in this specific clinical situation? The answer is based on assessment of the risk–benefit ratio for the patient. Benefits of imaging are often obvious. Risks, however, also exist, and include the effects of radiation (admittedly difficult to quantify), complications due to contrast agents or the technology (e.g., MRI-related accidents) or other medications, and the possible consequences of unexpected incidental findings that may require evaluation and intervention. The cost to society as well as top individuals must be considered.

There are clear steps in the development of any clinical guidelines. First, there must be a sound, reproducible, transparent methodology. Then, specific clinical conditions must be defined, including consideration of their incidence, impact (e.g., success of diagnosis, treatment, and outcomes), and cost to the system. There must be sufficient high-quality literature available to justify review and guideline creation. The literature must be comprehensively and systematically reviewed and summarized. The summary and the topic as a whole must be reviewed by a group that includes all relevant stakeholders. Recommendations must be based to as a great an extent as possible on the literature, supplemented by expert opinion. The guideline must be regularly updated. Any potential conflicts of interest must be clearly presented. Overall, the methodology must follow accepted norms and be reproducible and transparent.

M. Bettmann, M.D., F.A.C.R., F.S.A.R. (✉)
Wake Forest University School of Medicine,
Winston-Salem, NC, USA

American College of Radiology, Reston, VA, USA
e-mail: mabettmann@gmail.com

M. Hunink, M.D., Ph.D.
Erasmus University Medical Center, Rotterdam,
The Netherlands

Harvard T.H. Chan School of Public Health, Boston,
MA, USA

Netherlands Institute for Health Sciences (NIHES),
Rotterdam, The Netherlands
e-mail: m.hunink@erasmusmc.nl

Med Radiol Diagn Imaging (2018)
DOI 10.1007/174_2017_164, © Springer International Publishing AG
Published Online 24 April 2018

There are many challenges in developing and using CIG. In addition to accurate representation and synthesis of what is known, these include adaptation to specific groups of patients and medical systems—what is appropriate for a pediatric age group, for example, may not be appropriate for adults. What works in a fee-for-service developed nation with all imaging modalities available may not work in a rural society with limited equipment and expertise. Finally, the primary goal of CIG is to improve patient care, so they have some clear value for educational purposes, of trainees, non-imagers, patients, families, and regulators. Their greatest use lies in incorporation into the process of requesting imaging studies, to guide appropriate use. This includes prevention of overuse and also elimination of under-use. As such CIG are now widely used in the physician order entry component of electronic health records

The development of clinical imaging guidelines is, by consensus, based on several principles: there is sufficient data from high-quality literature on which to base guidelines, the clinical issues addressed are important, and quality of care can be improved by the development and use of guidelines (Eccles et al. 2012; Committee on Standards for Developing Trustworthy Clinical Practice Guidelines 2011; World Health Organization (WHO) 2012; Bettmann et al. 2015a). There are also several terms used for Clinical Imaging Guidelines (CIG): referral guidelines, appropriate use criteria, appropriateness criteria, and justification guidelines. Although there may be subtle differences, all refer to guidance documents that are developed using a widely accepted and well-defined methodology to provide advice on which specific imaging study, if any, is likely to be most useful in a specific clinical setting. Inherent in guidelines is the focus on balancing the possible benefit against the possible risk. The benefits of imaging range from improved care to reassurance, for the healthcare provider and the patient. There are also both real and potential risks, although in general they are more limited for an imaging study than for a medication or a surgical intervention. The real risks include those related to injury from a medication that may be necessary for the imaging study (e.g., a contrast agent or a sedative) and discovery of unexpected findings that may lead to further investigation or even to intervention but no real benefit to the patient. Findings such as an incidental thyroid nodule (Hoang and Nguyen 2017) or ovarian cyst or a benign liver lesion fall into this category. While significant incidental findings occur, nonsignificant but concerning ones are more frequent (Hoang and Nguyen 2017). Radiation is another risk (Tran et al. 2017; Mathews et al. 2013; Hendee and O'Connor 2012). Although the precise risk of a single imaging exam is essentially impossible to quantitate, and the risk of diagnostic level radiation continues to be debated, it is clear that there are at the very least potential negative consequences of radiation; the concerns are greater in younger patients, due to the latency of these potential adverse effects. Finally, the cost of the imaging exam is an important variable. Depending on the nature of the healthcare system, this may not be a concern to the individual undergoing the imaging exam, but it is always a concern to the system as a whole. If the likelihood is very low or negligible that a specific imaging exam in a specific clinical setting is going to provide useful information—for example a routine chest radiograph in an otherwise healthy young adult nonsmoker—then even a modest cost is hard to justify. Both cost and radiation, then, are always part of the risk-benefit equation. The aim of CIG is to provide the best possible advice in specific clinical settings, realising that with the clear limitations in knowledge, the many specific clinical variables (age, gender, medical history, environmental and familial risk factors), and available expertise and equipment, a definitive recommendation may not always be possible.

There are many reasons other than medical necessity to consider imaging (Schuur et al. 2014; New Report Reveals 19.7 Million Misdirected Physician Referrals in the U.S 2014). These include patient preference; a patient may want a CT scan for back pain, simply for personal reassurance. Also, many healthcare providers feel that they can both reassure themselves and their patients and perhaps lessen the risk of a malpractice accusation if an imaging exam is ordered even if there is no real concern for negligence. There may also be financial incentives to getting an imaging study, if the ordering provider has a fiduciary interest in the imaging equipment. It may simply be expeditious: it can be faster to get an imaging study than to carefully evaluate a patient in a busy emergency room, or explain at length to an anxious patient that an imaging study is unlikely to be clinically useful. The use of CIG is an effective means to deal with many of these non-medical reasons for obtaining imaging. Again, the entry point for CIG is the question: Which, *if any*, imaging exam is most likely to be helpful in the diagnosis and care of this patient in this clinical setting. Thus the overarching aims of CIGs are to educate healthcare personnel, patients, and patient families, and to improve the quality of care. To this end, readily available and accessible CIGs can be used as educational tools for medical students and other trainees, as a resource for patients, or as clinical decision support for healthcare providers. This latter is perhaps the most difficult but also the most important function of guidelines, as it speaks most directly to improving healthcare.

Clinical guidelines have been available for at least three decades, in various formats (Brook et al. 1986; Fitch et al. 2001). They are a natural tool in the focus on evidence-based medicine, and they have been developed by many different organisations. Several specialty societies, such as the American College of Pediatrics (American Academy of Pediatrics Subcommittee on Urinary Tract Infection, Steering Committee on Quality Improvement and Management 2011) and the American College of Otolaryngology-Head and Neck Surgery (Schwartz et al. 2009), have long produced guidelines on specific diseases, such as recurrent urinary tract infections in children and hoarseness. These guidelines generally take several years to develop, are very cost- and time-intensive, and cover the entire spectrum of a disease or disease process, from initial consideration through diagnosis, treatment and clinical outcome. Imaging guidelines, in contrast, have focused on the use of imaging in specific clinical situations-for example, imaging in patients with recurrent UTIs or acute onset of hoarseness (dysphonia). Conceptually imaging guidelines may be considered horizontal (covering imaging in many diseases and clinical scenarios), as compared to the broader, more vertical disease-based guidelines.

To create any medical guidelines, whether they focus on imaging specifically or on a broader illness or process, there must be a very well-defined approach that is thorough, transparent and includes a number of specific components and steps. The specific approach currently in wide use has evolved from the work of the Rand Corporation in the late 1980s (Brook et al. 1986). Numerous specialty societies have adopted and used the general approach, with variations. Subsequently, organisations including the Institute of Medicine in the US (Committee on Standards for Developing Trustworthy Clinical Practice Guidelines 2011), NICE in the UK (National Institute for Health and Care Excellence 2017) and the American College of Radiology (Methodology Documents 2017) and have defined the necessary approach, methodology and components. Although there are some differences, much of the approach is agreed by all the organisations that have addressed this topic. Furthermore, these steps are a reflection of the Appraisal of Guidelines for Research & Evaluation (AGREE) Instrument which is a tool to assess the methodological rigor and transparency of clinical practice guideline development (Table 1) (http://www.agreetrust.org/agree-ii/).

These are the accepted basic principles and steps that all guidelines must adhere to be generally accepted as valid:

1. The topic to be addressed by the guideline must have substantial clinical relevance and impact.
2. There must be clear definition of both the need for and the focus of the guideline. A guideline may be based on a specific disease or clinical problem, such as middle ear infections in children or head trauma. The motivation for the development of guidelines may be that a process is either clinically very important or very prevalent, that the approach is problematic, or that diagnosis or treatment

Table 1 Summary of the AGREE II domains and items that should be specifically described (http://www.agreetrust.org/resource-centre/agree-reporting-checklist/)

Domain	Items
1. Scope and purpose	Overall objective Health question Applicable population (patients / public)
2. Stakeholder involvement	Group membership How views and preferences of target population were sought/ considered Target users
3. Rigor of development	Details of the strategy used to search for evidence Criteria used to select evidence Strengths and limitations of the evidence Methods used to formulate the recommendations Health benefits, side effects, and risks that were considered Link between the recommendations and the evidence Methodology for external review Updating procedure
4. Clarity of presentation	Specific and unambiguous recommendations Management options Key recommendations
5. Applicability	Facilitators and barriers to application Advice and tools for implementation Resource implications Monitoring/auditing criteria
6. Editorial independence	Funding body's influence Group members' competing interests

is very resource intensive (either because of high cost per incident, or high incidence).

3. There must be sufficient high-quality literature to allow the development of the guideline, although supplementary incorporation of expert opinion is always necessary as the literature is essentially never entirely conclusive. One important illustration of the need to supplement high-quality studies with expert opinion is the diagnosis and treatment of UTIs, since there are so many relevant variables, such as the age and gender of the patient, the prior treatments and associated risk factors. Another example is the imaging of newly-diagnosed prostate cancer. Despite many studies and much experience, the optimal approach remains open to debate (NGC Prostate Guidelines 2016).
4. The literature must be systematically reviewed using sound, transparent and high-quality methodology. The method for reviewing, evaluating and synthesising the literature must be clear, well-defined and reproducible. There are many ways of rating publications, but all approaches must have a clear method for indicating the strengths and weaknesses of the individual article reviewed and cited as well as the strength of the cited literature as a body in supporting or refuting conclusions. This can be difficult, as the subject matter to be reviewed and synthesised is usually complex and technical, a further reason why expert opinion is a necessary part of the process.
5. All relevant stakeholders must have a role in the process. It is clear that expertise in a topic or modality is important. If, for example, an aspect of arthritis is the focus, rheumatologists, orthopedists, physiatrists and imagers must be involved. This specific topic is also important to general internists, likely to paediatricians, and certainly to patients. If the focus is imaging, individuals with expertise in the relevant modalities (e.g., MRI, CT, PET) must be part of the guideline-developing team. It is generally agreed that patients must be represented, but this is not straightforward as there is no universal prototypical patient or patient point-of-view.
6. All potential conflicts of interest must be clearly and transparently expressed. This includes potential financial conflicts, such as when an expert is a consultant or speaker for a device or pharmaceutical company, or may be more subtle. For example, a surgeon who specialises in joint replacement will have some bias in treating severe arthritis. This is acceptable, but must be clearly evident when the guideline is made available.
7. There must be a reproducible, transparent and well-defined definition of the entire process of progressing from literature review to guideline release. This includes a description of the role and membership of each of the groups involved in the process. Some guidelines are developed

using one group to review the literature and develop a narrative. A second group may then assume the responsibility for defining and voting on the recommendations, and a third for reviewing and approving them. Alternatively, all of these tasks may be assigned to a single group, with final review by a separate oversight group.

The process for the members of the group to review and rate the suggested conclusions, as well as the method for reaching consensus, must be well-defined, transparent and reproducible.

Most often, a single author or small group produces a draft narrative, including a set of recommendations. A panel that includes subject experts as well as other stakeholders then rates the recommendations. These ratings are generated for various specific clinical questions, such as for different laboratory investigations or other diagnostic approaches or for specific therapies. With CIG, the ratings are for the appropriateness of all relevant specific imaging studies in a particular clinical situation.

The most widely used rating scale is from 1 to 9, with 1–3 defined as "not usually appropriate," 4–6 defined as "may or may not be appropriate" and 7–9 defined as "usually appropriate." After initial rating, an attempt is made to reach consensus on the recommendations. This requires a clear definition not only of the rating system but also of what qualifies as consensus. That is, is consensus defined as the rating of all panellists falling within one of the three categories, or within two points in the rating? Further it is necessary to specify what per cent of the group must be in agreement to conclude that there is consensus: agreement of 60% or 75% or 90% of the group as a whole or of those members who vote, who are present on a call or are present at a meeting? The specifics of the rating and of what constitutes consensus vary among the different groups creating guidelines. There is no one correct approach, but consistency, reproducibility and transparency are all imperative (Fig. 1).

The most widely accepted methodology utilizes the modified Delphi approach (Fitch et al. 2001; Methodology Documents. First, individuals review the narrative and the suggested indications and independently rate them. If the ratings all fall within a designated range, this is considered acceptable agreement. Any that do not achieve consensus in a first rating round are then discussed by the rating group. Then a second round and, for some societies, a third round is held using the same rules. It is rare that it is not possible to reach consensus with discussions and two or three voting rounds, but if this does occur, the imaging study is rated as "no consensus." This is unusual in practice, but it may occur either because the group is unable to reach consensus on a rating (as defined), or because the rating panel has determined that there is insufficient high-quality information to support a recommendation.

<u>**Variant 1:**</u> **Chronic ankle pain. Initial imaging.**

Procedure	Appropriateness Category	Relative Radiation Level
X-ray ankle	Usually Appropriate	☢
Tc-99m bone scan ankle	Usually No t Appropriate	☢☢☢
US ankle	Usually Not Appropriate	O
CT ankle without IV contrast	Usually Not Appropriate	☢
CT ankle with IV contrast	Usually Not Appropriate	☢
CT ankle without and with IV contrast	Usually Not Appropriate	☢
MRI ankle without IV contrast	Usually Not Appropriate	O
MRI ankle without and with IV contrast	Usually Not Appropriate	O

Fig. 1 Overview of a variant from the American College of Radiology Appropriateness Criteria on Chronic Foot Pain

8. After rating, the topic is reviewed by an oversight committee, shared with other stakeholders and then widely distributed. Ideally, each new guideline is submitted to an oversight organisation, such as the AHRQ National Guidelines Clearinghouse (The AHRQs National Guideline Clearinghouse 2017), an NIH-funded organisation, for review, approval and inclusion.
9. There must be a plan and method for regular review and updating of each guideline. While this may add significant cost and effort, it is an imperative component of the whole process. Medicine changes rapidly so that regular updating is the only way to ensure that guidelines remain valid and relevant. Further the US Protecting Access to Medicare Act (PAMA) will require that for all Medicare-covered services, approved guidelines must be consulted for all advanced imaging exams (i.e., CT, MRI, PET), at least in certain critical medical areas (Protecting Access to Medicare Act of 2014.

The specific discrete steps in the development of a clinical imaging guideline are:

1. Selection and definition of the topic to be covered
2. Literature review, selection and rating
3. Synthesis of a narrative on the topic
4. Review and rating of specific imaging modalities
5. Re-review and discussion to achieve consensus (modified Delphi method)
6. Oversight review and approval
7. Wide distribution and adoption
8. Regular revision (every 1–3 years, or as needed based on evolving knowledge and experience).

As noted, to be valid and justify widespread acceptance and adoption, all guidelines including CIG must be based primarily on high quality, peer-reviewed research that is publically available. This refers primarily to work published in peer-reviewed journals but may encompass research presented at meetings, after peer review that can be effectively reviewed and validated. The databases used and any limitations on language or type of publication must be stated. For example, for the ACR Appropriateness Criteria, only articles with at least an English-language abstract are considered, and case reports or opinion articles are excluded. The literature that is reviewed must be rated as to type of report (e.g., prospective randomised clinical trial, review article, case control trial, retrospective review) and the strength and validity of the conclusions. The aim of this initial review of the literature is to define not only the type of study or report, but also the strengths and weaknesses of the study design and performance, and the extent to which the data support the conclusions.

In addition to selecting and then rating individual publications, it is necessary to rate the strength of the evidence overall. Usually, a systematic evaluation is made of the strength of the conclusion. That is, regardless of the rating generated by the panellists, how strongly are the final ratings, recommendations and conclusions supported by high quality studies? This is more relevant, and more accurate, for broader topics that have been investigated with multiple large-scale, prospective, double-blind clinical trials, such as acute myocardial infarction, or treatment for stage 1 Hodgkin's lymphoma. It is less meaningful for rating imaging studies, since true prospective clinical trials, sufficiently sized to achieve both clinical and statistical significance, are relatively unusual in the imaging literature.

There are several additional challenges in creating CIG, and more in using them. An overarching consideration is the harm to benefit ratio of a specific imaging study, which is hard to calculate. Key variables include the clinical setting, cost and radiation risk, but additional obvious concerns are availability of imaging modalities and expertise in their use and interpretation. If only a portable MRI unit is available, and that only on specific days, then another study may be appropriate, even though not rated as highly as an MRI. If there is no expertise with Ultrasound, even though ultrasound may have a higher rating, it may or may not be appropriate to use another imaging modality.

The clinical setting may dictate different approaches due to demographics as well as varying prevalence rates of diseases in different regions and populations. Often, this must be addressed by the healthcare provider requesting the study, the family and the imager. For example, to obtain a chest radiograph for a cough may be rated low in an economically advantaged region in a developed nation, but may be rated higher (i.e., more appropriate) in a region with endemic TB. Dealing with this variability, however, is inherent in high-quality CIGs. If cough, for example is the indication, good CIGs will address various presentations (e.g., acute vs. chronic, febrile, underlying major risk factors) and all major possible underlying pathologies, ranging from specific infectious agents to other etiologies, regardless of location. As the world effectively shrinks, disease prevalence is less a concern than availability of equipment and expertise, and these, again, are inherently considered in high-quality guidelines.

The cost of imaging is always a consideration, as it is for any medical intervention, but it is very hard to define. What constitutes cost varies with the point of view used. For example, if the societal viewpoint is adopted, costs that must be quantified include not what the reimbursement was, but rather the cost of the imaging equipment, the personnel to operate it and to interpret studies, the physical costs of the facilities and the support staff to maintain them, and the costs of individual patients to take time off from work and to travel to the imaging site. If the governmental point-of-view is used, the payment for the service is what is relevant. This does not necessarily reflect the cost to actually perform the imaging but rather what society is willing or able to pay. It usually includes the calculated institutional costs, with some overhead, but not additional societal expenses. Further, it is clear that in the US, the price quoted by an institution or imaging center for an imaging study is rarely actually paid, either by Medicare or private insurers, and does not necessarily have a direct relationship to the cost of performing the study. Ultimately, it is important to recognize that cost of imaging should always be considered as should the induced costs of treatment and the long-term costs saved by appropriate intervention. In general the costs of testing are small relative to the costs of missing an important diagnosis that may have detrimental consequences, especially when considered from the societal perspective.

Radiation exposure is similarly complex. It is generally (albeit not universally) accepted that ionising radiation at diagnostic levels may have deleterious effects, and that these are directly related to the dose to the patient, both a single exam and cumulative lifetime dose, and are inversely related to age -that is, the risk is assumed to be greater in children. Radiation exposure, then, must be considered in creating guidelines (Tran et al. 2017; Mathews et al. 2013; Hendee and O'Connor 2012; Radiation dose calculation in the ACR Appropriateness Criteria 2017). Beyond this, however, it is hard to reach consensus. If a study that does not use ionising radiation, such as MRI or Ultrasound, is likely to give information that is as valuable, then CT, radiographs and radionuclide studies should be avoided, especially in children. It is rare, however, that this situation occurs. It is more frequent that the information from different modalities gives different levels of information. The trade-off between the putative benefit of the imaging study and the risk to the patient must always be considered. Often this is not an easy task, because of variables (such as dose and radiation risk) that cannot be calculated with confidence (Fig. 2).

Another major consideration in the development of CIG is their actual use. CIG have been available for over 20 years, and there has been much discussion concerning when and how they are used. Until the last few years, despite encouragement including a mandate from the European Community in 2012 that CIG be available in all member countries (Bettmann et al. 2015b), at this time they have been used intermittently and most often for general educational purposes rather than to guide clinical decision making. This has begun to change due to IT advances, regulatory oversight and the wide recognition that imaging is often inappropriately used-it is both overused and underused, often in the same region or even clinic. Now, due to awareness of the cost, radiation, and inappropriate use considerations, as well as to the evolving regulatory mandate in the US, use of CIG is increasing dramatically. It remains unclear to what extent their use will alter clinical practice. One large study, the CMS Demonstration Project (Timbie et al. 2015) sug-

a

Sample Topic

Clinical Condition: Orbits, Vision and Visual Loss

Variant 1: Traumatic visual defect. Suspect orbital injury. Initial imaging.

Variant 2: Nontraumatic orbital asymmetry, exophthalmos, or enophthalmos. Initial imaging.

Variant 3: Suspected orbital cellulitis, uveitis, or scleritis. Initial imaging.

Variant 4: Suspected optic neuritis. Initial imaging.

Variant 5: Visual loss. Etiology identified on ophthalmologic examination or laboratory tests.

Variant 6: Visual loss. Intraocular mass, optic nerve, or pre-chiasm symptoms. Initial imaging.

Variant 7: Nonischemic visual loss. Chiasm or post-chiasm symptoms. Initial imaging.

Variant 8: Ophthalmoplegia or diplopia. Initial imaging.

b

Variant 1: **Traumatic visual defect. Suspect orbital injury. Initial imaging.**

Procedure	Appropriateness Category	RRL
CT orbits without IV contrast	Usually Appropriate	☢☢☢
CT head without IV contrast	Usually Appropriate	☢☢☢
MRI head without IV contrast	May Be Appropriate	O
MRI orbits without IV contrast	May Be Appropriate	O
CT orbits with IV contrast	May Be Appropriate (Disagreement)	☢☢☢
CTA head and neck with IV contrast	May Be Appropriate	☢☢☢
MRI head without and with IV contrast	May Be Appropriate	O
MRI orbits without and with IV contrast	May Be Appropriate (Disagreement)	O
MRA head and neck without and with IV contrast	May Be Appropriate	O
MRA head and neck without IV contrast	May Be Appropriate	O
Arteriography cervicocerebral	Usually Not Appropriate	☢☢☢
CT head with IV contrast	Usually Not Appropriate	☢☢☢
CT head without and with IV contrast	Usually Not Appropriate	☢☢☢
CT orbits without and with IV contrast	Usually Not Appropriate	☢☢☢
X-ray orbit	Usually Not Appropriate	☢

Fig. 2 Example of one Appropriateness Criteria, on Orbits, Vision and Visual Loss, with the table for variant 1, orbital trauma, suspect orbital injury, initial imaging. Note that some exams are rated as appropriate, some as may or may not be appropriate, and some inappropriate

gested that the use of CIG had relatively little effect on imaging utilisation. This study, however, required guidelines only for a limited number of clinical conditions, and the ability to avoid using the guidelines, and to ignore their advice, was built in to the study. It concluded that the system used was unable to assign appropriateness numbers to the majority of requested exams, and this provides an opportunity for improvement in and increased use of CIG in clinical decision support. This actually supports broader use of CIG and integration into the EMR and CPOE systems. An additional study, examining the use of two slightly different decision support systems supports this conclusion (Schneider et al. 2015). Other studies, in various venues have suggested that use of CIG does lead to a substantial reduction in inappropriate exams (Prevedello et al. 2013; Weilburg et al. 2017).

CIG are difficult, time consuming and costly to create and maintain. There is, however, a demonstrated ability to create and then use them, and there is emerging evidence to support the concept that their active use, as part of an electronic health care system, improves both the appropriate use of imaging and medical care. Over time, with improved electronic health records and IT availability, and increasing awareness of the need to consider and then balance risk and benefit for imaging and all medical care, the use of guidelines as part of clinical decision support systems is likely to increase.

References

ACR Appropriateness Criteria Methodology Documents (2017) https://www.acr.org/Quality-Safety/Appropriateness-Criteria. Accessed 6 June 2017

ACR Appropriateness Criteria, Radiation Dose Assessment Introduction (2017) https://www.acr.org/~/media/ACR/Documents/ppCriteria/RadiationDoseAssessmentIntro.pdf?la=en. Accessed 7 June 2017

American Academy of Pediatrics Subcommittee on Urinary Tract Infection, Steering Committee on Quality Improvement and Management (2011) Urinary tract infection: clinical practice guideline for the diagnosis and management of the initial UTI in febrile infants and children 2 to 24 months. Pediatrics 128:595–610

Bettmann MA, Holmberg O, Perez Rosario M, Remedios D, Malone J (2015a) International collaboration on clinical imaging guidelines: many hands make light work. J Am Coll Radiol 12(1):43–44

Bettmann MA, Oikarinen H, Rehani M, Holmberg O, del Rosario PM, Naidoo A, Do K-H, Dreyer K, Ebdon-Jackson S (2015b) Clinical imaging guidelines part 4: challenges in identifying, engaging and collaborating with stakeholders. J Am Coll Radiol 12: 370–375

Brook RH, Chassin MR, Fink A et al (1986) A method for the detailed assessment of the appropriateness of medical technologies. Int J Technol Assess Health Care 2(1):53–63

CMS.gov, Protecting Access to Medicare Act of 2014–2017 https://www.cms.gov/Medicare/Quality-Initiatives-Patient-Assessment-Instruments/Appropriate-Use-Criteria-Program/index.html. Accessed 7 June 2017

Committee on Standards for Developing Trustworthy Clinical Practice Guidelines (2011) Clinical practice guidelines we can trust. Institute of Medicine, Washington, DC

Eccles MP, Grimshaw JM, Shekelle P, Schünemann HJ, Woolf S (2012) Developing clinical practice guidelines: target audiences, identifying topics for guidelines, guideline group composition and functioning and conflicts of interest. Implementation Sci 7:60

Fitch K, Bernstein S, Aguilar MD et al (2001) The Rand/UCLA appropriateness method user's manual. Rand, Santa Monica, CA

Hendee WR, O'Connor MK (2012) Radiation risks of medical imaging: separating fact from fantasy. Radiology 264(2):312–321

Hoang JK, Nguyen XV (2017) Understanding the risks and harms of management of incidental thyroid nodules: a review. JAMA Otolaryngol Head Neck Surg 43(7):718–724. https://doi.org/10.1001/jamaoto.2017.0003

Mathews JD, Forsythe AV, Brady Z, Butler MW, Goergen SK, Byrnes GB, Giles GG, Wallace AB, Anderson PR, Guiver TA, McGale P, Cain TM, Dowty JG, Bickerstaffe AC, Darby SC (2013) Cancer risk in 680,000 people exposed to computed tomography scans in childhood or adolescence: data linkage study of 11 million Australians. BMJ 346:f2360. https://doi.org/10.1136/bmj.f2360

National Institute for Health and Care Excellence (2017) NHS: UK National Health Service. Available at: http://www.nice.org.uk/about/who-weare. Accessed 7 June 2017

New Report Reveals 19.7 Million Misdirected Physician Referrals in the U.S (2014) https://www.kyruus.com/new-report-reveals-19-7-million-misdirected-physician-referrals-u-s-year. Accessed 6 June 2017

NGC Prostate Guidelines (2016) https://www.guideline.gov/search?q=prostate+cancer+imaging. Accessed 6 June 2017

Prevedello LM, Raja AS, Ip IK, Sodickson S, Khorasani R (2013) Does clinical decision support reduce

unwanted variation in yield of CT pulmonary angiogram? Am J Med 126:975–981
Schneider E, Zelenka S, Grooff P, Alexa D, Bullen J, Obuchowski A (2015) Radiology order decision support: examination-indication appropriateness assessed using 2 electronic systems. J Am Coll Radiol 12: 349–357
Schuur JD, Carney DP, Lyn ET et al (2014) A top-five list for emergency medicine: a pilot project to improve the value of emergency care. JAMA Int Med 174:509–515
Schwartz SR, Cohen SM, Dailey SH et al (2009) Clinical practice guideline: hoarseness (dysphonia). Otolaryngol Head Neck Surg 141(3 Suppl 2):S1–31
The AHRQs National Guideline Clearinghouse (2017) https://www.guideline.gov/. Accessed 6 June 2017
Timbie JW, Hussey PS, Burgette LF, Wenger NS, Rastegar A, Brantley I, Khodyakov D, Leuschner KJ, Weidmer BA, Kahn KL (2015) Medicare imaging demonstration final evaluation report to congress. Rand Health Q 5(1):4
Tran V, Zablotska LB, Brenner AV, Little MP (2017) Radiation-associated circulatory disease mortality in a pooled analysis of 77,275 patients from the Massachusetts and Canadian tuberculosis fluoroscopy cohorts. Sci Rep 7:44147. https://doi.org/10.1038/srep44147
Weilburg JB, Sistrom CL, Rosenthal DI, Stout MB, Dreyer KJ, Rockett HR, Baron JM, Ferris TG, Thrall JH (2017) Utilization management of high-cost imaging in an outpatient setting in a large stable patient and provider cohort over 7 years. Radiology 284(3):766–776. https://doi.org/10.1148/radiol.2017160968
World Health Organization (WHO) (2012) WHO handbook for guideline development. http://apps.who.int/iris/bitstream/10665/75146/1/9789241548441_eng.pdf. Accessed 6 June 2017

Clinical Decision Support Tools for Order Entry

Laila Cochon and Ramin Khorasani

Contents

Abbreviations

AUC	Appropriate use criteria
CDS	Clinical decision support
CPOE	Computerized physician order entry system
EHR	Electronic health record
IT	Information technology

Abstract

Medical imaging has helped to transform healthcare and will continue to advance the understanding and treatment of disease. Despite the substantial benefits of medical imaging, there is wide variation in the use of imaging (especially high-cost imaging) and concern about it's inappropriate use persists. Inappropriate use may result in suboptimal quality of care and wasteand may harm patients by exposure to unnecessary ionizing radiation, the risks of over-diagnosis and over-treatment, including unnecessary additional tests and treatments provided in follow-up of incidental or ambiguous imaging findings.

Clinical decision support tools for order entry provide an opportunity to embed evidence/ clinical best practices in the workflow of providers requesting imaging examinations to reduce inappropriate use of imaging. In this chapter, we define clinical decision support for order entry, review trends in imaging use and describe general features of effective clinical decision support including experience from large-scale implementations. We conclude by reviewing some of the emerging challenges and opportunities for imaging clinical decision support and future directions.

L. Cochon, M.D. • R. Khorasani, M.D., M.P.H. (✉)
Department of Radiology, Center for Evidence-Based Imaging, Brigham and Women's Hospital, Harvard Medical School, Boston, MA, USA
e-mail: rkhorasani@bwh.harvard.edu

Med Radiol Diagn Imaging (2018)
DOI 10.1007/174_2017_162, © Springer International Publishing AG
Published Online 05 April 2018

Key Points

- Despite the substantial benefits that medical imaging confers, there is wide variation in use of imaging (especially high-cost imaging) and concern about inappropriate use persists.
- Although reports on impact of imaging Clinical Decision Support (CDS) have been inconsistent, clinical decision support (CDS)-enabled interventions have been shown to improve adherence to evidence, including clinical practice guidelines, and to reduce the rate of inappropriate imaging and increase its yield.
- Imaging decision support is most effective when based on clinically relevant and trustworthy evidence, embedded in provider workflow, efficient, and actionable, and avoids redundant data entry.
- Beginning on January 1, 2020, the United States Protecting Access to Medicare Act (PAMA) will require ordering providers to consult appropriate use criteria (AUC) prior to ordering certain outpatient advanced diagnostic imaging tests (CT, MR, and nuclear medicine exams) for Medicare fee-for-service beneficiaries, as a requirement of payment for such services.
- PAMA presents a substantial opportunity to improve the quality and value of diagnostic imaging while reducing waste and improving patient experience.
- Imaging CDS as an Information Technology (IT) implementation alone is unlikely to optimize care. CDS-enabled multifaceted quality improvement interventions are more likely to improve clinical decision making.

  Future research is needed to evaluate the impact of various CDS interventions and help define best practices for design and implementation of this promising tool to promote evidence-based care.

1 Definitions

- Imaging CDS represents an online, iterative interaction between a user (ordering provider) and a computer software system to provide evidence-based feedback in real time (at the time of ordering) to improve clinical decision making (Fig. 1).
- A CDS application is comprised of two components, the "syringe" and the "medicine." The "syringe" refers to the information technology mechanism that interacts with the user and the CPOE system to deliver the evidence (i.e., the "medicine") to improve the ordering provider's clinical decision; the "medicine" refers to the evidence/clinical logic/rules embedded in CDS.
- AUC are defined as evidence-based criteria to enhance appropriate use of diagnostic imaging tests for a given condition/diagnosis. Their primary purpose is to aid in the clinical decision-making process, guiding the ordering physician to make the most appropriate treatment decision given a specific patient's clinical condition or presentation. The source and/or publisher of the AUCs presented to the user in the CDS application may include professional society guidelines, peer-reviewed publications, and clinical decision rules, or local best practices.
- Strength of evidence: The quality or grade of evidence underlying an AUC varies from evidence based on expert opinion only to evidence based on rigorous science. The grade of evidence is an important contributor to the "trustworthiness" of the AUC as defined by the Institute of Medicine (Ransohoff et al. 2013). The sources and strength of evidence presented in CDS should optimally be transparently available to the user at the time of clinical decision making (Fig. 2).

2 Trends in Imaging Use and Costs

Medical imaging has helped to transform health care and will continue to advance the understanding and treatment of disease (Tempany 2001; Jolesz and Blumenfeld 1994; Weissleder 1999). But despite the substantial benefits of medical imaging in many clinical situations, there is wide variation in the use of

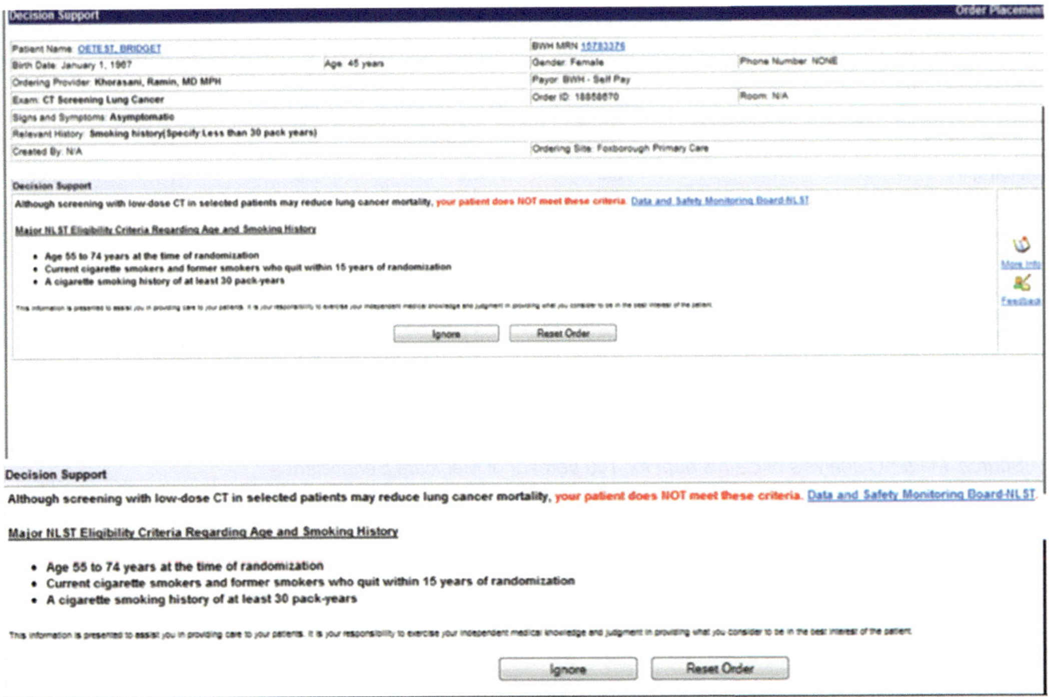

Fig. 1 Interactive CDS alert displays actionable advice to an ordering provider in the process of ordering a lung cancer screening CT on a 45-year-old asymptomatic women with <30 pack-year smoking history. These clinical attributes are necessary for CDS to determine if the patient will not benefit from screening based on available evidence

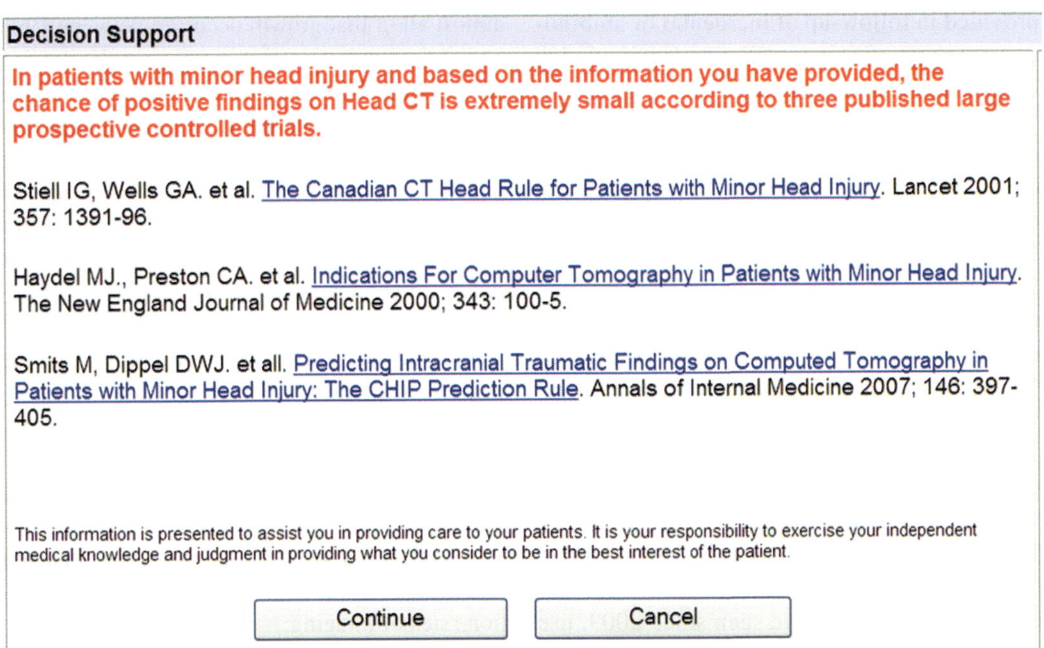

Fig. 2 CDS feedback provides sources of evidence to the ordering user

Type of service	Change in units of service per beneficiary: Average annual 2009–2013	Change in units of service per beneficiary: 20013–2014	Change in volume per beneficiary: Average annual 2009–2013	Change in volume per beneficiary: 20013–2014	Percent of 2014 allowed charges
All services	**–0.1%**	**0.3%**	**N/A**	**0.4%**	**100%**
Imaging	**–0.9**	**–1.0**	**–2.3**	**–1.1**	**11.0**
Advanced–CT: other	1.2	4.2	0.3	3.2	1.6
Echography–heart	1.0	–0.5	–4.1	–1.5	1.1
Advanced–MRI: other	0.1	2.0	–1.7	1.0	0.9
Echography–other	3.8	1.9	3.0	1.9	0.9
Standard–musculoskeletal	–0.2	0.2	–0.7	–0.6	0.9
Standard–nuclear medicine	–7.7	–5.8	–11.6	–7.9	0.8
Standard–breast	0.5	–2.3	–0.4	–2.6	0.7
Imaging/procedure–other	–5.8	–4.2	–1.7	–1.5	0.6
Advanced–MRI: brain	–1.8	1.2	–3.7	–0.8	0.4
Advanced–CT: head	0.2	2.2	–1.2	1.6	0.4
Standard–chest	–2.6	–3.6	–3.0	–4.0	0.4
Echography–abdomen and pelvis	0.5	–1.2	0.3	–1.2	0.4

Source: MedPAC analysis of claims data for 100 percent of Medicare Beneficiaries

Fig. 3 Imaging utilization among medicare beneficiaries. Source: MedPAC analysis of claims data for 100% of Medicare Beneficiaries

imaging (especially high-cost imaging) and concern about inappropriate use persists. Inappropriate use may result in waste (Hendee et al. 2010) and suboptimal quality of care, and may harm patients by exposure to unnecessary ionizing radiation (Sodickson et al. 2009; Smith-Bindman et al. 2009; Lin 2010) or unnecessary additional tests and treatments provided in follow-up of incidental or ambiguous imaging findings (Black 1998; Welch et al. 2011).

Imaging has been identified as a potential driver for rising United States healthcare expenditures although recent reports suggest that utilization levels have moderated or even declined slightly. In 2003, approximately 206 million imaging services were provided to a total of 34.8 million Part B Medicare beneficiaries. By 2006, that number increased 58.4% to 326 million services for 35.9 million beneficiaries (Harvey 2012). By 2013–2014, across all services, Medicare volume per beneficiary grew by 0.4%; but at −1.1% for imaging services (Fig. 3). The Medicare Payment Advisory Commission observed that "While the imaging decrease continues the downward trend we have seen since 2009, use of imaging services remains much higher than it was in 2000" (Medicare Payment Advisory Commission 2016).

In a population-based study utilizing data for one million to two million patients annually from 1996 to 2010 in six large integrated health systems across the United States, the number of CT scans tripled over the study period, to 149 per 1000 patients in 2010, while the number of MRIs quadrupled, to 65 per 1000 patients in 2010 (Smith-Bindman et al. 2012). However, almost all of that growth occurred between 1996 and 2006, and after that time, overall slowing (MRI), or stabilization (CT) in medical imaging utilization was observed. It should be noted that increase in utilization does not necessarily equate waste. For example, increased use of abdominal CT in the emergency room for patients suspected of acute appendicitis has reduced the negative appendectomy rate, particularly for women. In one study, the use of CT was associated with a >10-fold decline in the negative appendectomy rate (portion of appendectomies with a normal appendix at pathology), from >20% to less than 2% (Raja et al. 2010). Future research is needed to explicitly evaluate the impact of imaging in various clinical settings so that quality and value deliberations focus on evidence of clinical impact rather than utilization rates of imaging.

Wide, likely unwarranted, variation also exists in the utilization of CT and MRI across the United States (Fig. 4). For 34 million Medicare

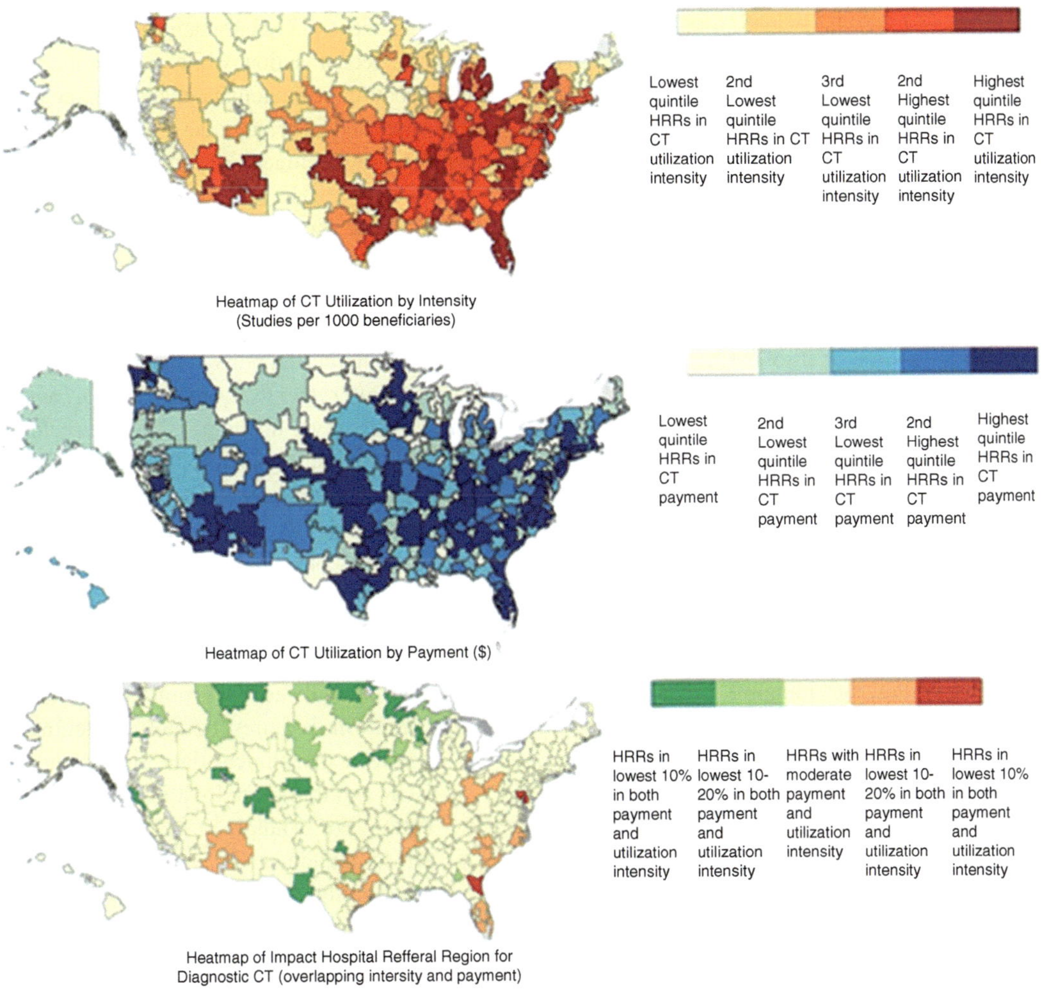

Published in: Ivan K. Ip; Ali S. Raja; Steven E. Seltzer; Atul A. Gawande; Karen E. Joynt; Ramin Khorasani;
Radiology **2015**, 275 718-24
DOI: 10.1148/radiol. 15141964
2015 by the Radiological Society of Northt America, Inc.

Fig. 4 Heat map of CT utilization by intensity (#tests per 1000 Medicare beneficiaries) and by payment, as well as by impact (defined as high utilization *and* payment), demonstrates substantial, likely unwarranted, variation among the 600 Health Referral Regions in the United States (Ip et al. 2015a)

beneficiaries, 124 million unique diagnostic imaging services (totaling $5.6 billion) were performed in 2012. The average adjusted CT utilization intensity ranged from 330.4 studies per 1000 beneficiaries in the lowest decile to 684.0 in the highest decile (relative risk, 2.1); adjusted MR imaging utilization intensity varied from 105.7 studies per 1000 beneficiaries to 256.3 (relative risk, 2.4) (Ip et al. 2015a). The most common CT and MRI procedures were head CT and lumbar spine MRI.

3 General Features of Effective Clinical Decision Support During Radiology Order Entry

Best practices for implementation of imaging CDS are debated and remain uncertain. However, experience to date from implementation of CDS in various domains including in imaging highlights a number of key features (Khorasani et al. 2014; Bates et al. 2003; Ip et al. 2013)

1. *Efficient*: CDS should be optimally embedded in provider workflow. Every computer "mouse click," scroll, or new screen counts should be vigilantly minimized. The speed at which the user gets through the workflow also matters. Redundant data entry in CDS, whether from need to reauthenticate in the CDS application (enter username and password separately from the EHR) or reenter clinical information already captured elsewhere within the EHR, is a major source of user frustration, contributing to provider burnout, (Health Affairs 2017) and creates additional risk of a user entering erroneous data in CDS just to get through the workflow in a busy clinical practice. A clinically useful electronic radiology requisition should optimally capture and communicate the patient's relevant signs and symptoms, known diagnoses, differential diagnostic considerations, and targeted laboratory results necessitating the imaging procedure being requested (e.g., "left lower quadrant pain, 5 days' duration, fever, elevated WBC count, ?diverticulitis"). Relying solely on a single billing *ICD-9-* or *ICD-10*-coded data in the EHR will likely be inadequate to convey the clinical indication and justification for an imaging examination (the primary purpose of CPOE) and thus may hinder a clinically effective CDS program. Any data obtained as part of the imaging CDS interaction should flow back to the EHR and the physician's note when relevant. Such clinical workflows may be implemented by a single-vendor solution, or will require enhanced interoperability between the EHR and imaging CDS system, a feature generally lacking and suboptimally pursued by most vendors to date.

   System design must enable the ordering physician to act on CDS recommendations efficiently. A suboptimal integration of imaging CDS systems with EHR products can result in confusing and inefficient workflows when ordering providers attempt to modify or cancel an imaging order based on a CDS recommendation. For example, if the CDS recommendation is to change a head CT order to a head MRI order, then the provider should be able to accept the recommendation (i.e., click "Accept") while viewing the CDS recommendation. The provider's Accept action while interacting with CDS should then automatically cancel the head CT order and generate a new head MRI order with the same clinical information entered for head CT in the EHR without any further requirement for the user to interact with CDS for the new MRI request. Workflow inefficiencies encourage the ordering provider to ignore the imaging CDS recommendation, creating waste and resulting in suboptimal quality of care.
2. *Educational (rather than punitive) and evidence-based:* Effective imaging CDS interactions need to provide a clinically useful experience in a very limited time span in the middle of provider workflow. This requires the educational experience, and more specifically the clinical content of the CDS alert visible on the computer screen to the user, to have some unique features.
   (a) The clinical feedback must be *clinically valid*. This requires thoughtful integration between the clinical data entered in the EHR and that shared with the CDS application. For example, it has become popular to launch a CDS alert based on a structured indication (a clinical indication selected from a predetermined menu in the EHR) while allowing a user to then enter free text comments to communicate the clinical reason for the examination to the radiologist. Figures 5 and 6 highlight the challenge of presenting a clinically valid alert to the user if the structured indication is broad, ambiguous, or does not otherwise describe the patient's presentation adequately to help determine appropriateness of the order.
   (b) The clinical feedback presented in the CDS should be clinically relevant and "**trustworthy**." Evidence delivered through imaging CDS essentially represents a practice or institution's standard of care and should be consistent with the best practices the clinical leadership can support. The Institute of Medicine has published standards for developing practice guidelines (Institute of Medicine (US) Committee on Standards for

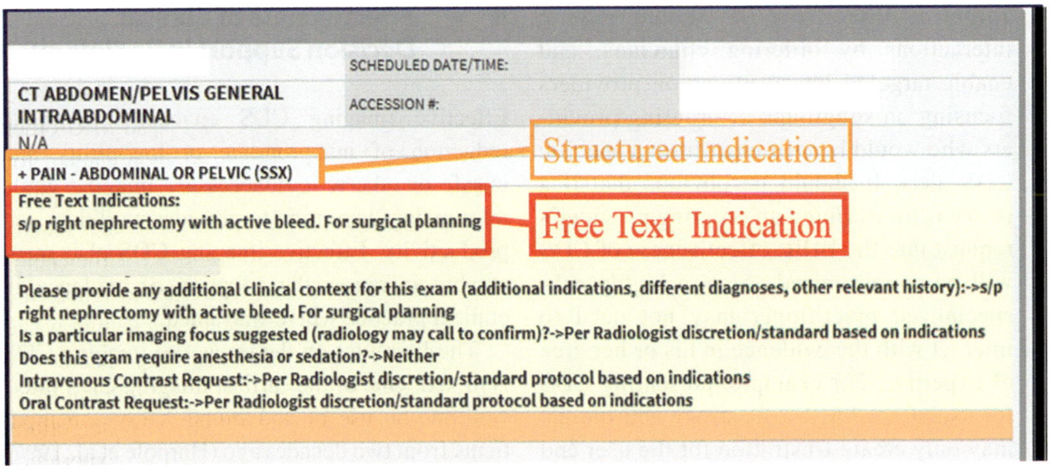

Fig. 5 An electronic requisition for an abdominal CT highlights the potential discrepancy between structured and free text indications selected by the ordering user in the EHR. Providing feedback on the appropriateness of this request based on the selected structured indication alone will likely be viewed as clinically irrelevant by the ordering user

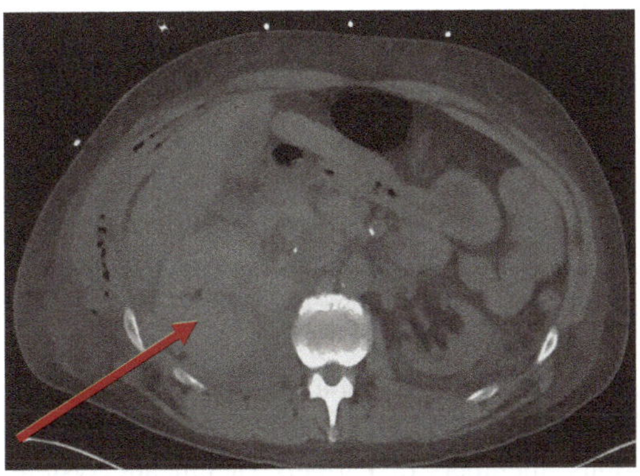

Fig. 6 An image from the CT scan requested in Fig. 5 demonstrated hemorrhage in the right nephrectomy bed (*arrow*)

Developing Trustworthy Clinical Practice Guidelines 2011) which highlight the importance of assessing the strength of each unique piece of evidence or recommendation, (Ransohoff et al. 2013) using the "level of evidence" and "grade of recommendation" frameworks (OCEBM Levels of Evidence - CEBM [Internet] 2009; Grade Definitions - US Preventive Services Task Force [Internet] 2012) as a key factor in determining the trustworthiness of the clinical recommendation. Grading evidence is also useful when comparing overlapping or potentially conflicting evidence from multiple sources. The strength of evidence is also essential to inform policy makers, healthcare delivery systems, and providers as to the relative merit of each recommendation embedded in imaging CDS. Finally, ordering providers are more likely to modify their clinical decision based on strong evidence or those endorsed by national professional societies and local thought leaders to represent institution's best practices.

(c) The alert's educational content must be **brief, unambiguous, and actionable** (suggesting an alternate decision to the one the user is contemplating in the ordering process). Given the need for efficient workflow, the use of ambiguous or elaborate language to communicate recommendations can confuse and frustrate busy providers and decrease system effectiveness. Presenting low-value information (superfluous information not directly relevant to the immediate ordering decision being executed by the user) can create alert fatigue and may even cause providers to ignore relevant CDS recommendations by simply learning to click "ignore" each time a CDS alert displays without making the time to consume the information being presented.

3. *Targeted*: Effective CDS should require interactions by ordering clinicians, and enable targeted interventions on providers focusing on subgroups of ordering providers who would benefit most from a specific CDS alert. It should be obvious that if a proxy is transcribing an ordering provider's request into the EHR, effectiveness of CDS will be compromised. Also, a highly subspecialized practitioner may not need to interact with the evidence in his or her area of expertise. For example, presenting CDS for use of head MRI to a stroke neurologist may only create frustration for the user and undermine the effectiveness of CDS.
4. IT intervention alone, even if based on strong evidence, is unlikely to optimize ordering practices. Consequences of ignoring clinically valid, trustworthy CDS alerts may include required synchronous (at the time of order) peer-to-peer consultation (Ip et al. 2014) or asynchronous feedback (practice pattern variation reports comparing a provide to his or her colleagues) (Raja et al. 2015). Such multifaceted CDS-enabled quality improvement initiatives (including consequences of ignoring alerts) are more likely to reduce inappropriate use of imaging (Raja et al. 2015; Ip et al. 2013; O'Connor et al. 2014; Weilburg et al. 2017; Blackmore et al. 2011). It is thus more helpful to think of effective CDS implementation as a clinical transformation initiative rather than an IT implementation alone. Large-scale CDS-enabled utilization management and medical management interventions (Ip et al. 2013; Weilburg et al. 2017) have shown significant impact on the use of high-cost imaging in large academic medical centers.
5. *Measure, monitor impact*, and adjust CDS interventions based on desired outcomes of improving appropriateness of imaging. Assuming impact is likely to eliminate the possibility of sustainable clinical improvement in your practice.

4 Effectiveness of Clinical Decision Support in Radiology

Effective imaging CDS enables measurable reduction of inappropriate or low-utility and unsafe or otherwise unnecessary imaging while minimizing disruption to provider workflow and productivity. Effective imaging CDS also measurably increases the adoption of evidence in clinical practice where warranted.

The literature on the impact of imaging CDS is mixed. One of the earliest imaging CDS interventions on use of abdominal X-rays on inpatients from two decades ago (Harpole et al. 1997) showed that providers were unwilling to cancel their order but were more willing to modify their request (e.g., change supine KUB order to supine and upright KUB including the hemidiaphragms if clinical concern is perforated viscus). The first description of Web-enabled ambulatory CPOE and CDS in 2001 (Khorasani 2001) was followed by early reports of impact (Ip et al. 2013; Sistrom et al. 2009), as well as meaningful use and adoption (Ip et al. 2012) (Vartanians et al. 2010) across the healthcare enterprise by pioneers and early adopters of this approach at Brigham and Women's Hospital (BWH) and Massachusetts General Hospital (MGH) at Harvard Medical School in Boston. Both institutions, members of Partners Healthcare System, instituted multifaceted CDS-enabled interventions (including CDS, distribution of feedback reports on use of high-cost imaging to ordering providers, and financial incentives to ordering providers to reduce high-cost imaging) as part of a pay-for-performance contract with several local payers in Massachusetts to avoid onerous payer-initiated pre-authorization programs beginning in 2005. A study at Virginia Mason using CDS-enabled, targeted (to specific clinical conditions) multifaceted interventions with local best practices embedded as evidence in imaging CDS showed significant reduction in use of lumbar spine MRI, head MRI, and sinus CT (Blackmore et al. 2011). Tables 1–3 summarize the results of several select interventions at

Table 1 CDS implementation and high-cost imaging use at BWH

Setting	Outcome
Outpatients (2005–2009)	12% decrease in high-cost imaging/1000 member-months, sustained over 4 years in a commercial payer population (Ip et al. 2013)
Emergency department (ED) (2007–2012)	33% decrease in CT; 21% decrease in MRI per 1000 ED visits (Raja et al. 2014a)
Inpatient (2009–2012)	21% decrease in CT/1000 admissions; adjusted for severity of disease (Shinagare et al. 2014)
Overall	7.5% decrease in repeat CTs (approx. 22% of all CTs are repeated within 90 days) (O'Connor et al. 2014; Wasser et al. 2013)

Table 2 Impact of effective CDS based on high-quality, condition-specific evidence *"Choosing Wisely"*

Setting	Outcome
CT for suspected pulmonary embolism (ACEP)	ED use decreases 20%; yield up 69% over 2 years (Raja et al. 2012)/inpatient use decreases 13% over 1 month, then stable (Dunne et al. 2015)
MRI for low back pain (ACP)	Outpatients: MRI use decreases 30% on the day of primary care provider (PCP) visit; 12.3% within 30 days of index PCP visit (Ip et al. 2014)
CT for minor traumatic brain injury (ACEP)	13.4% decrease in use of CT in ED (Ip et al. 2015b)

ACEP American College of Emergency Physicians, *ACP* American College of Physicians

BWH to help highlight broad conclusions on the impact of imaging CDS on use of high-cost imaging.

5 Experience from Large Scale Implementation of Imaging CDS

Concerned with the potential contribution of high-cost imaging to the rising costs of health care, Congress enacted the Medicare Improvement for Patients and Providers Act (MIPPA) in 2008 (Medicare C for, Baltimore MS 7500 SB, Usa M 2013). MIPPA mandated that the Centers for Medicare and Medicaid Services (CMS) undertake a demonstration project (named Medicare Imaging Demonstration or MID) in lieu of a federal pre-authorization program for high-cost imaging. The MID was designed as a 2-year demonstration and launched in October 2011 to assess the impact of preselected professional society guidelines embedded in CDS on use of ambulatory high-cost imaging for outpatient Medicare fee-for-service patients (Medicare the USC for, Boulevard MS 7500 S, Baltimore, Baltimore M 21244 7500 SB, Usa M 21244 2017). Designed as an alternative to prior authorization, the MID project evaluated the impact of two processes on use of 12 high-cost image procedures for ambulatory fee-for-service Medicare patients: a) CDS that was primarily based on AUC created by the American College of Radiology and the American College of Cardiology, and b) practice

Table 3 Impact of CDS-enabled Interventions on documented adherence to evidence

Imaging/condition	Reference	Type	Control (%)	Intervention (%)	*P*-value
Head CT/ED minor trauma (ACEP)	Gupta JAMIA 2014 (Gupta et al. 2014)	Education only	49	76	<0.001
Chest CT/ED PE (NQF)	Raja Acad Rad 2014 (Raja et al. 2014b)	Education only	57	76	<0.01
Chest CT/ED PE (NQF)	Raja AJR 2015 (Raja et al. 2015)	Add MD feedback	78	85	<0.05
LS MRI/ambulatory (ACP)	Ip Am J Med 2014 (Ip et al. 2014)	Add peer to peer, MD feedback	78	96	<0.005

pattern variation reporting to providers. MID was carried out across five geographically and organizationally diverse groups of practices (conveners). With 139,757 orders placed by 3916 physicians at 363 practice sites from October 2012 to September 2014, it was the largest implementation of CDS for imaging to date.

Pooled national data across all conveners was analyzed independently by the RAND corporation and the results were submitted by CMS to Congress in the fall of 2014 (Medicare Imaging Demonstration Evaluation Report to Congress [Internet] 2014). There was no significant change in utilization of high-cost imaging when comparing post-CDS intervention data to pre-intervention (control) among MID participants or when comparing utilization of high-cost imaging in the post-intervention MID practices to concurrent controls selected by CMS and RAND from practices that were not enrolled in the MID. Most orders (63.3% of orders during the baseline period and 66.5% during the intervention period) were unable to be matched by the CDS systems to appropriateness criteria (Hussey et al. 2015). There was a slight (though not statistically significant) improvement in observed appropriateness of imaging as assessed by CDS scores (11.1% of orders were scored inappropriate during baseline vs. 6.4% during the intervention period; 73.7% of baseline orders were scored appropriate vs. 81.0% during the intervention period).

A subsequent analysis of MID data from a single convener including data from delivery systems in three states (Massachusetts, New York, and Pennsylvania) showed that nearly 99% of CDS alerts were ignored by ordering providers. Providers were >20 times more likely to modify an order than to cancel it, similar to a previously published study in 1997 (Harpole et al. 1997). However, actionability of alerts, as well as prior experience with CDS, were identified as important predictors of provider response to CDS alerts (Ip et al. 2017). Actionable alerts (those that could generate an immediate order behavior change in the ordering physician) had a tenfold higher rate of modification (8.1 vs. 0.7%; $p < 0.0001$) or cancellation (0.2 vs. 0.02%; $p < 0.0001$) compared with orders with nonactionable alerts. Orders from institutions with preexisting imaging CDS had a sevenfold lower rate of cancellation or modification than was seen at sites with newly implemented CDS (1.4 vs. 0.2%; $p < 0.0001$).

Although reports of impact of imaging CDS implementation are not entirely consistent, some general conclusions can be made.

1. Imaging CDS-enabled interventions can improve adherence to evidence (Table 3), including clinical practice guidelines, reduce inappropriate use of imaging (Ip et al. 2013, 2015b; Blackmore et al. 2011; Vartanians et al. 2010), increase its yield (Raja et al. 2012; Dunne et al. 2015), and improve quality of care and patient experience. However, there is little empirical evidence that imaging CDS alone, as an IT implementation, will reduce inappropriate use of imaging. Multifaceted CDS-enabled clinical quality improvement interventions, such as those including ordering provider feedback, will likely be needed to improve appropriate use of imaging (Ip et al. 2013; Weilburg et al. 2017).
2. It is likely that CDS based on higher grades of evidence or endorsed by national professional societies *and* supported by local thought leaders as clinical best practices will have higher impact on altering ordering provider behavior. However, more research is needed to understand best practices for design and implementation of imaging CDS to improve its clinical impact while reducing unnecessary distractions for ordering providers.

6 Emerging Challenges and Opportunities for Imaging Clinical Decision Support

In an effort to improve quality of health care and reduce waste through meaningful use of health IT, CDS was a fundamental component of Stage II of the meaningful use criteria for health information technology (HIT) set out in the federal Health Information Technology for Economic and Clinical Health (HITECH) Act of 2009 regulations (Health Information Technology for Economic and Clinical Health (HITECH) Act 2009; Jha 2010; Blumenthal and Tavenner 2010). More recently, Section 218b of the Protecting Access to Medicare Act (PAMA) of 2014, aptly named Promoting Evidence-Based Care, requires that healthcare ordering providers use approved CDS systems to consult specified AUC when ordering certain ambulatory advanced imaging procedures (Table 4) as a requirement for payment for such services to furnishing providers (for both technical and professional components of radiology services) (Protecting Access to Medicare Act of 2014 2014). Per the resulting CMS regulations, beginning on January 1, 2019, PAMA will require ordering providers to consult AUC prior to ordering outpatient CT, MR, and nuclear medicine exams for certain "priority clinical areas" for Medicare fee-for-service beneficiaries. PAMA represents a major opportunity for radiology practices to create value in health care but many implementation challenges remain (Hentel et al. 2017). Under these regulations, no radiology practice will receive Medicare payment for these "certain" advanced imaging procedures unless the claim submitted to CMS for payment includes documentation of ordering provider consultation with a certified CDS mechanism containing AUCs created by a qualified provider-led entity (QPLE).

CMS has created a process for certifying CDS mechanisms (the IT tool or the "syringe"), and a separate process for creation of the AUCs (the "medicine" or the rules to be embedded in CDS)—by delegating the creation of AUCs to QPLEs.

Table 4 CMS priority clinical areas (Hentel et al. 2017)

• Coronary artery disease (suspected or diagnosed)
• Suspected pulmonary embolism
• Headache (traumatic and nontraumatic)
• Hip pain
• Low back pain
• Shoulder pain (to include suspected rotator cuff injury)
• Cancer of the lung (primary or metastatic, suspected or diagnosed)
• Cervical or neck pain

CMS has created an annual application process for national professional societies and other provider-led entities (such as healthcare delivery systems) to receive delegated authority from CMS to become a QPLE. QPLEs have the authority to publish AUCs which if implemented, at least for the priority clinical areas identified by CMS, will allow any provider group to meet PAMA requirements. As of mid-2017, there are 16 QPLEs. Each must meet rigorous requirements, including literature review, multidisciplinary expert panel review of existing literature, grading of each unique piece of evidence in the AUC set using a well-accepted evidence grading framework, and publication of the AUC set in a public website for public scrutiny.

CMS intends to expand the clinical priority areas over time. The priority clinical areas are also intended to be targets for identifying outlier ordering providers, and to potentially expose such outliers to additional pre-authorization programs beginning in 2020. Based on the imaging program experience, CMS may extend the program beyond imaging.

Successfully implemented and adopted, these new regulations have the potential to help improve quality of care, promote evidence-based practice, and reduce waste. However, national implementation of such a program faces several challenges (Hentel et al. 2017). These challenges include enhancing and operationalizing the claims submission process between providers and CMS, establishing the process for private radiology practices who receive imaging requests from many varied referring provider practices, each of which may decide on implementation of a different CDS mechanism based on their own EHR, or conceivably a different set of rules ("medicine") as envisioned under PAMA and its related regulations. As written, the regulation's workflow burden resides primarily in the referring provider domain while the financial burden resides solely in radiology. Attempts to align these varied incentives would likely be helpful in achieving the intended goals of the law.

7 Future Direction

Despite substantial progress in use of imaging CDS to enable evidence-based practice to improve quality and reduce waste, much remains unknown. It remains unclear whether in the current healthcare environment, imaging CDS will achieve its promise of enabling evidence-based practice beyond the leading healthcare delivery institutions which have demonstrated its early effectiveness. It is crucial that maturation of imaging CDS solutions accelerates, buoyed by the looming opportunity created under PAMA. Several streams of improvements and innovation are worth highlighting below.

1. Workflow interactions between EHR vendors and CDS mechanisms need much improvement. Efficient and clinically relevant CDS alerts require sharing of a patient's clinical presentation (beyond a billing code) among systems exposed to providers. It is unclear whether such CDS functions will be ultimately incorporated into EHR modules or whether interoperability standards, many of which exist already, will spur much-needed innovations and improvements in the CDS vendor space. Workflow optimization must consider the impact of each "click" and "scroll," and each distraction, on provider burnout.
2. Policies and regulations, including healthcare financing changes to pay for value rather than volume, would be helpful to align the diverse and at times conflicting incentives of all stakeholders, most importantly including patients, to motivate the needed clinical transformation for promoting evidence-based care.
3. Funding for research to accelerate creation of evidence-based decision rules, using either traditional methodologies (Gupta et al. 2014; Stiell et al. 1992; Wells et al. 2001; Alper et al. 2017) or promising new avenues such as machine learning, deep learning, or artificial intelligence, is sorely needed to improve the usefulness of CDS to clinicians.
4. A public repository of transparently graded (CEBM 2009), publicly available evidence, akin to an "iTunes" library for music, could accelerate the creation of AUCs by QPLEs, may help improve collaboration among QPLEs, identify knowledge gaps in current literature, and allow QPLEs and end users to compare AUCs from different publishers of AUCs when such rules contradict or overlap. Such initiatives can focus on the accumulation, curation, organization, and functionalization of medical evidence rather than on the creation of new evidence (Lacson et al. 2016; Yan et al. 2016).
5. Evaluation of the impact of implementations will be critical in understanding best practices for design and implementation of imaging CDS. Resourcing assessment of impact and sharing results publicly and in peer-reviewed literature will help advance this important tool in effectuating the promise of health information technology in healthcare delivery.

References

Alper EA, Ip IK, Silveira PC, Piazza G, Goldhaber SZ, Benson CB, Lacson R, Khorasani R (2017) Risk stratification model: lower extremity ultrasonography for hospitalized patients suspected of deep vein thrombosis. J Gen Intern Med 1–5

Bates DW, Kuperman GJ, Wang S, Gandhi T, Kittler A, Volk L et al (2003) Ten commandments for effective clinical decision support: making the practice of evidence-based medicine a reality. J Am Med Inform Assoc 10(6):523–530

Black WC (1998) Advances in radiology and the real versus apparent effects of early diagnosis. Eur J Radiol 27(2):116–122

Blackmore CC, Mecklenburg RS, Kaplan GS (2011) Effectiveness of clinical decision support in controlling inappropriate imaging. J Am Coll Radiol 8(1):19–25

Blumenthal D, Tavenner M (2010) The "meaningful use" regulation for electronic health records. N Engl J Med 363(6):501–504

CEBM (2009) Oxford Centre for Evidence-based Medicine - Levels of Evidence (March 2009) [Internet]. [cited 2017 Aug 29]. http://www.cebm.net/oxford-centre-evidence-based-medicine-levels-evidence-march-2009/

Dunne RM, Ip IK, Abbett S, Gershanik EF, Raja AS, Hunsaker A et al (2015) Effect of evidence-based clinical decision support on the use and yield of CT pulmonary angiographic imaging in hospitalized patients. Radiology 276(1):167–174

Grade Definitions—US Preventive Services Task Force [Internet] (2012) [cited 2017 Jun 19]. https://www.uspreventiveservicestaskforce.org/Page/Name/grade-definitions
Gupta A, Ip IK, Raja AS, Andruchow JE, Sodickson A, Khorasani R (2014) Effect of clinical decision support on documented guideline adherence for head CT in emergency department patients with mild traumatic brain injury. J Am Med Inform Assoc 21(e2):e347–e351
Harpole LH, Khorasani R, Fiskio J, Kuperman GJ, Bates DW (1997) Automated evidence-based critiquing of orders for abdominal radiographs: impact on utilization and appropriateness. J Am Med Inform Assoc 4(6):511–521
Harvey L (2012) Medical Imaging: Is the Growth Boom Over? [Internet]. Neiman Health Policy Institute; [cited 2017 Jun 19]. (Neiman Report). Report No.: 1. https://www.acr.org/~/media/ACR/Documents/PDF/Research/Brief-01/PolicyBriefHPI092012.pdf
Health Affairs (2017) Physician Burnout Is A Public Health Crisis: A Message To Our Fellow Health Care CEOs [Internet]. [cited 2017 May 14]. http://healthaffairs.org/blog/2017/03/28/physician-burnout-is-a-public-health-crisis-a-message-to-our-fellow-health-care-ceos/
Health Information Technology for Economic and Clinical Health (HITECH) Act (2009) Public Law 111–5 Feb, 2009
Hendee WR, Becker GJ, Borgstede JP, Bosma J, Casarella WJ, Erickson BA et al (2010) Addressing overutilization in medical imaging. Radiology 257(1):240–245
Hentel K, Menard A, Khorasani R (2017) New CMS clinical decision support regulations: a potential opportunity with major challenges. Radiology 283(1):10–13
Hussey PS, Timbie JW, Burgette LF, Wenger NS, Nyweide DJ, Kahn KL (2015) Appropriateness of advanced diagnostic imaging ordering before and after implementation of clinical decision support systems. JAMA 313(21):2181–2182
Institute of Medicine (US) Committee on Standards for Developing Trustworthy Clinical Practice Guidelines (2011) Graham R, Mancher M, Miller Wolman D, Greenfield S, Steinberg E (eds) Clinical Practice Guidelines We Can Trust [Internet]. Washington, DC: National Academies Press (US); [cited 2017 Jun 19]. http://www.ncbi.nlm.nih.gov/books/NBK209539/
Ip IK, Schneider LI, Hanson R, Marchello D, Hultman P, Viera M et al (2012) Adoption and meaningful use of computerized physician order entry with an integrated clinical decision support system for radiology: ten-year analysis in an urban teaching hospital. J Am Coll Radiol 9(2):129–136
Ip IK, Schneider L, Seltzer S, Smith A, Dudley J, Menard A et al (2013) Impact of provider-led, technology-enabled radiology management program on imaging. Am J Med 126(8):687–692
Ip IK, Gershanik EF, Schneider LI, Raja AS, Mar W, Seltzer S et al (2014) Impact of IT-enabled intervention on MRI use for back pain. Am J Med 127(6):512–518.e1
Ip IK, Raja AS, Seltzer SE, Gawande AA, Joynt KE, Khorasani R (2015a) Use of public data to target variation in providers' use of CT and MR imaging among Medicare beneficiaries. Radiology 275(3):718–724
Ip IK, Raja AS, Gupta A, Andruchow J, Sodickson A, Khorasani R (2015b) Impact of clinical decision support on head computed tomography use in patients with mild traumatic brain injury in the ED. Am J Emerg Med 33(3):320–325
Ip IK, Lacson R, Hentel K, Malhotra S, Darer J, Langlotz C et al (2017) Predictors of provider response to clinical decision support: lessons learned from the Medicare imaging demonstration. AJR Am J Roentgenol 208(2):351–357
Jha AK (2010) Meaningful use of electronic health records: the road ahead. JAMA 304(15):1709–1710
Jolesz FA, Blumenfeld SM (1994) Interventional use of magnetic resonance imaging. Magn Reson Q 10(2):85–96
Khorasani R (2001) Computerized physician order entry and decision support: improving the quality of care. Radiographics 21(4):1015–1018
Khorasani R, Hentel K, Darer J, Langlotz C, Ip IK, Manaker S et al (2014) Ten commandments for effective clinical decision support for imaging: enabling evidence-based practice to improve quality and reduce waste. Am J Roentgenol 203(5):945–951
Lacson R, Raja AS, Osterbur D, Ip I, Schneider L, Bain P et al (2016) Assessing strength of evidence of appropriate use criteria for diagnostic imaging examinations. J Am Med Inform Assoc 23(3):649–653
Lin E (2010) Radiation risk from medical imaging. Mayo Clin Proc 85(12):1142–1146
Medicare C for, Baltimore MS 7500 SB, Usa M (2013) 2008-10-30(2) [Internet]. [cited 2017 Aug 28]. https://www.cms.gov/Newsroom/MediaReleaseDatabase/Fact-sheets/2008-Fact-sheets-items/2008-10-302.html
Medicare Imaging Demonstration Evaluation Report to Congress [Internet] (2014) [cited 2017 Jun 19]. https://innovation.cms.gov/Files/reports/MedicareImagingDemoRTC.pdf
Medicare Payment Advisory Commission (2016) Report to the Congress: Medicare Payment Policy [Internet]. [cited 2017 Jun 19]. march-2016-report-to-the-congress-medicare-payment-policy.pdf
Medicare the USC for, Boulevard MS 7500 S, Baltimore, Baltimore M 21244 7500 SB, Usa M 21244 (2017) Medicare Imaging Demonstration | Center for Medicare & Medicaid Innovation [Internet]. [cited 2017 Jun 19]. https://innovation.cms.gov/initiatives/Medicare-Imaging/
O'Connor SD, Sodickson AD, Ip IK, Raja AS, Healey MJ, Schneider LI et al (2014) Journal club: requiring clinical justification to override repeat imaging decision support: impact on CT use. AJR Am J Roentgenol 203(5):W482–W490
OCEBM Levels of Evidence—CEBM [Internet] (2017) [cited 2017 Jun 19]. http://www.cebm.net/ocebm-levels-of-evidence/

Protecting Access to Medicare Act of 2014 (2014) Public Law 113-93 Apr 1, 2014 p. Congressional Record Vol 160

Raja AS, Wright C, Sodickson AD, Zane RD, Schiff GD, Hanson R et al (2010) Negative appendectomy rate in the era of CT: an 18-year perspective. Radiology 256(2):460–465

Raja AS, Ip IK, Prevedello LM, Sodickson AD, Farkas C, Zane RD et al (2012) Effect of computerized clinical decision support on the use and yield of CT pulmonary angiography in the emergency department. Radiology 262(2):468–474

Raja AS, Ip IK, Sodickson AD, Walls RM, Seltzer SE, Kosowsky JM et al (2014a) Radiology utilization in the emergency department: trends of the past 2 decades. AJR Am J Roentgenol 203(2):355–360

Raja AS, Gupta A, Ip IK, Mills AM, Khorasani R (2014b) The use of decision support to measure documented adherence to a national imaging quality measure. Acad Radiol 21(3):378–383

Raja AS, Ip IK, Dunne RM, Schuur JD, Mills AM, Khorasani R (2015) Effects of performance feedback reports on adherence to evidence-based guidelines in use of CT for evaluation of pulmonary embolism in the emergency department: a randomized trial. AJR Am J Roentgenol 205(5):936–940

Ransohoff DF, Pignone M, Sox HC (2013) How to decide whether a clinical practice guideline is trustworthy. JAMA 309(2):139–140

Shinagare AB, Ip IK, Abbett SK, Hanson R, Seltzer SE, Khorasani R (2014) Inpatient imaging utilization: trends of the past decade. AJR Am J Roentgenol 202(3):W277–W283

Sistrom CL, Dang PA, Weilburg JB, Dreyer KJ, Rosenthal DI, Thrall JH (2009) Effect of computerized order entry with integrated decision support on the growth of outpatient procedure volumes: seven-year time series analysis. Radiology 251(1):147–155

Smith-Bindman R, Lipson J, Marcus R, Kim K-P, Mahesh M, Gould R et al (2009) Radiation dose associated with common computed tomography examinations and the associated lifetime attributable risk of cancer. Arch Intern Med 169(22):2078–2086

Smith-Bindman R, Miglioretti DL, Johnson E, Lee C, Feigelson HS, Flynn M et al (2012) Use of diagnostic imaging studies and associated radiation exposure for patients enrolled in large integrated health care systems, 1996-2010. JAMA 307(22):2400–2409

Sodickson A, Baeyens PF, Andriole KP, Prevedello LM, Nawfel RD, Hanson R et al (2009) Recurrent CT, cumulative radiation exposure, and associated radiation-induced cancer risks from CT of adults. Radiology 251(1):175–184

Stiell IG, Greenberg GH, McKnight RD, Nair RC, McDowell I, Worthington JR (1992) A study to develop clinical decision rules for the use of radiography in acute ankle injuries. Ann Emerg Med 21(4):384–390

Tempany CMC (2001) Advances in biomedical imaging. JAMA 285(5):562–567

Vartanians VM, Sistrom CL, Weilburg JB, Rosenthal DI, Thrall JH (2010) Increasing the appropriateness of outpatient imaging: effects of a barrier to ordering low-yield examinations. Radiology 255(3):842–849

Wasser EJ, Prevedello LM, Sodickson A, Mar W, Khorasani R (2013) Impact of a real-time computerized duplicate alert system on the utilization of computed tomography. JAMA Intern Med 173(11):1024–1026

Weilburg JB, Sistrom CL, Rosenthal DI, Stout MB, Dreyer KJ, Rockett HR et al (2017) Utilization management of HIGH-COST IMAGING in an outpatient setting in a large stable patient and provider cohort over 7 years. Radiology 284(3):766–776

Weissleder R (1999) Molecular imaging: exploring the next frontier. Radiology 212(3):609–614

Welch HG, Schwartz L, Woloshin S (2011) Overdiagnosed: making people sick in the pursuit of health. Beacon Press, Boston, MA, p 228

Wells PS, Anderson DR, Rodger M, Stiell I, Dreyer JF, Barnes D et al (2001) Excluding pulmonary embolism at the bedside without diagnostic imaging: management of patients with suspected pulmonary embolism presenting to the emergency department by using a simple clinical model and d-dimer. Ann Intern Med 135(2):98–107

Yan Z, Lacson R, Ip I, Valtchinov V, Raja A, Osterbur D et al (2016) Evaluating terminologies to enable imaging-related decision rule sharing. AMIA Annu Symp Proc 2016:2082–2089

Part III

Imaging Protocols

Informed Use of Medical Radiation in Diagnostic Imaging

Donald P. Frush

Contents

D.P. Frush
Pediatric Radiology, Duke Medical Center,
Box 3808, Room 1905 CHC, Erwin Road, Durham,
NC 27710, USA
e-mail: donald.frush@duke.edu

Abstract

Examinations that use medical ionizing radiation consisting of radiography, fluoroscopy, computed tomography, and nuclear imaging are essential tools in healthcare. This recognition however is accompanied by the risks of radiation which at doses very much greater than used in diagnostic imaging has known biological effects. The potential risk at diagnostic levels of radiation is the stochastic effect of cancer. Because of the connotations of the term radiation, doses and risks are often misunderstood by patients/caregivers and referring providers. This results in the "safety" aspect of radiation safety and quality often being the prevailing focus. In order to address the growing accountability of the imaging team, experts must understand doses delivered and what is known about risks, and develop a practice based on the tenets of radiation protection relevant to medical use: justification and optimization. This practice should include a dose-monitoring program. In addition, one should be able to have conversations across many different levels of understanding that are balanced and informed with respect to content, and appropriately delivered.

Med Radiol Diagn Imaging (2017)
DOI 10.1007/174_2017_84,
Published Online 27 June 2017

1 Introduction

Diagnostic imaging is an invaluable tool for medical care. Exemplifying this is computed tomography (CT) which has been heralded in a survey of medical practitioners as one of the foremost advancements in medical care in the preceding three decades (Fuchs and Sox 2001); ranked together with MR, CT was #1 out of 30 advancements that included coronary artery bypass grafting, endoscopy, calcium channel blockers, statins, and mammography. Inclusive of CT, however, the majority of diagnostic medical examinations depend on the use of ionizing radiation. These consist of radiography, fluoroscopy, CT, and nuclear imaging. Ionizing radiation in high doses, much higher than his routinely used in medical diagnostic imaging, has recognized biological risks and effects. Because the word "radiation" has a generic implication of harm, there is a heightened awareness/concern by patients, caregivers, and the public about radiation exposure, whether medical or not. Together with a clear increase in the use of medical imaging modalities over the past 20–30 years, and acknowledgment that there should not be variability in similar examinations with respect to delivered radiation doses, the use of medical radiation has become a much more visible accountability for medical providers. Early recognition of the harm from X-ray radiation dates back to Clarence Dally, the first martyr of ionizing radiation exploration and science (Brown 1995) in whom the damage from ionizing radiation was evident by 1900. Nevertheless, there continues to be misunderstanding of how much radiation is delivered during medical imaging examinations, and what is the potential impact of this radiation (Steele et al. 2016; Steele et al. 2017; Lam et al. 2015; Ditkofsky et al. 2016; Sadigh et al. 2014; Rehani and Berris 2012; Boutis et al. 2013; Puri et al. 2012; Hartwig et al. 2013; Robey et al. 2014). Paralleling this is an increasing call for awareness, accountability, and action in the use of medical radiation (Frush et al. 2013). To this end, review of the use of ionizing radiation in the context of safety and quality is warranted. Content consists of clarification of the language of radiation used in the medical imaging, review of trends in use, current perspectives on and prevailing positions in radiation risk, general constructs of radiation protection (CT examples will be emphasized as a large contributor to medical dose), and use of radiation especially in the vulnerable populations in children and with fetal exposure. The value of communication strategies relevant to medical radiation use and potential risk will be summarized. The subject of informed use of ionizing radiation considering all the above factors is broad and deep, including somewhat contentious view on actual risk. The text is amply cited to enhance those areas where more in-depth discussion is desired.

2 The Association of Safety and Quality for Medical Radiation

Radiation is requisite in performing much of diagnostic imaging and cautious use has long been the model, whether under the label of radiation safety or radiation protection. There has been a call for increased accountability by the medical community in the use of medical radiation, especially for diagnostic purposes (Frush et al. 2013). This accountability can be monitored under a comprehensive safety and quality program. "Quality" according to Webster's dictionary is a degree of excellence, and often, including in the familiar pairing of the phrase "safety and quality" implies that the degree is actually excellent, rather than acceptable or good. "Safety" can be considered the absence of harm. Since harm would not generally be in harmony with care that is excellent quality, safety is a requisite component for achieving quality. However, the two are neither interchangeable nor independent. Arguably, a high-quality medical imaging practice should strive to be as safe as possible, but a safe program may not be sufficient for the label of excellent quality, as there are many other attributes of quality (e.g., efficient, service oriented, diagnostically accurate, patient-centered). Why, then not just use the more inclusive word of "quality"? An explanation is that safety is such a dominant and fundamental requisite of the medical landscape, underscored by the recognition and importance of minimizing unsafe medical practice in the 1999 Institute of Medicine report "To Err is Human" (http://www.nationalacademies.org/hmd/Reports/1999/To-Err-is-Human-Building-A-Safer-Health-System.aspx), that it comes to occupy a defensibly conjugal position with quality as a familiar designation. The following material then subscribes to this perspective. There is a potential downfall of this pairing of safety and quality with respect to ionizing radiation and that is the potential overemphasis on the safety aspect of the use of ionizing radiation at the expense of the quality component. Radiation protection through reduction can be the consuming objective rather than informed use of radiation to obtain the necessary diagnostic yield; this may necessitate relatively higher patient doses. Support for this elevation of "radiation dose reduction" above all else is partly embodied in diagnostic reference levels (DRLs), which are based only on radiation dose estimates, generally above which measures should be taken. But relatively low levels of radiation, considered "safer" in the pure sense of the word, may not be of appropriate quality. Radiation protection then as a phrase is not as encompassing as (appropriate) radiation management, more inclusive of both radiation risk and quality elements: that is, the right amount of radiation. DRLs—diagnostic (more aptly dose) reference levels—then might be more fittingly hybridized with measures of image quality under a broader denomination of performance reference levels (PRLS) (performance = dose + quality). Similarly, efforts for a comprehensive and balanced approach to radiation safety and quality may be more appropriately under the rubric *informed* use of radiation than radiation *protection* (Frush et al. 2016).

A few additional clarifications on the subject of medical radiation and safety and quality are warranted. First radiation when used alone implies ionizing type radiation. "Dose" as a term, almost invariably implies dose estimates when used in the clinic arena. "Risk" when discussed often embodies potential risk as some risks with respect to low levels of radiation are uncertain. The phrase "low-dose," in the context of medical radiation, is not an absolute, and in fact is somewhat fluid given technical and technique advances resulting in radiation reduction, such as iterative reconstruction; low-dose signifies a relatively lower doses than is customary. The following information applies to quality and safety for the patient, recognizing that occupational protection is an obligatory component of a comprehensive radiation safety and quality program. Finally, and most importantly, while the majority of the diagnostic of the following material will be dealing with discussions related to radiation use and safety, one must be mindful of the greater context of radiation use in medical imaging: the opportunity to provide valuable information for delivering high-quality medical care. This added value should be really a keystone in discussions with care providers, patients, and caregivers (e.g., parents) when discussing radiation use and potential risk irrespective of specialty.

3 Factors Contributing to the Current Profile for Radiation (and Risk) in Medical Imaging

There is a variety of factors that contribute to the current profile of a radiation used in medical imaging. These factors include an increasing frequency of examinations; examinations with relatively high doses of radiation; potential cumulative exposures; an increase in patient, caregiver, public, and even healthcare provider awareness and concern for radiation (risks) paired with misunderstanding of radiation doses delivered during medical imaging; increased scrutiny by health authorities, regulatory agencies, and other body such as a accrediting organizations; and alarming information in the lay press.

There are nearly 4,000,000,000 examinations performed each year globally that use ionizing radiation (UNSCEAR 2008). In the United States, the per capita increase in radiation from medical imaging increased about 600% in the last 30 years (NCRP 2009). This was largely due to CT examinations, which constitute about 25%

of all radiation exposure, including background exposure, to the US population. Increases in frequency have also been observed more globally based on information from the Atomic Radiation (UNSCEAR) (2013). While the use of imaging over time depends on the type, overall the frequency of examinations that use radiation has leveled off recently or decreased in the past few years (Levin et al. 2007, 2017), especially in children (Parker et al. 2015; Menoch et al. 2012; Miglioretti et al. 2013). Still, the overall use over the past generation has clearly increased. Moreover, radiation doses between the different modalities can vary by orders of magnitude (UNSCEAR 2000; Mettler et al. 2008, 2009; Perez et al. 2015). While this relative range of exposures may be well recognized by imaging experts, the difference in dose for radiation in radiography versus the use of radiation in computed tomography may not be well understood. There may also be a great deal of variability in radiation doses that may result from similar imaging examinations (Hopkins et al. 2013; Smith-Bindman et al. 2009; Demb et al. 2017; Mileto et al. 2017; PiDRL). Some variability in examinations of identical body regions is reasonable based on factors such as indication, or the patient characteristics (i.e., size). Investigators have argued that the variation in doses is greater than it should be (Miglioretti et al. 2013).

There is also increase in the public awareness of radiation; this is exemplified through several portals in the United States. Some of this was due to material in the lay press a number of years ago, including articles in the New York Times regarding CT doses, radiography doses in children, and doses from cone beam CT (Redberg and Smith-Bindman 2014; http://www.nytimes.com/2011/02/28/health/28radiation.html; http://www.nytimes.com/2010/11/23/us/23scan.html; http://www.nytimes.com/2009/10/16/us/16radiation.html; http://articles.latimes.com/2009/oct/14/local/me-cedars-sinai14), and some overexposures in a radiation therapy. For CT, two events also resulted in increased public scrutiny. One was an over exposure of a young child in California following failures in performing an appropriate CT examination (http://www.nytimes.com/2009/10/16/us/16radiation.html). The second example was found in the performance of perfusion CT scans at a number of institutions resulting in tissue reactions (previously referred to as deterministic effects) in several hundred individuals (http://articles.latimes.com/2009/oct/14/local/me-cedars-sinai14). Partly from these events, the state of California enacted dose-reporting requirements (The State of California SB 1237 2010). In addition, other regulatory and accrediting agencies such as The Joint Commission (http://www.jointcommission.org/assets/1/18/AHC_DiagImagingRpt_MK_20150806.pdf) and the American College of Radiology (ACR) (https://www.acr.org/Quality-Safety/Accreditation) established standards for accreditation of programs using diagnostic imaging relative to radiation use. The FDA also promoted more informed use and requirements for reporting of doses that exceeded thresholds in fluoroscopy (https://www.fda.gov/radiation-emittingproducts/radiationemittingproductsandprocedures/medicalimaging/medicalx-rays/ucm115354.htm). The Environmental Protection Agency provided information on use of radiation in medical imaging (https://www3.epa.gov/radtown/medical-xrays.html), and the Centers for Medicare and Medicaid Services (CMS) enacted radiation guidance through the Revised Hospital Radiologic and Nuclear Medicine Services Interpretive Guidelines(https://www.cms.gov/Medicare/Provider-Enrollment-and-Certification/SurveyCertificationGenInfo/Downloads/Survey-and-Cert-Letter-15-38.pdf). Industry also responded, such as a Manufactures Imaging Technology Association XR 29 for CT (http://www.medicalimaging.org/policy-and-positions/mita-smart-dose/) and interventional radiology (http://www.medicalimaging.org/policy-and-positions/mita-smart-dose/mita-smart-dose-interventional/) and other aspects of radiation safety (http://www.medicalimaging.org/policy-and-positions/radiation-dose-safety/). Globally, the International Atomic Agency (IAEA) Basic Safety Standards (http://www-ns.iaea.org/standards/review-of-the-bss.asp?s=11&l=88) also deal with aspects of safe use of radiation in medical imaging. In 2012, the World Health Organization and IAEA cosponsored a radiation protection conference resulting in the Bonn Call for Action (https://rpop.iaea.org/RPOP/RPoP/Content/AdditionalResources/Bonn_Call_for_Action_Platform/), with ten action items relative to the medical use of ionizing radiation. The World Health Organization has also endeavored to increase awareness and education of radiation used in diagnostic imaging (http://www.who.int/ionizing_radiation/about/med_exposure/en/index1.html). In December 2017, a follow-up conference to the Bonn conference occurred in Vienna. Moreover, recognition of the importance of that informed views of radiation is also found with the development of multiple national and trans non-regulatory national organizations for radiation protection. These began with the Image Gently Alliance in 2007, followed by Image Wisely in 2010, EuroSafe (www.eurosafeimaging.org), AFROSAFE (www.afrosaferad.org) Japan Safe Imaging, Canada Safe Imaging (www.canadasafeimaging.ca/en/homepage), LatinSafe (www.latinsafe.org/espanol/), and most recently in May of 2017, ArabSafe. Together, these organizations are a testimonial to the global recognition of the need for radiation safety through education and awareness.

There continues to be a misunderstanding of radiation doses form various modalities, as well as the potential biological effects, particularly cancer induction, from imaging modalities. These include across populations of patients, parents and other care providers, the public, and other healthcare providers. In one study of trainees, Sadigh et al., only 17% of surgical residents had a discussion of radiation safety at least once in the prior 6 months of residency. In addition, only 39% of medical, surgical, obstetrical and gynecological, and radiology trainees combined had a similar discussion (Sadigh et al. 2014). Less than half of all the surveyed trainees had discussion of radiation safety in the pregnant patient at least once in the prior 6 months in residency and radiation safety in children at least once in 6 months of residency. In an international study through the Atomic Energy Agency, Rehani and Berris in surveying referring physicians from 28 countries found that 26% of physicians gave incorrectly high estimates of radiation dose for chest CT (30 mSv) and just under 35% could provide the equivalent number of chest X-rays for an abdomen CT examination (Rehani and Berris 2012). While the numbers are small, 2.2% of all physicians thought that old age was relatively higher radiation sensitivity than childhood and that MRI produced ionizing radiation. Boutis et al. in a survey of parents at a tertiary care pediatric emergency department reported that less than half of parents surveyed knew of issues related to potential malignancy risk associated with head CT imaging. A *moderate* risk of cancer from radiography was felt to be present by 5.4% of parents surveyed versus 5.1% for head CT and a *large* risk of cancer was similar between radiography and CT, 0.8% versus 1.1%, respectively (Boutis et al. 2013). Finally, Ditkofsky et al. (2016) reported that just under 50% of attending physicians and 72% of emergency department residents were either not very comfortable, uncomfortable, or extremely uncomfortable discussing the amount of radiation used in certain patients. In the same group surveyed, only 17.1% of attending physicians and 9.3% of resident physicians were extremely comfortable in explaining risks of radiation exposure to the patient (Ditkofsky et al. 2016).

The current profile of radiation at use of medical imaging has also been underscored by a call for obtaining signed informed consent for a diagnostic medical radiation use. For example, a recent point counterpoint outlined the contrary positions on the need for a consent and the reader is referred for details on both sides of the issue (Harvey et al. 2015; Armao et al. 2015; Nievelstein and Frush 2012). Suffice it to say that in the US there is not a prevailing call, nor is there a substantive practice for obtaining this consent.

Finally, the unbalanced promotion of radiation risk was recently well reviewed by Cohen (2015), related to a publication where CT examinations in childhood were associated with a risk of developing a brain tumor (1:10,000 risk). In this opinion piece, Cohen correctly pointed out the emphasis on the alarming aspects rather than the consensus opinion on this level of radiation and risk. However, there have also been efforts to implicate various education and awareness campaigns, including those in the US [Image Gently www.imagegently.org (Goske et al. 2008a, b) and Image Wisely www.imagewisely.org (Brink and Amis 2010)] whose mission is to inform a variety of audiences about radiation doses, potential risks, and methods to assure appropriate use. These organizations and similar efforts have been challenged as contributing to the public fear and should be terminated. This position is contested (Frush 2016; Cohen 2016).

4 Radiation and Risk

In order to gauge the significance of safety with respect to medical ionizing radiation, and potential strategies to mitigate the risk, it is necessary to understand the presence and magnitude of risks. Recall that we think of safety as the absence of harm, or with radiation the minimization of potential harm (the ALARA principle). The harm, or detriment, of ionizing radiation is divided into tissue reactions, cell death, (seen beginning with relatively high doses) and stochastic effects, DNA injury and altered cell function, (seen beginning with relatively low doses). However detriment can also be psychological, such as guilt for having a child undergo an examination that exposes them to radiation and concern (unwarranted or otherwise), over the long-term consequences of that exposure. A detriment could also be a practice that uses, for example, 50% more dose for extremity radiography than standards established for like practices. The biological risk increase is arguable zero, but the perception of that practice as a "high dose" practice, and lack of attention to patient welfare, may be a detriment to the administrators as well as referring physicians, the latter who may send business elsewhere. It is just important that one is mindful of the spectrum of detriment that may occur, and the detriment is not always isolated to the patient.

Be that as it may, most of the discussion of risk and dose deals with the real and potential biological effects categorized above. It is not the intent of this chapter to fully explore this range of detriment; it is just important for the reader to recognize that the classification of safety and risk are often distilled to clear a biological harm that is not necessarily the only consideration. A few additional points need to be made with respect to radiation use and these biological effects. First, the risk of a procedure is warranted if the examination is justified. Moreover, the occurrence of biological effects from radiation, such as during a complex or life-saving interventional procedures such as skin erythema maybe obligatory. That is, the presence of a biological effect does not indicate that this was an accidental or negligent use of radiation.

In radiology practices, this biological harm may be either a tissue reaction or stochastic effect. For the overwhelming majority of diagnostic imaging procedures, doses are well below threshold for tissue effects (outside of accidental or other inadvertent exposures as previously noted). In more complicated interventional procedures, often with therapeutic manipulations, there may be both tissue reactions and stochastic risks. The concept of misuse of radiation dose as well has not traditionally been considered within the spectrum of medical error. Perhaps this is because the medium, radiation, has no immediate physical (i.e., sensory activating such as taste, or pain) properties. In addition, the potential biological effects from a stochastic standpoint may take years, even decades to manifest. This is much different from risks associated with other interventions and medicine such as administration of antibiotics or narcotics, surgical procedures, or chemotherapy for cancer where the risks are more immediately evident and associative as they are proximal to the event. Nevertheless, it is worth considering that overdosing (as well as under dosing) radiation in the context of medical imaging could be considered a medical error, and unsafe practice.

The consensus statement of the majority of scientific and medical professionals related to ionizing radiation used in medical imaging is that the risk of cancer below 50–100 mSv is uncertain (https://rpop.iaea.org/RPOP/RPoP/Content/InformationFor/Patients/information-public/index.htm; WHO 2016; http://www.aapm.org/org/policies/details.asp?id=318&type=PP; http://

hps.org/documents/risk_ps010-3.pdf; Jolly and Meyer 2009). Above 100 mSv, there are data that demonstrates a significant, albeit small, risk of developing cancer. Given this uncertainty, the labeling of any amount of radiation as having risk may be better achieved by using *potential* as a modifier for risk, as this is more a presumptive and reflects this uncertainty. It is possible to find a wide variation in the positions with respect to diagnostic levels of radiation and stochastic cancer risks. These range from a perspective of hormesis, where a small amount of radiation is helpful (Jolly and Meyer 2009) to positions that there is no evidence of risk, to positions that even a small amounts of radiation can result in a potential increased risk of cancer (Pearce et al. 2012; Mathews et al. 2012; Huang et al. 2014; Hendee and O'Connor 2012; Krille et al. 2015; Journy et al. 2015; Boice 2015). For example, in children, one group of investigators concluded that the risk of leukemia was increased in children who had three or more a neonatal chest X-rays (Bartley et al. 2010). It is not the purpose of this chapter to promote the merits of one position or another but merely to reemphasize that at this point in time, the linear no threshold model, although challenged even recently, is still the most widely accepted model, and the position that the risk of cancer below 50–100 mSv is uncertain is the most prevalent.

With respect to the pediatric population and low-level radiation from medical imaging from CT, there have been three investigations, which have associated cancer from these examinations performed in childhood. A frequently cited report is by Pearce in which they conclude that for a head CT examinations in childhood, there was a 1:10,000 chance of developing a brain tumor (Pearce et al. 2012). Since that time of that publication, two other investigations have a called into question the association of cancer and CT examinations in childhood, and a recent summary by Boice addressed other difficulties with investigations that are making this connection (Boice 2015). There have been ranges of fatal cancer risk from about 1:150 to 1:10,000 with a general age-independent risk 1:1000 (= to 5% per Sievert fatal cancer risk) (Pearce et al. 2012; Einstein and Henzlova 2007).

The mechanisms and factors associated with the development of cancer are obviously quite complex. What is known is that children are a more vulnerable population than adults are. This is for several reasons. First, a similar exposure to a small child as a larger (i.e., cross section) adult results in higher organ doses to that child. In addition, tissues and organs in children are in general more vulnerable to radiation due to the fact they are growing. However, this is not true for all cancers. About 35% of a childhood cancers are more vulnerable to ionizing radiation. For about 25% of cancers, this difference between children and adults is unknown. In about 10% of cancers (e.g., lung cancer), adults are more vulnerable to radiation (UNSCEAR 2013). Finally, there is a longer lifetime to manifest the potential radiation-induced DNA perturbations, a fundamental element in carcinogenesis that could result in the development of cancer. That is, a relatively high dose in an individual who is 89 years of age is likely not to have the same significance in terms of latency of a solid malignancy as the same organ dose to a child who is 8.9 years of age.

Radiation safety in pregnancy has been recently comprehensively addressed by NCRP report 174 (http://ncrponline.org/publications/reports/ncrp-report-174/). This outlines what is known about dose risks, risk mitigation, and development of programs and policies for radiation protection and pregnant or potentially a pregnant woman. It is important to recognize that exposure is not only an issue for the fetus, as some examinations, such as a chest CT can provide relatively high breast doses, tissue which is are more sensitive during gestation. The American College of Radiology provides a practice paradigm and technical standard for use of radiation in pregnancy which can service a guideline in establishing a program (https://www.acr.org/~/media/9E2ED55531FC4B4FA53EF3B6D3B25DF8.pdf) as there is no national consensus document.

In summary, the most widely recognized risk discussions with ionizing radiation deal with biological effects, and in diagnostic imaging those consist almost exclusively of stochastic, potential cancer risks. However, it is important when developing a safety and quality program to consider a broader scope of what is considered detriment that may include such factors as adherence to standards of practice, potential psychological harm, and practice reputation among considerations.

5 Strategies for Safe Use of Ionizing Radiation in Medical Imaging

The following material is not intended to provide modality specific information on dose management strategies across all ages. This is well beyond the scope of this chapter. What will be emphasized are general considerations in radiation does accountability through a management program that addresses the fundamental requirements in medical practice. The intent is to discuss generic approaches to radiation management.

The principles of radiation protection in medical imaging consist of justification and optimization. Justification is that the examination is appropriate and optimization signifies that the performance of the examination is done to some standard.

Justification is a shared responsibility between two or more services, one of which is the imaging service. Generally, the other is the referring service but may be or be in addition to a consultant service. The definition of an appropriate examination is sometimes difficult and there are multiple factors that contribute to a justification examination, beyond the simple evidence-based medical benefit. Some of these have been recently reviewed and consist of, in US practice, defensive medicine, availability of imaging services (and expertise) off hours, and referrer preference (Frush 2014). A congress report from 2012 that dealt with justification in medical outlined several strategies for improving medical utilization including point of care decision support, evidence-based, guidelines, increased use of practice guidelines, facility accreditation, management of self-referral, management of defensive medicine, Stakeholder education, and payment reform (Hendee et al. 2010). Currently, in the United States, one of the biggest strategies is the migration to use electronic decision support. With this, the appropriateness of the examination and or other guidance such as decision rules may be available at the point of care to assist healthcare providers in deeming whether an examination is warranted or not. The optimization of examinations is beyond the scope of this chapter. Suffice it to say that this is the responsibility of the imaging team. From the safety and quality standpoint, performing the examination should adhere to the ALARA principle and be programmatic. The fundamentals of safe and high-quality imaging program with respect to the use of ionizing radiation should include the following: (1) developed, implemented and maintained, and audited as a consensus; that is, stakeholders may include information technology experts, radiologists, technologists, medical physicists, health physicists (e.g., radiation safety officers), and administrators; (2) consistency between all areas of the enterprise as well as between all providers who use modalities that employee ionizing radiation; (3) informed and developed based on best practices, including evidence-based information, and/or established relevant professional standards including achieving justification and optimization of examinations; (4) designed (e.g., data generation, analysis, and discussion) with multiple "customers" in mind and that includes patients, caregivers, the public, healthcare refers, imaging experts, administration, appropriate regulatory, and other health authority individuals; (5) considered a component of a high reliability organization which emphasizes attention to both work culture and adherence to a culture of safety (Sexton et al. 2009; Schein 2004).

Current requirements for TJC accreditation in the US require a dose-monitoring program that consists of guidelines for the performance of CT and nuclear imaging (http://www.jointcommission.org/assets/1/18/AHC_DiagImagingRpt_MK_20150806.pdf). Challenges in developing, implementing, maintaining, and auditing this program include what are benchmarks (especially as dose standards may drift downwards with medical advancements), what is considered nonstandard dosing including to vulnerable populations, who overseas this, what are penalties, who leverages the penalties, what to do with potentially massive amounts of data, differences in equipment and ability to provide consistent state of the art medical imaging (Frush and Samei 2015).

Also important in dose-monitoring programs will be the development of diagnostic reference levels (PiDRL; International Commission on Radiological Protection 2007; McCullough 2010; Vassileva and Rehani 2015) for all modalities. These may serve as benchmarks for a performance of examination. However, limitations with diagnostic reference levels include the absence of a quality metric. That is, these relate only to dose and have no information relative to the capability for the adherence to quality measures related to diagnostic capabilities.

With respect to pediatric imaging, size should be a consideration in administering ionizing radiation, including administered doses for radionuclide imaging, and altered parameters for radiography (appropriate number of projections, lower radiation exposures, collimation, use of grids), fluoroscopy (limited fluoroscopy time, filters, pulsed fluoroscopy with low frame rate, frame hold, video recording, collimation, grids), and CT (lower kilovoltage-kV, and lower time tube current product-mAs). There are additional dose management strategies for children that are more standard than in adults such as increased use of nonionizing modalities (e.g., ultrasound for neck masses, possible appendicitis), and less frequent use of multiphase CT examinations. Many of these dose reduction opportunities in children were relatively recently reviewed (Khong et al. 2013); many of these strategies overlap with adult populations as this size is also encountered in the pediatric age-range. Training in medical physics, radiation biology, and testing for certification as well as assessing abilities during practice (continuous certification) should contain quality and safety material content related to dose management and risk assessment.

6 Radiation Risk Dialogues

A fundamental component of any safety program for ionizing radiation is the ability for adequate communication. Risk communication depends on knowledge of the both the certainties and uncertainties of risks related to the use radiation, emphasizing the value of the imaging modality. The content should be delivered appropriate for the level of understanding of the relative party or discussants.

Multiple resources for informed use of radiation in medical imaging exist including Image Gently for children, Image Wisely for adults, radiologyinfo.org, and a recent release by the World Health Organization, Communicating Radiation Risk in Pediatric Imaging to support risk-benefit dialogue. This is a comprehensive communication resource that covers all modalities that use ionizing radiation and is intended primarily for children but much of the information is applicable to adults (Perez et al. 2015). In addition, the websites for global organizations/campaigns listed earlier offer information of radiation management in children and adults.

Fundamentally, patients and their caregivers want to know that they will be well taken care of, that they have been given the opportunity to ask questions, you have answered those questions to a reasonable level of completeness and sophistication, and have given them the option for additional resources if necessary. Implicit in this conversation again is the reinforcement of the high value of medical imaging. This is often dismissed in light of more complex discussions of risk and risk reduction. Fundamentals of good communication involve being informed, sensitive, and engaged (Levetown 2008). I avoid the discussion of risk numbers. Other communication resources from the patients' perspective in the emergence setting have been provided by Broder (Broder and Frush 2014), and an excellent discussion for radiation use in medical imaging, emphasizing a balanced discussion of risk by McCullough (McCollough et al. 2015).

Through the use of balanced resources, imagers and other provider should be able to have a dialogue that is appropriate to the conversants with respect to (estimated) doses from medical imaging examinations, including what is (and isn't known) about radiation risk communication in healthcare, and to assure informed awareness of the need for justification and optimization and taking appropriate and necessary measures to be resonant with safe and high-quality imaging practice (Abujudeh 2017).

References

Abujudeh H, Kaewlai R, Shaqdan K, Bruno MA (2017) Key principles in quality and safety in radiology. AJR 208:W101–W109

Armao DM, Smith JK, Semelka RC (2015) Debriefing the brief: it is time for the provision of informed consent before pediatric CT. Radiology 275:326–330

Bartley K, Metayer C, Selvin S, Ducore J, Buffler P (2010) Diagnostic X-rays and risk of childhood leukaemia. Int J Epidemiol 39:1628–1637

Boice JD (2015) Radiation epidemiology and recent paediatric computed tomography studies. Ann ICRP 44:236–248

Boutis K, Cogollo W, Fischer J et al (2013) Parental knowledge of potential cancer risks from exposure to computed tomography. Pediatrics 132:305–311

Brink JA, Amis ES (2010) Image wisely: a campaign to increase awareness about adult radiation protection. Radiology 257:601–602

Broder JS, Frush DP (2014) Content and style of radiation risk communication for the pediatric patients. J Am Coll Radiol 11:238–242

Brown P (1995) American martyrs to radiology. Clarence Madison Dally (1865–1904). Am J Roentgenol 164(1):237–239

Cohen MD (2015) ALARA, Image Gently and CT-induced cancer. Pediatr Radiol 45:465–470

Cohen MD (2016) Point: should the ALARA concept and Image Gently Campaign be terminated? J Am Coll Radiol 13:1195–1198

Demb J, Chu P, Nelson T et al (2017) Optimizing radiation doses for computed tomography across institutions: dose auditing and best practices. JAMA Intern Med. Epub ahead of print. Accessed 17 Apr 2017

Ditkofsky N, Shekhani HN, Cloutier M et al (2016) Ionizing radiation knowledge among emergency department providers. J Am Coll Radiol 13:1044–1049

Einstein AJ, Henzlova MJ Rajagopalan S, Estimating risk of cancer associated with radiation exposure from 64-slice computed tomography coronary angiography. JAMA 298:317–323

Frush DP (2014) Whats and whys with neonatal CT. Pediatrics 133(6):e1738–e1739

Frush DP (2016) Counterpoint: Image Gently: should it end or endure? J Am Coll Radiol 13:1199–1202

Frush D.P., Samei E. (2015) CT radiation dose monitoring: current state and new prospects CME. http://www.medscape.org/viewarticle/839485. Accessed 17 Apr 2017

Frush DP, Denham CR, Goske MJ et al (2013) Radiation protection and dose monitoring in medical imaging: a journey from awareness, through accountability, ability and action…but where will we arrive? J Patient Saf 9(4):232–238

Frush DP, Benjamin LS, Kadom N et al (2016) The Think A-Head campaign: an introduction to Image Gently 2.0. Pediatr Radiol 46:1774–1779

Fuchs VR, Sox HC (2001) Physicians' views of the relative importance of thirty medical innovations. Health Aff 20:30–42

Goske MJ, Applegate KE, Frush DP et al (2008a) Image Gently: a national education and communication campaign in radiology using the science of social marketing. J Am Coll Radiol 12:1200–1205

Goske MJ, Applegate KE, Frush DP et al (2008b) The image gently campaign: increasing CT radiation dose awareness through a national education and awareness program. Pediatr Radiol 38:265–269

Hartwig HD, Clingenpeel J, Perkins AM, Rose W, Abdullah-Anyiwo J (2013) Parental knowledge of radiation exposure in medical imaging used in the pediatric emergency department. Pediatr Emerg Care 29:705–709

Harvey HB, Brink JA, Frush DP (2015) Informed consent for radiation risk from CT is unjustified based on the current scientific evidence. Radiology 275:321–325

Hendee WR, O'Connor MK (2012) Radiation risks of medical imaging: separating fact from fantasy. Radiology 264:312–321

Hendee WR, Becker GJ, Borgstede JP et al (2010) Addressing overutilization in medical imaging. Radiology 257:240–245

Hopkins KL, Pettersson DR, Koudelka CW et al (2013) Size-appropriate radiation doses in pediatric body CT: a study of regional community adoption in the United States. Pediatr Radiol 43:1128–1135

Huang WY, Muo CH, Lin CY et al (2014) Paediatric head CT scan and subsequent risk of malignancy and benign brain tumour: a nation-wide population-based cohort study. Br J Cancer 110:2354–2360

International Commission on Radiological Protection (ICRP) (2007) Radiological protection in medicine. ICRP publication 105. Ann ICRP 37(6):1–6

Jolly D, Meyer JA (2009) A brief review of radiation hormesis. Australas Phys Eng Sci Med 32:180–187

Journy N, Rehel J-L, Ducou Le Pointe H et al (2015) Are the studies on cancer risk from CT scans biased by indication Elements of answer from a large-scale cohort study in France. Br J Cancer 112:185–193

Khong P, Ringertz H, Frush D et al (2013) ICRP publication 121: radiological protection in paediatric diagnostic and interventional radiology. Ann ICRP 42(2):1–63

Krille L, Dreger S, Schindel R et al (2015) Risk of cancer incidence before the age of 15 years after exposure to ionising radiation from computed tomography: results from a German cohort study. Radiat Environ Biophys 54:1–12

Lam DL, Larson DB, Eisenberg JD, Forman HP, Lee CI (2015) Communicating potential radiation-induced cancer risks from medical imaging directly to patients. J Am Coll Radiol 205:962–970

Levetown M (2008) Communicating with children and families: from everyday interactions to skill in conveying distressing information. Pediatrics 121:e1441–e1460

Levin DC, Rao VM, Parker L, Frangos AJ, Sunshine JH (2007) Recent trends in utilization rates of noncardiac thoracic imaging: an example of how imaging growth might be controlled. J Am Coll Radiol 4(12):886–889

Levin DC, Laurence Parker L, Palit CD, Rao VM (2017) After nearly a decade of rapid growth, use and complexity of imaging declined, 2008–14. Health Aff 36(4):663–670

Mathews J, Forsythe A, Brady Z et al (2012) Cancer risk in 680000 people exposed to computed tomography scans in childhood or adolescence: data linkage study of 11 million Australians. BMJ 346:1–18

McCollough CH, Bushberg JT, Fletcher JG, Eckel LJ (2015) Answers to common questions about the use and safety of CT scans. Mayo Clin Proc 90:1380–1392

McCullough CH (2010). Diagnostic reference levels. http://www.imagewisely.org/~/media/ImageWisely-Files/Medical-Physicist-Articles/IW-McCullough-Diagnostic-Reference-Levels.pdf. Accessed 17 Apr 2017

Menoch MJA, Hirsh DA, Khan N et al (2012) Trends in computed tomography utilization in the pediatric emergency department. Pediatrics 129:e690–e697

Mettler FA, Huda W, Yoshizumi TT, Mahesh M (2008) Effective doses in radiology and diagnostic nuclear medicine: a catalog. Radiology 248:254–263

Mettler FA, Bhargavan M, Faulkner K et al (2009) Radiologic and nuclear medicine studies in the United States and worldwide: frequency, radiation dose, and comparison with other radiation sources—1950–2007. Radiology 253(2):520–531

Miglioretti DL, Johnson E, Williams A et al (2013) The use of computed tomography in pediatrics and the associated radiation exposure and estimated cancer risk. JAMA Pediatr 167:700–707

Mileto A, Nelson RC, Larson DG et al (2017) Variability in radiation dose from repeat identical CT examinations: longitudinal analysis of 2851 patients undergoing 12,635 thoracoabdominal CT scans in an academic health system. Am J Roentgenol 28:1–12

NCRP (2009) Ionizing radiation exposure of the population of the United States. National Council on Radiation Protection and Measurements, Bethesda, MD. Report No. 160

Nievelstein RJ, Frush DP (2012) Commentary. Should we obtain informed consent for examinations that expose patients to radiation? Am J Roentgenol 199:664–669

Parker MW, Shah SS, Hall M et al (2015) Computed tomography and shifts to alternate imaging modalities in hospitalized patients. Pediatrics 136:e573–e581

PiDRL—European Diagnostic Reference Levels for Paediatric Diagnostic Imaging. http://www.eurosafeimaging.org/pidrl. Accessed 17 Apr 2017

Pearce MS, Salotti JA, Little MP et al (2012) Radiation exposure from CT scans in childhood and subsequent risk of leukemia and brain tumors: a retrospective cohort study. Lancet 380:499–505

Perez M, Miller D, Frush DP, et al. 2015 Communicating radiation risks in pediatric imaging to support risk-benefit dialogue. Who Health Organization. http://www.who.int/ionizing_radiation/pub_meet/radiation-risks-paediatric-imaging/en/. Accessed 17 Apr 2017

Puri S, Hu R, Quazi RR et al (2012) Physicians' and midlevel providers' awareness of lifetime radiation—attributable cancer risk associated with commonly performed CT studies: relationship to practice behavior. Am J Roentgenol 199:1328–1336

Redberg R.F., Smith-Bindman R. (2014) We are giving ourselves cancer. The New York Times. http://www.nytimes.com/2014/01/31/opinion/we-are-giving-ourselves-cancer.html. Accessed 17 Apr 2017

Rehani MM, Berris T (2012) International Atomic Energy Agency study with referring physicians on patient radiation exposure and its tracking: a prospective survey using a web-based questionnaire. BMJ 2:1–10

Robey TE, Edwards K, Murphy MK (2014) Barriers to computed tomography radiation risk communication in the emergency department: a qualitative analysis of patient and physician perspectives. Acad Emerg Med 21:122–129

Sadigh G, Khan R, Kassin MT, Applegate KE (2014) Radiation safety knowledge and perceptions among residents. Acad Radiol 21:869–878

Schein EH (2004) Organizational culture and leadership, 3rd edn. John Wiley and Sons, Inc., San Francisco

Sexton JB, Grillo S, Fullwood C, Pronovost PJ. (2009) Assessing and improving safety culture. In: Frankel A, Leonard M, Simmonds T, Haraden C, Vega KB (eds) The essential guide for patient safety officers, vol 2009. Chicago, IL: Joint Commission Resources with the Institute for Healthcare Improvement: pp 11–20

Smith-Bindman R, Lipson J, Marcus R et al (2009) Radiation dose associated with common computed tomography examinations and the associated lifetime attributable risk of cancer. Arch Intern Med 169:2078–2086

Steele JR, Jones AK, Clarke RK et al (2016) Oncology patient perceptions of the use of ionizing radiation in diagnostic imaging. J Am Coll Radiol 13:768–774

Steele JR, Jones AK, Clarke RK et al (2017) Use of an online education platform to enhance patients' knowledge about radiation in diagnostic imaging. J Am Coll Radiol 14:382–392

The State of California SB 1237 (2010). http://www.leginfo.ca.gov/pub/09-10/bill/sen/sb_1201-1250/sb_1237_bill_20100929_chaptered.html. Accessed 17 Apr 2017

United Nations Scientific Committee on the Effects of Atomic Radiation (2013) UNSCEAR report sources, effects and risks of ionizing radiation. Vol. II: scientific annex B: effects of radiation exposure in children

UNSCEAR (2000) Sources and effects of ionizing radiation. Vol. 1: sources

UNSCEAR (2008) UNSCEAR report Vol. I: sources and effects of ionizing radiation
Vassileva J, Rehani M (2015) Diagnostic reference levels. Am J Roentgenol 204:W1–W3
WHO Factsheet (2016) Ionizing radiation, health effects and protective measures. http://www.who.int/mediacentre/factsheets/fs371/en/. Accessed 17 Apr 2017
http://www.nationalacademies.org/hmd/Reports/1999/To-Err-is-Human-Building-A-Safer-Health-System.aspx. Accessed 17 Apr 2017
http://www.nytimes.com/2011/02/28/health/28radiation.html. Accessed 17 Apr 2017
http://www.nytimes.com/2010/11/23/us/23scan.html. Accessed 17 Apr 2017
http://www.nytimes.com/2009/10/16/us/16radiation.html. Accessed 17 Apr 2017
http://articles.latimes.com/2009/oct/14/local/me-cedars-sinai14. Accessed 17 Apr 2017
http://www.jointcommission.org/assets/1/18/AHC_DiagImagingRpt_MK_20150806.pdf. Accessed 17 Apr 2017
https://www.acr.org/Quality-Safety/Accreditation. Accessed 17 Apr 2017
https://www.fda.gov/radiation-emittingproducts/radiationemittingproductsandprocedures/medicalimaging/medicalx-rays/ucm115354.htm. Accessed 17 Apr 2017
https://www3.epa.gov/radtown/medical-xrays.html. Accessed 17 Apr 2017
https://www.cms.gov/Medicare/Provider-Enrollment-and-Certification/SurveyCertificationGenInfo/Downloads/Survey-and-Cert-Letter-15-38.pdf. Accessed 17 Apr 2017
http://www.medicalimaging.org/policy-and-positions/mita-smart-dose/. Accessed 17 Apr 2017
http://www.medicalimaging.org/policy-and-positions/mita-smart-dose/mita-smart-dose-interventional/. Accessed 17 Apr 2017
http://www.medicalimaging.org/policy-and-positions/radiation-dose-safety/. Accessed 17 Apr 2017
http://www-ns.iaea.org/standards/review-of-the-bss.asp?s=11&l=88. Accessed 17 Apr 2017
https://rpop.iaea.org/RPOP/RPoP/Content/AdditionalResources/Bonn_Call_for_Action_Platform/. Accessed 17 Apr 2017
http://www.who.int/ionizing_radiation/about/med_exposure/en/index1.html. Accessed 17 Apr 2017
https://rpop.iaea.org/RPOP/RPoP/Content/InformationFor/Patients/information-public/index.htm. Accessed 17 Apr 2017
http://www.aapm.org/org/policies/details.asp?id=318&type=PP. Accessed 17 Apr 2017
http://hps.org/documents/risk_ps010-3.pdf. Accessed 17 Apr 2017
http://ncrponline.org/publications/reports/ncrp-report-174/. Accessed 17 Apr 2017
https://www.acr.org/~/media/9E2ED55531FC4B4FA53EF3B6D3B25DF8.pdf. Accessed 17 Apr 2017

Approach to CT Dose Optimization: Role of Registries and Benchmarking

Mannudeep K. Kalra

Contents

M.K. Kalra, M.D.
Divisions of Thoracic and CardioVascular Imaging, Department of Radiology, Webster Center for Quality and Safety, Massachusetts General Hospital, 55 Fruit Street, Boston, MA 02114, USA
e-mail: mkalra@mgh.harvard.edu

Past two decades have seen remarkable improvements in both hardware and software technologies related to computed tomography (CT) (Tabari et al. 2017). Starting from the addition of multiple detector rows to the single-detector-row helical CT scanners in the late 1990s to the ensuing embellishment with powerful X-ray tubes and efficient detectors, CT has come a long way. These technological advances helped multidetector row CT scanners cement an indispensable role in patient care but also led to concerns over associated radiation doses.

To address radiation concerns, the CT industry introduced or advanced multiple solutions such as automatic exposure control, automatic tube potential selection, pre-patient beam collimation, and iterative reconstruction techniques. In parallel, investigations highlighted variability in radiation doses between same and different institutions for similar clinical indications. Although European institutions and organizations took the lead in benchmarking of CT radiation doses for various procedures based on surveys, the American College of Radiology (ACR) dose index Registry (DIR) represented a pioneering effort to collect actual radiation doses associated with CT examinations.

This chapter presents a brief review of scan factors that affect CT radiation dose and adopts a scenario-based approach to highlight strategies to accomplish CT radiation dose optimization.

Med Radiol Diagn Imaging (2017)
DOI 10.1007/174_2017_85, © Springer International Publishing AG
Published Online 14 June 2017

1 Factors Affecting CT Radiation Doses

Amongst different factors affecting CT radiation doses, the most important one is the determination of appropriateness or justification for performing the examination. Fortunately, robust guidelines and recommendations are available from the America to Australia addressing this key aspect. The ACR Appropriateness Criteria are available for different body regions and clinical indications to help radiologists and referring physicians to select and recommend the most appropriate imaging examination. Some proprietary and commercial software have adopted these guidelines in their radiology order entry (ROE) decision support systems. Several studies have demonstrated the value of these decision support systems to reduce inappropriate radiology examinations including CT (Sistrom 2008; Sistrom et al. 2009, 2015; Sistrom and Honeyman 2002; Vartanians et al. 2010; Brink 2014; Gimbel et al. 2013; Gupta et al. 2014; Hendee et al. 2010).

Several patient factors affect radiation doses associated with CT (Kalra et al. 2015). For the same clinical indication and the body region, a patient with larger cross-sectional dimensions in the imaged region requires higher radiation dose as compared to one with smaller dimensions. This reasoning should also apply to the reduction of radiation doses for vulnerable children as compared to larger adult patients.

Certain body regions with lower attenuation can be imaged at lower radiation doses as compared to other regions with similar cross-sectional dimension but higher attenuation (Kalra et al. 2004a, 2008; Maher et al. 2004). A chest CT, for example, can be performed at substantially lower radiation dose as compared to the abdominal CT due to lower attenuation of the chest structures versus the abdominal organs. Likewise, organs and lesions with higher inherent contrast can also be imaged at lower doses compared to those with lower contrast. Thus, CT for lung nodules can be performed at substantially lower radiation doses compared to CT for routine examination of the chest where mediastinum also needs to be assessed. In the abdomen, CT for kidney stones and CT colonography can be adequately performed at reduced radiation doses due to their high inherent contrast compared to CT for evaluation of low contrast organs like liver and pancreas.

CT protocols requiring more than one image series through the same body part are associated with higher radiation dose as compared to dose needing a single series examination. Several abdominal CT protocols, for example, for evaluation of liver, pancreas, and adrenal masses, require multi-series imaging. Routine acquisition of the contrast or non-contrast images prior to post-contrast image series must be discouraged. Furthermore, scan length for additional series must be limited to a localized region of interest. If all other scan factors are held constant, the radiation dose is directly proportional to the scan length, a fact that can be utilized for optimizing radiation dose for multi-series CT examinations.

Several technical factors have a profound effect on CT radiation doses (Kalra et al. 2011; Lira et al. 2015; Padole et al. 2015a). Tube current (measured in milliamperes or mA) has a direct linear relationship with the associated radiation dose. Consequently, it is the most frequently modified scan factor for optimization of radiation doses. Automatic exposure control (AEC) techniques, also known as automatic tube current modulation, should be employed for adapting tube current for most CT protocols. These techniques require the user to specify the required image quality reference parameter for AEC (such as standard deviation, Toshiba; noise index, GE; quality reference mAs, Siemens). Then, based on the patient's regional attenuation and size, AEC automatically selects and modulates the tube current to achieve the user-specified image quality reference parameter. Some AEC techniques allow a user to specify the range of tube current to avoid inadvertently lower or higher radiation doses. Others enable users to select the strength of modulation from very weak to very strong to control the extent of tube current modulation. The anatomic AEC includes angular tube current modulation, longitudinal tube current modulation, and combined angular and longitudinal current modulation techniques. Several studies have reported substantial radiation dose reduction with use of

AEC techniques in both children and adults (Kalra et al. 2004b, c, d, e, 2005a, b; Matsubara et al. 2009; Peng et al. 2009; Shen et al. 2015).

The organ-based tube current modulation techniques available on some CT scanners allow users to reduce radiation dose to certain radiosensitive structures such as eye lenses and breasts (Euler et al. 2015; Lungren et al. 2012; Reimann et al. 2012; Wang et al. 2011). These techniques either reduce the tube current or turn off the X-ray tube for projections where X-rays are directly incident on the radiosensitive structures. This is based on the premise that most radiation dose to the superficial organs such as eye lenses and breasts is contributed from the directly incident X-rays. Several studies have shown that these organ-based tube current modulation techniques can substantially reduce radiation doses to eye lenses and breasts (Reimann et al. 2012; Nikupaavo et al. 2015). In-plane shielding devices based on bismuth have been assessed in prior studies to reduce radiation doses to eye lenses, thyroid, and breasts (Einstein et al. 2012; Kalra et al. 2009; Kim et al. 2013; Vollmar and Kalender 2008; Wang et al. 2012). In the opinion of the author and the practice at his institution, these shielding devices should be discouraged since their inappropriate use can increase artifacts and measured CT attenuation values (Kalra et al. 2009). Furthermore, when these devices are placed prior to the acquisition of the planning radiograph, the AEC techniques may employ higher than necessary tube current.

For retrospective electrocardiographically (ECG) gated cardiac CT, there is temporal modulation of the tube current to reduce the tube current in less important cardiac phases compared to the more important phases of reduced movement of the coronary arteries. Compared to fixed tube current, ECG-based tube current modulation can help reduce the radiation dose associated with coronary CT angiography by up to 50% based on the heart rate and the selected minimum tube current (Tabari et al. 2017; Ghoshhajra et al. 2014; De Cecco et al. 2011; Gosling et al. 2013; Sabarudin et al. 2012; Ünal et al. 2015; Kalra and Brady 2008). In prospective ECG-triggered cardiac CT, the X-ray tube is simply turned off during phases where data acquisition is not necessary for coronary CT examinations; therefore, it is often associated with lower radiation dose compared to the retrospective ECG-gated cardiac CT (Husmann et al. 2009; Khan et al. 2011; Park et al. 2015; Sun et al. 2012; Tang et al. 2016; Xu et al. 2013; Zhang et al. 2015).

Tube potential (measured in kilovoltage or KV) has a profound effect on radiation dose as well as the appearance of iodine-based contrast in the CT images (Lira et al. 2015). A reduction in tube potential not only decreases the radiation dose but also is associated with a substantial increase in attenuation of the iodine-based contrast media. Most children less than about 80 kg can be and possibly should be scanned at lower tube potential (such as 70–100 KV) regardless of the image reconstruction technique (Ben-David et al. 2014; Dion et al. 2004; Eller et al. 2012, 2013, 2014; Ghafourian et al. 2012; Gnannt et al. 2012a; Gonzalez-Guindalini et al. 2013). Non-obese adults undergoing CT angiography or contrast-enhanced chest CT can also be scanned at lower tube potential (i.e., less than 120 KV). Availability of more powerful X-ray tubes (capable of generating more than 500 mA and as much as 1300 mA) and iterative reconstruction techniques have made reduction of tube potential an attractive method for reducing radiation dose as well as the required volume of intravenous contrast media in both adults and children (Park et al. 2015; Chen et al. 2016; Haubenreisser et al. 2015; Itatani et al. 2013; Kaul et al. 2014; Andrabi et al. 2015; Pan et al. 2016; Pontana et al. 2013; Rompel et al. 2016; Sun et al. 2015a, b; You et al. 2015; Zhang et al. 2013, 2016).

Most CT scanners require users to manually specify the required tube potential for CT examinations. Several CT vendors have now introduced automatic tube potential selection techniques (for example, Care kV, Siemens; kV Assist, GE) to help select the most appropriate tube potential for a given patient's size and type of CT examination. These techniques require users to specify the type of CT examination (such as non-contrast, post-contrast, and CT angiography). The technique estimates the patient size information from the planning radiograph like AEC techniques and then selects the most appropriate tube potential and if necessary modifies AEC to maintain or improve contrast to noise ratio in the images. Several studies have reported the value of automatic tube potential selection techniques for reducing radiation doses for chest, cardiac, abdominal, and vascular applications (Ben-David et al. 2014; Eller et al. 2013; Zhang et al. 2016; Beeres et al. 2014; Ebner et al. 2014; Hou et al. 2016; Niemann et al. 2013; Faggioni et al. 2012; Fuentes-Orrego et al. 2013; Gnannt et al. 2012b).

Gantry rotation time (measured in seconds) refers to the time taken for the X-ray tube to complete one 360° revolution around the patient. If other scan factors are held constant, shorter gantry rotation time implies lower radiation dose and vice versa. Pitch is a unitless entity which refers to the ratio of table feed per gantry rotation (mm) to the total nominal width of the X-ray beam. Like the gantry rotation time, pitch affects the scan time, with lower values requiring longer time if all other scan parameters are held constant. For some scanners (Siemens and Philips), a change in pitch (up to 1.5:1) brings about a change in tube current to offset any change in radiation dose. Others (such as GE and Toshiba) are associated with higher dose at a lower pitch and lower dose at a higher pitch. Choice of the pitch should depend on the requirement of scan time. A pitch greater than 1.6:1 is possible on dual source CT scanners where the two helices from each X-ray tube-detector combination fill the gaps in acquisition data in the other helix. Such high non-overlapping pitch (i.e., greater than 1.6:1) has been applied for rapid acquisition of CT images at substantially reduced radiation doses in chest, cardiac, and vascular applications (Ghoshhajra et al. 2014; Sun et al. 2012; Chinnaiyan et al. 2014; den Harder et al. 2016; Guberina et al. 2016; Korn et al. 2013; Lim et al. 2016; Paul et al. 2013; Schulz et al. 2012).

Detector configuration is another important scan factor, particularly for the multidetector-row CT scanners. The detector configuration is represented by the product of the number of detector rows and the thickness of each detector row in millimeter. Choice of detector configuration is based on the required scan length and the section thickness for given clinical indications. For CT scanners with matrix array type of detector configuration (i.e., identical thickness of all detector rows), the latter is not a factor in determining the detector configuration. CT scanners with variable detector row thicknesses require a use of thinner detector configuration for reconstruction of thinner sections. Conversely, when thicker sections are acceptable for evaluation, detector beam collimation or wider detector configuration can be used. For longer scan lengths, a wider detector configuration is more dose efficient as compared to a narrow detector configuration. When the scan length is short, such as for head CT, a narrow detector configuration is more dose efficient as compared to a wider detector configuration. Some advanced multidetector row CT scanners now employ adaptive shielding mechanism to reduce X-ray beam falling beyond the detectors and thereby enhance the dose efficiency (Tabari et al. 2017; Chatterson et al. 2014).

Although seemingly a reconstruction parameter rather than a scan factor, section thickness does influence radiation dose for some scanners (such as GE and Toshiba) which use objective noise as image quality metric for AEC. On other scanners, section thickness does not influence the AEC. Modern multidetector row CT scanners offer an opportunity for acquiring submillimeter section thickness which however should be used conscientiously since thinner sections have more noise compared to thicker sections and may thus tempt use of higher radiation dose. For lungs, and CT angiography, submillimeter sections are paramount but often do not require higher doses as these structures have higher inherent contrast which offsets the disadvantage of increased noise in thinner sections. For other low contrast organs, such as brain and liver, one can acquire thinner sections but interpret at thicker sections to decrease the noise content in the images.

Thanks to the video gaming industry, modern CT scanners now have iterative reconstruction techniques that require higher and faster computation power to generate images with less noise, and artifacts as compared to conventional filtered back projection techniques of image reconstruction. Most vendors offer more than one proprietary iterative reconstruction techniques on their line of CT scanners. These techniques empower users to alter scan factors to reduce radiation dose while maintaining or improving image quality versus filtered back projection. Most techniques require users to select its strength for a specific clinical protocol. This, unfortunately, adds a subjective element which varies wildly based on radiologists preference. At higher strengths, the images assume a rather distinctive pixelated or paintbrush appearance, while at lower strengths, image quality improvements may not be fully realized. Regardless, several studies have reported that iterative reconstruction techniques can help users to reduce radiation doses substantially versus their predecessor filtered back projection (Padole et al. 2015a, b, 2016; Kalra et al. 2012, 2013; Khawaja et al. 2014, 2015a, b, c; Pourjabbar et al. 2015; Prakash et al. 2010a, b, c; Singh et al. 2010, 2012, 2013; Abdullah et al. 2016; Arapakis et al. 2014; Benz et al. 2016; Berta et al. 2014; Cho et al. 2014; Hwang et al. 2012a; b; Jensen et al. 2016; Kalmar et al. 2014). Image quality improvements with these newer techniques are especially apparent when using lower tube potential, obtaining thinner sections, and imaging larger patients.

2 CT Dose Descriptors

CT dose index volume (CTDIvol, mGy) and dose length product (DLP, mGy.cm) are the main CT descriptors that represent radiation doses in 16 cm (for head CT) and 32 cm (for body CT) homogeneous phantoms. The former represents average dose at a given section position whereas the latter is the total absorbed dose over the entire scan series. The DLP is derived from multiple lying CTDIvol with the scan length. These descriptors do not represent actual patient doses but enable users to compare radiation doses across different CT protocols and CT scanners.

Since patients rarely have a homogeneous diameter of 32 cm, the American Association of Physicists in Medicine (AAPM) has proposed a size-specific dose estimate (SSDE) to convert CTDIvol into a patient size-specific dose descriptor (Khawaja et al. 2015d; Larson 2014). The patient size is derived either from the planning radiograph or the cross-sectional CT images by measuring the anteroposterior or lateral dimension of the body. The lookup tables provide a conversion factor based on these dimensions which are then multiplied with the CTDIvol to obtain SSDE.

Currently, there is no place of effective dose or estimated effective dose (represented in millisieverts or mSv) in CT radiation dose monitoring or optimization. This metric is frequently and often quite erroneously obtained by multiplying the DLP with a conversion coefficient. Subsequently, the derived estimated effective doses are used to represent or calculate associated risk of radiation dose. Neither DLP represents actual patient dose nor does a single conversion coefficient encompasses different patient age, gender, size, and body composition. Sophisticated software is available for estimating absorbed organ doses for CT scanning but provides substantially different values based on their method of estimation. To date, it is difficult to extrapolate practical applications for these multiple organ doses from a single CT examination in CT radiation dose optimization.

3 ACR DIR and European Guidelines

As of July 2016, there were close to 30 million CT examinations from over 1500 facilities in the ACR DIR, which was launched in 2011 to collect information related to CT radiation doses (Kanal et al. 2017; Robinson et al. 2013). Currently, the ACR DIR houses information pertaining to CTDIvol, DLP, and SSDE (for centers providing planning radiographs) (Murugan et al. 2015a, b). Several commercial third party software is also available for radiation dose monitoring and tracking for CT (Cook et al. 2011).

The Joint Commission, a critical accrediting and certifying organization for nearly 21,000 healthcare organizations and programs in the United States, recommends that CT centers participate in CT dose registry for tracking and monitoring of radiation doses. Kanal et al. have recently published body region- and patient size-based dose reference levels (representing doses used in 75th percentile of doses used in participating institutions) and achievable doses (representing doses used in 50th percentile of doses used in participating institutions) for the top 10 CT protocols in adults (Table 1) (Kanal et al. 2017). The European DRLs for pediatric CT have also become available from the European Society of Radiology (ESR) (Table 2) (European Guidelines on DRLs for Paediatric Imaging 2017).

Table 1 DRL and AD for different chest and abdominal CT protocols from the ACR DIR (adapted from Kanal et al. 2017)

	CTDIvol (mGy)		SSDE (mGy)	
CT protocol	AD	DRL	AD	DRL
Non-contrast chest CT	9	12	11	15
Post-contrast chest CT	10	13	11	15
CT pulmonary angiography	11	14	13	17
Non-contrast abdomen and pelvis CT	13	16	15	19
Post-contrast abdomen and pelvis CT	12	15	15	18
Non-contrast abdomen, pelvis, and kidney CT	12	15	14	19
Post-contrast chest, abdomen, and pelvis CT	12	15	14	18

Table 2 Pediatric CT DRL from the European guidelines on DRL for pediatric imaging (adapted from European Guidelines on DRLs for Paediatric Imaging 2017)

Body region	Age or weight	CTDIvol (mGy) DRL
Head	0 to <3 months	24
	3 months to 1 year	28
	1 to <6 years	40
	≥6 years	50
Chest	<5 kg	1.4
	5 to <15 kg	1.8
	15 to <30 kg	2.7
	30 to <50 kg	3.7
	50 to <80 kg	5.4
Abdomen	<5 kg	
	5 to <15 kg	3.5
	15 to <30 kg	5.4
	30 to <50 kg	7.3
	50 to <80 kg	13

The ADs and DRLs can help users to assess radiation doses associated with their CT practices. However, users should realize that these recommendations help in the initial setup of an ideal CT practice from a radiation dose optimization point of view. The granularity in terms of each specific CT examination dose is missing as is the information stratification based on the scanner capabilities. Neither ACR DIR nor ESR publications provide recommendations for liver or pancreas or lung nodule follow-up CT protocols. Neither provides information regarding CT scanner-specific guidelines to empower users to use the scanner capabilities to its maximum. If participation in dose monitoring and/or tracking is the beginning of a journey to "dose-perfection," meeting and/or beating of the DRL and AD are important but not the ultimate step which involves use of specific scanner capabilities to deliver body region-, size-, and clinical indication-based radiation doses while obtaining image quality sufficient for diagnostic evaluation.

4 Scenarios for CT Dose Optimization

A series of plausible scenario are presented in this section based on several years of author experience in the field. While none may apply to some CT centers, these can serve as learning exercises towards CT radiation dose optimization.

In an ideal center, CT is utilized for relevant or appropriate clinical reasons based on some guidelines via a radiology order entry and decision support interface. One or more radiologists lead the efforts of clinical indication- and body region-specific CT protocols. Thus, within each body regions, such as chest, there are at least a few clinical indication-specific protocols for pulmonary embolism, diffuse lung diseases, lung nodule follow-up, lung cancer screening, and airway evaluation. Specific clinical indications, starting and ending landmarks for each scan phase, the number of scan phases, section thickness, and their timing, as well as details for oral and intravenous contrast injection, are stated for each protocol. This work is implemented with one or more specified CT technologists who help in implementation and monitoring of compliance. CT protocols are formally created and archived in electronic format with or without hard copies for easy reference since protocols archived in CT user interface protocols only can sometimes change or disappear! Radiologists and technologists then work as a team with a medical physicist to fill in the scan factors for each protocol. Techniques such as AEC, automatic tube potential selection, and iterative reconstruction are employed where available to enable dose reduction. The latter also helps set the alert and notification values for CTDIvol and/or DLP for different protocols. These values warn the technologists if radiation doses for any CT examinations exceed them. CT doses are monitored by the medical physicist while the radiologists flag issues with image quality. Radiation doses are monitored with a commercial dose-tracking system which enables scanner and patient-specific granularity not afforded in the ACR DIR. Protocols are reviewed on a quarterly basis.

The aforementioned scenario might not exist even in tertiary well-staffed centers. Workload, priorities, and lack of familiarity with scan factors and radiation dose often prevent radiologists and CT technologists from substantial participation in dose optimization efforts. Likewise, medical physicists may not be available full time or when available may not be as well verse or interested in CT protocols as in MR or mammography. Referring physicians may not be receptive to imposing radiology order entry decision support systems adding to their clinical burden and forcing them to reconcile with guidelines they did not help create. Finally, finances may not be available for dose-tracking or monitoring resources and/or modern CT equipment with more bells and whistles to accomplish lower radiation doses.

Without will exists no way to radiation dose optimization. Yet without means, there are opportunities to deliver safety. Education though is a prerequisite for any meaningful effort. In a worst-case scenario, all or most of the limitations in preceding paragraph can befall on a CT practice making dose optimization extremely challenging. Such centers should consider at least some participation in the ACR DIR, which will send regular dose audits comparing the center to the rest of the country. Such quarterly reports inform the center about their doses compared to the rest of the country and identify protocols in most need of repair. CT vendor can then be contacted for advice and guidance regarding options for dose optimization. There are also several freeware programs to track and monitor CT radiation doses which can be networked to provide information on radiation doses.

With a complete lack of any dose-tracking and monitoring software, manual labor becomes imperative. For such scenario, users should at least strive for minimum possible goals. Foremost, users must ensure that children receive lower radiation doses compared to adults in terms of CTDIvol and DLP. Smaller children should receive lower doses than larger kids. AEC and/or automatic tube potential selection techniques can help substantially. Putting up benchmark doses or DRLs and AD in the CT suite can help motivate towards maintaining radiation dose level. Next, evaluation of patients undergoing chest and abdominal CT examinations can be looked at to assess if chest doses are at least a third to half of abdominal doses. Unfortunately, the ACR DIR (Table 1) data on DRL and AD does not demonstrate this but European Guidelines and recommendations for children elegantly capture this remarkable difference. A quick review of the graphic user interface of scanners can tell if there are clinical indication-specific protocols. One should then look into the creation of at least a few clinical indication-based CT protocols for each body region. For example, routine abdomen, liver mass, kidney stone protocol and CT urography protocols in the abdomen. Creation of electronic or hard copies of CT protocols helps in streamlining the optimization of protocols and radiation doses. Dose adjustment for clinical indications requires users to modify AEC and automatic tube potential selection techniques to accomplish radiation dose optimization based on clinical indications.

This section will be incomplete if stress is not placed on the fact that dose optimization is a team effort which requires patient participation too. Patients should ask for the reasons for CT requisition and techniques. Patients though should not deny themselves of this imaging modality when there is clinical justification for CT scanning. When the indications are right, CT can save lives and provide meaningful information which affects treatment and outcome.

5 Summary

From the perspective of CT radiation dose optimization, CT radiation dose tracking and monitoring is an important step. Participation in dose registries and knowledge of benchmark doses for CT can help tremendously in dose reduction. Ultimately, dose optimization requires a team of the willing and the able spanning from referring physicians, radiologists, CT technologists to medical physicists. Means of CT radiation dose optimization are now available; their optimal application is paramount.

References

Abdullah KA, McEntee MF, Reed W, Kench PL (2016) Radiation dose and diagnostic image quality associated with iterative reconstruction in coronary CT angiography: a systematic review. J Med Imaging Radiat Oncol 60(4):459–468

Andrabi Y, Saadeh TS, Uppot RN, Arellano RS, Sahani DV (2015) Impact of dose-modified protocols on radiation doses in patients undergoing CT examinations following image-guided catheter placement. J Vasc Interv Radiol 26(9):1339–1346.e1

Arapakis I, Efstathopoulos E, Tsitsia V, Kordolaimi S, Economopoulos N, Argentos S et al (2014) Using "iDose4" iterative reconstruction algorithm in adults' chest-abdomen-pelvis CT examinations: effect on image quality in relation to patient radiation exposure. Br J Radiol 87(1036):20130613

Beeres M, Romer M, Bodelle B, Lee C, Gruber-Rouh T, Mbalisike E et al (2014) Chest-abdomen-pelvis CT for staging in cancer patients: dose effectiveness and image quality using automated attenuation-based tube potential selection. Cancer Imaging 14:28

Ben-David E, Cohen JE, Nahum Goldberg S, Sosna J, Levinson R, Leichter IS et al (2014) Significance of enhanced cerebral gray-white matter contrast at 80 kVp compared to conventional 120 kVp CT scan in the evaluation of acute stroke. J Clin Neurosci 21(9):1591–1594

Benz DC, Gräni C, Mikulicic F, Vontobel J, Fuchs TA, Possner M et al (2016) Adaptive statistical iterative reconstruction-V: impact on image quality in ultralow-dose coronary computed tomography angiography. J Comput Assist Tomogr 40(6):958–963

Berta L, Mascaro L, Feroldi P, Maroldi R (2014) Optimisation of an MDCT abdominal protocol: image quality assessment of standard vs. iterative reconstructions. Physica Medica 30(3):271–279

Brink JA (2014) Clinical decision-making tools for exam selection, reporting and dose tracking. Pediatr Radiol 44(Suppl 3):418–421

Chatterson LC, Leswick DA, Fladeland DA, Hunt MM, Webster S, Lim H (2014) Fetal shielding combined with state of the art CT dose reduction strategies during maternal chest CT. Eur J Radiol 83(7):1199–1204

Chen CM, Lin YY, Hsu MY, Hung CF, Liao YL, Tsai HY (2016) Performance of adaptive iterative dose reduction 3D integrated with automatic tube current modulation in radiation dose and image noise reduction compared with filtered-back projection for 80-kVp abdominal CT: anthropomorphic phantom and patient study. Eur J Radiol 85(9):1666–1672

Chinnaiyan KM, Bilolikar AN, Walsh E, Wood D, DePetris A, Gentry R et al (2014) CT dose reduction using prospectively triggered or fast-pitch spiral technique employed in cardiothoracic imaging (the CT dose study). J Cardiovasc Comput Tomogr 8(3):205–214

Cho YJ, Schoepf UJ, Silverman JR, Krazinski AW, Canstein C, Deak Z et al (2014) Iterative image reconstruction techniques: cardiothoracic computed tomography applications. J Thorac Imaging 29(4):198–208

Cook TS, Zimmerman SL, Steingall SR, Maidment AD, Kim W, Boonn WW (2011) RADIANCE: an automated, enterprise-wide solution for archiving and reporting CT radiation dose estimates. Radiographics 31(7):1833–1846

De Cecco CN, Buffa V, Fedeli S, Vallone A, Ruopoli R, Luzietti M et al (2011) Dual-source CT coronary angiography: prospective versus retrospective acquisition technique. Radiol Med 116(2):178–188

Dion AM, Berger F, Helie O, Ott D, Spiegel A, Cordoliani YS (2004) Dose reduction at abdominal CT imaging: reduced tension (kV) or reduced intensity (mAs)? J Radiol 85(4 Pt 1):375–380

Ebner L, Knobloch F, Huber A, Landau J, Ott D, Heverhagen JT et al (2014) Feasible dose reduction in routine chest computed tomography maintaining constant image quality using the last three scanner generations: from filtered back projection to Sinogram-affirmed iterative reconstruction and impact of the novel fully integrated detector design minimizing electronic noise. J Clin Imaging Sci 4:38

Einstein AJ, Elliston CD, Groves DW, Cheng B, Wolff SD, Pearson GD et al (2012) Effect of bismuth breast shielding on radiation dose and image quality in coronary CT angiography. J Nucl Cardiol 19(1):100–108

Eller A, May MS, Scharf M, Schmid A, Kuefner M, Uder M et al (2012) Attenuation-based automatic kilovolt selection in abdominal computed tomography: effects on radiation exposure and image quality. Investig Radiol 47(10):559–565

Eller A, Wuest W, Scharf M, Brand M, Achenbach S, Uder M et al (2013) Attenuation-based automatic kilovolt (kV)-selection in computed tomography of the chest: effects on radiation exposure and image quality. Eur J Radiol 82(12):2386–2391

Eller A, Wuest W, Kramer M, May M, Schmid A, Uder M et al (2014) Carotid CTA: radiation exposure and image quality with the use of attenuation-based, automated kilovolt selection. Am J Neuroradiol 35(2):237–241

Euler A, Szucs-Farkas Z, Falkowski AL, Kawel-Bohm N, D'Errico L, Kopp S et al (2016) Organ-based tube current modulation in a clinical context: dose reduction may be largely overestimated in breast tissue. Eur Radiol 26:2656–2662

European Guidelines on DRLs for Paediatric Imaging (2017). http://www.eurosafeimaging.org/wp/wp-content/uploads/2014/02/European-Guidelines-on-DRLs-for-Paediatric-Imaging_Revised_18-July-2016_clean.pdf. Accessed 1 May 2017

Faggioni L, Neri E, Sbragia P, Pascale R, D'Errico L, Caramella D et al (2012) 80-kV pulmonary CT angiography with 40 mL of iodinated contrast material in lean patients: comparison of vascular enhancement with iodixanol (320 mg I/mL)and iomeprol (400 mg I/mL). Am J Roentgenol 199(6):1220–1225

Fuentes-Orrego JM, Hayano K, Kambadakone AR, Hahn PF, Sahani DV (2013) Dose-modified 256-MDCT of the abdomen using low tube current and hybrid iterative reconstruction. Acad Radiol 20(11):1405–1412

Ghafourian K, Younes D, Simprini LA, Weigold WG, Weissman G, Taylor AJ (2012) Scout view X-ray attenuation versus weight-based selection of reduced peak tube voltage in cardiac CT angiography. JACC Cardiovasc Imaging 5(6):589–595

Ghoshhajra BB, Lee AM, Engel LC, Celeng C, Kalra MK, Brady TJ et al (2014) Radiation dose reduction in pediatric cardiac computed tomography: experience from a tertiary medical center. Pediatr Cardiol 35(1):171–179

Gimbel RW, Fontelo P, Stephens MB, Olsen CH, Bunt C, Ledford CJ et al (2013) Radiation exposure and cost influence physician medical image decision making: a randomized controlled trial. Med Care 51(7):628–632

Gnannt R, Winklehner A, Goetti R, Schmidt B, Kollias S, Alkadhi H (2012a) Low kilovoltage CT of the neck with 70 kVp: comparison with a standard protocol. Am J Neuroradiol 33(6):1014–1019

Gnannt R, Winklehner A, Eberli D, Knuth A, Frauenfelder T, Alkadhi H (2012b) Automated tube potential selection for standard chest and abdominal CT in follow-up patients with testicular cancer: comparison with fixed tube potential. Eur Radiol 22(9):1937–1945

Gonzalez-Guindalini FD, Ferreira Botelho MP, Tore HG, Ahn RW, Gordon LI, Yaghmai V (2013) MDCT of chest, abdomen, and pelvis using attenuation-based automated tube voltage selection in combination with iterative reconstruction: an intrapatient study of radiation dose and image quality. Am J Roentgenol 201(5):1075–1082

Gosling O, Morgan-Hughes G, Iyengar S, Strain W, Loader R, Shore A et al (2013) Computed tomography to diagnose coronary artery disease: a reduction in radiation dose increases applicability. Clin Radiol 68(4):340–345

Guberina N, Lechel U, Forsting M, Ringelstein A (2016) Efficacy of high-pitch CT protocols for radiation dose reduction. J Radiol Prot 36(4):N57–N66

Gupta A, Ip IK, Raja AS, Andruchow JE, Sodickson A, Khorasani R (2014) Effect of clinical decision support on documented guideline adherence for head CT in emergency department patients with mild traumatic brain injury. J Am Med Inform Assoc 21(e2):e347–e351

den Harder AM, Willemink MJ, de Jong PA, Schilham AM, Rajiah P, Takx RA et al (2016) New horizons in cardiac CT. Clin Radiol 71(8):758–767

Haubenreisser H, Meyer M, Sudarski S, Allmendinger T, Schoenberg SO, Henzler T (2015) Unenhanced third-generation dual-source chest CT using a tin filter for spectral shaping at 100kVp. Eur J Radiol 84(8):1608–1613

Hendee WR, Becker GJ, Borgstede JP, Bosma J, Casarella WJ, Erickson BA et al (2010) Addressing overutilization in medical imaging. Radiology 257(1):240–245

Hou QR, Gao W, Zhong YM, Sun AM, Wang Q, Qiu HS et al (2016) A prospective evaluation of contrast and radiation dose and image quality in cardiac CT in children with complex congenital heart disease using low-concentration iodinated contrast agent and low tube voltage and current. Br J Radiol 90:20160669

Husmann L, Herzog BA, Burkhard N, Valenta I, Burger IA, Gaemperli O et al (2009) Low-dose coronary CT angiography with prospective ECG triggering: validation of a contrast material protocol adapted to body mass index. Am J Roentgenol 193(3):802–806

Hwang HJ, Seo JB, Lee JS, Song JW, Kim SS, Lee HJ et al (2012a) Radiation dose reduction of chest CT with iterative reconstruction in image space—part II: assessment of radiologists' preferences using dual source CT. Korean J Radiol 13(6):720–727

Hwang HJ, Seo JB, Lee JS, Song JW, Kim SS, Lee HJ et al (2012b) Radiation dose reduction of chest CT with iterative reconstruction in image space—part I: studies on image quality using dual source CT. Korean J Radiol 13(6):711–719

Itatani R, Oda S, Utsunomiya D, Funama Y, Honda K, Katahira K et al (2013) Reduction in radiation and contrast medium dose via optimization of low-kilovoltage CT protocols using a hybrid iterative reconstruction algorithm at 256-slice body CT: phantom study and clinical correlation. Clin Radiol 68(3):e128–e135

Jensen K, Andersen HK, Tingberg A, Reisse C, Fosse E, Martinsen AC (2016) Improved liver lesion conspicuity with iterative reconstruction in computed tomography imaging. Curr Probl Diagn Radiol 45:291–296

Kalmar PI, Quehenberger F, Steiner J, Lutfi A, Bohlsen D, Talakic E et al (2014) The impact of iterative reconstruction on image quality and radiation dose in thoracic and abdominal CT. Eur J Radiol 83(8):1416–1420

Kalra MK, Brady TJ (2008) Current status and future directions in technical developments of cardiac computed tomography. J Cardiovasc Comput Tomogr 2(2):71–80

Kalra MK, Maher MM, Toth TL, Hamberg LM, Blake MA, Shepard JA et al (2004a) Strategies for CT radiation dose optimization. Radiology 230(3):619–628

Kalra MK, Maher MM, Toth TL, Kamath RS, Halpern EF, Saini S (2004b) Radiation from "extra" images acquired with abdominal and/or pelvic CT: effect of automatic tube current modulation. Radiology 232(2):409–414

Kalra MK, Maher MM, Kamath RS, Horiuchi T, Toth TL, Halpern EF et al (2004c) Sixteen-detector row CT of abdomen and pelvis: study for optimization of Z-axis modulation technique performed in 153 patients. Radiology 233(1):241–249

Kalra MK, Maher MM, Toth TL, Kamath RS, Halpern EF, Saini S (2004d) Comparison of Z-axis automatic tube current modulation technique with fixed tube current CT scanning of abdomen and pelvis. Radiology 232(2):347–353

Kalra MK, Maher MM, Toth TL, Schmidt B, Westerman BL, Morgan HT et al (2004e) Techniques and applications of automatic tube current modulation for CT. Radiology 233(3):649–657

Kalra MK, Maher MM, D'Souza RV, Rizzo S, Halpern EF, Blake MA et al (2005a) Detection of urinary tract stones at low-radiation-dose CT with z-axis automatic tube current modulation: phantom and clinical studies. Radiology 235(2):523–529

Kalra MK, Rizzo S, Maher MM, Halpern EF, Toth TL, Shepard JA et al (2005b) Chest CT performed with z-axis modulation: scanning protocol and radiation dose. Radiology 237(1):303–308

Kalra MK, Singh S, Blake MA (2008) CT of the urinary tract: turning attention to radiation dose. Radiol Clin N Am 46(1):1–9, v

Kalra MK, Dang P, Singh S, Saini S, Shepard JA (2009) In-plane shielding for CT: effect of off-centering, automatic exposure control and shield-to-surface distance. Korean J Radiol 10(2):156–163

Kalra MK, Singh S, Thrall JH, Mahesh M (2011) Pointers for optimizing radiation dose in abdominal CT protocols. J Am Coll Radiol 8(10):731–734

Kalra MK, Woisetschlager M, Dahlstrom N, Singh S, Lindblom M, Choy G et al (2012) Radiation dose reduction with Sinogram Affirmed Iterative Reconstruction technique for abdominal computed tomography. J Comput Assist Tomogr 36(3):339–346

Kalra MK, Woisetschlager M, Dahlstrom N, Singh S, Digumarthy S, Do S et al (2013) Sinogram-affirmed iterative reconstruction of low-dose chest CT: effect on image quality and radiation dose. Am J Roentgenol 201(2):W235–W244

Kalra MK, Sodickson AD, Mayo-Smith WW (2015) CT radiation: key concepts for gentle and wise use. Radiographics 35(6):1706–1721

Kanal KM, Butler PF, Sengupta D, Bhargavan-Chatfield M, Coombs LP, Morin RL (2017) U.S. diagnostic reference levels and achievable doses for 10 adult CT examinations. Radiology:161911. doi: 10.1148/radiol.2017161911. [Epub ahead of print]

Kaul D, Grupp U, Kahn J, Ghadjar P, Wiener E, Hamm B et al (2014) Reducing radiation dose in the diagnosis of pulmonary embolism using adaptive statistical iterative reconstruction and lower tube potential in computed tomography. Eur Radiol 24(11):2685–2691

Khan A, Nasir K, Khosa F, Saghir A, Sarwar S, Clouse ME (2011) Prospective gating with 320-MDCT angiography: effect of volume scan length on radiation dose. Am J Roentgenol 196(2):407–411

Khawaja RD, Singh S, Gilman M, Sharma A, Do S, Pourjabbar S et al (2014) Computed tomography (CT) of the chest at less than 1 mSv: an ongoing prospective clinical trial of chest CT at submillisievert radiation doses with iterative model image reconstruction and iDose4 technique. J Comput Assist Tomogr 38(4):613–619

Khawaja RD, Singh S, Blake M, Harisinghani M, Choy G, Karaosmanoglu A et al (2015a) Ultra-low dose abdominal MDCT: using a knowledge-based Iterative Model Reconstruction technique for substantial dose reduction in a prospective clinical study. Eur J Radiol 84(1):2–10

Khawaja RD, Singh S, Blake M, Harisinghani M, Choy G, Karaosmanoglu A et al (2015b) Ultralow-dose abdominal computed tomography: comparison of 2 iterative reconstruction techniques in a prospective clinical study. J Comput Assist Tomogr 39(4):489–498

Khawaja RD, Singh S, Otrakji A, Padole A, Lim R, Nimkin K et al (2015c) Dose reduction in pediatric abdominal CT: use of iterative reconstruction techniques across different CT platforms. Pediatr Radiol 45(7):1046–1055

Khawaja RD, Singh S, Vettiyil B, Lim R, Gee M, Westra S et al (2015d) Simplifying size-specific radiation dose estimates in pediatric CT. Am J Roentgenol 204(1):167–176

Kim YK, Sung YM, Choi JH, Kim EY, Kim HS (2013) Reduced radiation exposure of the female breast during low-dose chest CT using organ-based tube current modulation and a bismuth shield: comparison of image quality and radiation dose. Am J Roentgenol 200(3):537–544

Korn A, Fenchel M, Bender B, Danz S, Thomas C, Ketelsen D et al (2013) High-pitch dual-source CT angiography of supra-aortic arteries: assessment of image quality and radiation dose. Neuroradiology 55(4):423–430

Larson DB (2014) Optimizing CT radiation dose based on patient size and image quality: the size-specific dose estimate method. Pediatr Radiol 44(Suppl 3):501–505

Lim HK, Ha HI, Hwang HJ, Lee K (2016) Feasibility of high-pitch dual-source low-dose chest CT: reduction of radiation and cardiac artifacts. Diagn Interv Imaging 97(4):443–449

Lira D, Padole A, Kalra MK, Singh S (2015) Tube potential and CT radiation dose optimization. AJR Am J Roentgenol 204(1):W4–10

Lungren MP, Yoshizumi TT, Brady SM, Toncheva G, Anderson-Evans C, Lowry C et al (2012) Radiation dose estimations to the thorax using organ-based dose modulation. Am J Roentgenol 199(1):W65–W73

Maher MM, Kalra MK, Toth TL, Wittram C, Saini S, Shepard J (2004) Application of rational practice and technical advances for optimizing radiation dose for chest CT. J Thorac Imaging 19(1):16–23

Matsubara K, Takata T, Koshida K, Noto K, Shimono T, Horii J et al (2009) Chest CT performed with 3D and z-axis automatic tube current modulation technique: breast and effective doses. Acad Radiol 16(4):450–455

Murugan VA, Bhargavan-Chatfield M, Rehani M, Kalra MK (2015a) American College of Radiology Dose Index Registry: a user's guide for cardiothoracic radiologists part 1: dose index registry (DIR)-what it means and does for CT? J Thorac Imaging 30(6):W66–W68

Murugan VA, Chatfield MB, Rehani M, Kalra MKACRDIR (2015b) A user's guide for cardiothoracic radiologists: part 2: how to interpret your DIR report. J Thorac Imaging 30(6):W69–W72

Niemann T, Henry S, Faivre JB, Yasunaga K, Bendaoud S, Simeone A et al (2013) Clinical evaluation of automatic tube voltage selection in chest CT angiography. Eur Radiol 23(10):2643–2651

Nikupaavo U, Kaasalainen T, Reijonen V, Ahonen SM, Kortesniemi M (2015) Lens dose in routine head CT: comparison of different optimization methods with anthropomorphic phantoms. Am J Roentgenol 204(1):117–123

Padole A, Ali Khawaja RD, Kalra MK, Singh S (2015a) CT radiation dose and iterative reconstruction techniques. Am J Roentgenol 204(4):W384–W392

Padole A, Singh S, Lira D, Blake MA, Pourjabbar S, Khawaja RD et al (2015b) Assessment of filtered back projection, adaptive statistical, and model-based iterative reconstruction for reduced dose abdominal computed tomography. J Comput Assist Tomogr 39(4):462–467

Padole A, Sainani N, Lira D, Khawaja RD, Pourjabbar S, Lo Gullo R et al (2016) Assessment of sub-millisievert abdominal computed tomography with iterative reconstruction techniques of different vendors. World J Radiol 8(6):618–627

Pan YN, Li AJ, Chen XM, Wang J, Ren DW, Huang QL (2016) Coronary computed tomographic angiography at low concentration of contrast agent and low tube voltage in patients with obesity: a feasibility study. Acad Radiol 23(4):438–445

Park CH, Lee J, Oh C, Han KH, Kim TH (2015) The feasibility of sub-millisievert coronary CT angiography with low tube voltage, prospective ECG gating, and a knowledge-based iterative model reconstruction algorithm. Int J Cardiovasc Imaging 31(Suppl 2):197–203

Paul J, Mbalisike EC, Nour-Eldin NE, Vogl TJ (2013) Dual-source 128-slice MDCT neck: radiation dose and image quality estimation of three different protocols. Eur J Radiol 82(5):787–796

Peng Y, Li J, Ma D, Zhang Q, Liu Y, Zeng J et al (2009) Use of automatic tube current modulation with a standardized noise index in young children undergoing chest computed tomography scans with 64-slice multidetector computed tomography. Acta Radiologica 50(10):1175–1181

Pontana F, Pagniez J, Duhamel A, Flohr T, Faivre JB, Murphy C et al (2013) Reduced-dose low-voltage chest CT angiography with Sinogram-affirmed iterative reconstruction versus standard-dose filtered back projection. Radiology 267(2):609–618

Pourjabbar S, Singh S, Kulkarni N, Muse V, Digumarthy SR, Khawaja RD et al (2015) Dose reduction for chest CT: comparison of two iterative reconstruction techniques. Acta Radiologica 56(6):688–695

Prakash P, Kalra MK, Ackman JB, Digumarthy SR, Hsieh J, Do S et al (2010a) Diffuse lung disease: CT of the chest with adaptive statistical iterative reconstruction technique. Radiology 256(1):261–269

Prakash P, Kalra MK, Digumarthy SR, Hsieh J, Pien H, Singh S et al (2010b) Radiation dose reduction with chest computed tomography using adaptive statistical iterative reconstruction technique: initial experience. J Comput Assist Tomogr 34(1):40–45

Prakash P, Kalra MK, Kambadakone AK, Pien H, Hsieh J, Blake MA et al (2010c) Reducing abdominal CT radiation dose with adaptive statistical iterative reconstruction technique. Investig Radiol 45(4):202–210

Reimann AJ, Davison C, Bjarnason T, Thakur Y, Kryzmyk K, Mayo J et al (2012) Organ-based computed tomographic (CT) radiation dose reduction to the lenses: impact on image quality for CT of the head. J Comput Assist Tomogr 36(3):334–338

Robinson TJ, Robinson JD, Kanal KM (2013) Implementation of the ACR dose index registry at a large academic institution: early experience. J Digit Imaging 26(2):309–315

Rompel O, Glockler M, Janka R, Dittrich S, Cesnjevar R, Lell MM et al (2016) Third-generation dual-source 70-kVp chest CT angiography with advanced iterative reconstruction in young children: image quality and radiation dose reduction. Pediatr Radiol 46(4):462–472

Sabarudin A, Sun Z, Ng KH (2012) A systematic review of radiation dose associated with different generations of multidetector CT coronary angiography. J Med Imaging Radiat Oncol 56(1):5–17

Schulz B, Potente S, Zangos S, Friedrichs I, Bauer RW, Kerl M et al (2012) Ultra-low dose dual-source high-pitch computed tomography of the paranasal sinus: diagnostic sensitivity and radiation dose. Acta Radiologica 53(4):435–440

Shen H, Dai G, Luo M, Duan C, Cai W, Liang D et al (2015) Image quality and radiation dose of CT coronary angiography with automatic tube current modulation and strong adaptive iterative dose reduction three-dimensional (AIDR3D). PLoS One 10(11):e0142185

Singh S, Kalra MK, Hsieh J, Licato PE, Do S, Pien HH et al (2010) Abdominal CT: comparison of adaptive statistical iterative and filtered back projection reconstruction techniques. Radiology 257(2):373–383
Singh S, Kalra MK, Shenoy-Bhangle AS, Saini A, Gervais DA, Westra SJ et al (2012) Radiation dose reduction with hybrid iterative reconstruction for pediatric CT. Radiology 263(2):537–546
Singh S, Khawaja RD, Pourjabbar S, Padole A, Lira D, Kalra MK (2013) Iterative image reconstruction and its role in cardiothoracic computed tomography. J Thorac Imaging 28(6):355–367
Sistrom CL (2008) In support of the ACR Appropriateness Criteria. J Am Coll Radiol 5(5):630–635. discussion 636–637
Sistrom CL, Honeyman JC (2002) Relational data model for the American College of Radiology Appropriateness Criteria. J Digit Imaging 15(4):216–225
Sistrom CL, Dang PA, Weilburg JB, Dreyer KJ, Rosenthal DI, Thrall JH (2009) Effect of computerized order entry with integrated decision support on the growth of outpatient procedure volumes: seven-year time series analysis. Radiology 251(1):147–155
Sistrom CL, Weilburg JB, Dreyer KJ, Ferris TG (2015) Provider feedback about imaging appropriateness by using scores from order entry decision support: raw rates misclassify outliers. Radiology 275(2):469–479
Sun K, Han RJ, Ma LJ, Wang LJ, Li LG, Chen JH (2012) Prospectively electrocardiogram-gated high-pitch spiral acquisition mode dual-source CT coronary angiography in patients with high heart rates: comparison with retrospective electrocardiogram-gated spiral acquisition mode. Korean J Radiol 13(6):684–693
Sun G, Hou YB, Zhang B, Yu L, Li SX, Tan LL et al (2015a) Application of low tube voltage coronary CT angiography with low-dose iodine contrast agent in patients with a BMI of 26–30 kg/m^2. Clin Radiol 70(2):138–145
Sun J, Zhang Q, Hu D, Duan X, Peng Y (2015b) Improving pulmonary vessel image quality with a full model-based iterative reconstruction algorithm in 80kVp low-dose chest CT for pediatric patients aged 0–6 years. Acta Radiologica 56(6):761–768
Tabari A, Lo Gullo R, Murugan V, Otrakji A, Digumarthy S, Kalra M (2017) Recent advances in computed tomographic technology: cardiopulmonary imaging applications. J Thorac Imaging 32(2):89–100
Tang PH, BJ D, Fang XM, XY H, Qian PY, Gao QS (2016) Submillisievert coronary CT angiography with adaptive prospective ECG-triggered sequence acquisition and iterative reconstruction in patients with high heart rate on the dual-source CT. J Xray Sci Technol 24(6):807–820
Ünal E, Yıldız AE, Güler E, Karcaaltıncaba M, Akata D, Kılınçer A et al (2015) Comparison of image quality and radiation dose between prospectively ECG-triggered and retrospectively ECG-gated CT angiography: establishing heart rate cut-off values in first-generation dual-source CT. Anatol J Cardiol 15(9):759–764
Vartanians VM, Sistrom CL, Weilburg JB, Rosenthal DI, Thrall JH (2010) Increasing the appropriateness of outpatient imaging: effects of a barrier to ordering low-yield examinations. Radiology 255(3):842–849
Vollmar SV, Kalender WA (2008) Reduction of dose to the female breast in thoracic CT: a comparison of standard-protocol, bismuth-shielded, partial and tube-current-modulated CT examinations. Eur Radiol 18(8):1674–1682
Wang J, Duan X, Christner JA, Leng S, Yu L, McCollough CH (2011) Radiation dose reduction to the breast in thoracic CT: comparison of bismuth shielding, organ-based tube current modulation, and use of a globally decreased tube current. Med Phys 38(11):6084–6092
Wang J, Duan X, Christner JA, Leng S, Grant KL, McCollough CH (2012) Bismuth shielding, organ-based tube current modulation, and global reduction of tube current for dose reduction to the eye at head CT. Radiology 262(1):191–198
Xu L, Yang L, Zhang Z, Wang Y, Jin Z, Zhang L et al (2013) Prospectively ECG-triggered sequential dual-source coronary CT angiography in patients with atrial fibrillation: comparison with retrospectively ECG-gated helical CT. Eur Radiol 23(7):1822–1828
You J, Dai Y, Huang N, Li JJ, Cheng L, Zhang XL et al (2015) Low-dose computed tomography with adaptive statistical iterative reconstruction and low tube voltage in craniocervical computed tomographic angiography: impact of body mass index. J Comput Assist Tomogr 39(5):774–780
Zhang WL, Li M, Zhang B, Geng HY, Liang YQ, Xu K et al (2013) CT angiography of the head-and-neck vessels acquired with low tube voltage, low iodine, and iterative image reconstruction: clinical evaluation of radiation dose and image quality. PLoS One 8(12):e81486
Zhang JL, Liu BL, Zhao YM, Liang HW, Wang GK, Wan Y et al (2015) Combining coronary with carotid and cerebrovascular angiography using prospective ECG gating and iterative reconstruction with 256-slice CT. Echocardiography 32(8):1291–1298
Zhang F, Yang L, Song X, Li YN, Jiang Y, Zhang XH et al (2016) Feasibility study of low tube voltage (80kVp) coronary CT angiography combined with contrast medium reduction using iterative model reconstruction (IMR) on standard BMI patients. Br J Radiol 89(1058):20150766

Part IV

Modality Operations

Clinical Audit

Jane Adam

Contents

J. Adam
Department of Radiology, St. George's Hospital, London, UK
e-mail: drjaneadam@gmail.com

1 Definition of Clinical Audit

The word 'audit' has unfortunate connotations from the financial world where it is defined as 'an official inspection of an organization's accounts, typically by an independent body'. This implies an outside inspection which is seeking to uncover errors, omissions and concealment or fraud. Clinical audit in medicine is better defined as a mechanism for quality improvement and is perhaps best defined as 'a quality improvement process that seeks to improve patient care and outcomes through systematic review of care against explicit criteria and the implementation of change'. An early adopter in Europe was the National Health Service (NHS) in Great Britain, where it was introduced by a 1989 Government White Paper (Department of Health 1989). Clinical audit activity must now be published via quality accounts, and provided to the Care Quality Commission, and audit work is increasingly being linked to reimbursement. Since 2012, all doctors have been obliged to take part in quality improvement initiatives to retain their right to practice and this may include clinical audit data (Jutley et al. 2001).

On a Europe-wide level, clinical audit specific to radiology and nuclear medicine has

Med Radiol Diagn Imaging (2017)
DOI 10.1007/174_2017_122,
Published Online 11 November 2017

been defined and elaborated in a European Commission (EC) guideline for clinical audit, summarised by the European Society of Radiology (ESR) (2011). This distinguishes audit from research, inspection, quality assurance and other regulatory activities and firmly defines it as a multidisciplinary process designed to improve and maintain the quality of patient care.

Although the guideline focuses on the important role of audit in any investigation involving ionising radiation, it recommends auditing all services and processes.

In practice, there is much variation in Europe. Some counties, such as Finland, have instituted 5-yearly audit programmes with external multidisciplinary visits to radiology departments in order to ensure uniformity of practice and regular monitoring of performance; beneficial effects of this approach have been published (Hirvonen-Kari et al. 2009). However, carrying out audit does involve the investment of time and resources, and some countries have undoubtedly lagged behind. There is now more urgency to address the issue of audit in the updated EU radiation protection legislation which comes into force in 2018 and which makes the carrying out of audit in relation to investigations involving radiation mandatory, to ensure its appropriate use (Council Directive 2013). Audit of optimisation of radiation dose and use of dose reference levels is also coming to the fore.

2 The Purpose and Role of Audit

If it is accepted that audit is an agent for improvement, it follows that it is not a 'pass or fail' process, but one of monitoring and awareness of performance, and a striving for improvement (National Institute of Clinical Excellence 2002). However, there have to be benchmarks/targets against which departments or individuals can assess their performance to see where improvement is required, or could be achieved. It is easy to assume that our personal performance or that of our institution is satisfactory, but if it is never measured then that remains an unproven assumption. In many respects, the main benefit of audit is that it requires objective assessment of whatever is being audited. Here, however, there is an important distinction with research. Audit is a sampling process, and does not have the requirement to be statistically valid. It is an indicator of performance at one point in time, and does not require the statistical vigour of a research exercise. It is indicative, not definitive, pointing to areas where performance may need to be improved, or which can be broadly accepted as satisfactory. Where there seems to be underperformance, more detailed analysis will be required to uncover the reasons, or a more extensive or detailed audit process may be required to see if the underperformance is indeed real. This is important if the results of the audit may have important implications for a department, or individual employees, and concerns that audit data will be used indiscriminately or as a basis for punitive action will limit uptake and engagement (Johnston et al. 2000). The potential overlap with inspection or licensing is problematic. Inspection can have a 'pass or fail' element, and this is important for the protection of patients if practice is unsafe or unsatisfactory. In radiology the safety aspects are focused particularly on radiation exposure, but in practice both audit and inspection have the same goal, which is the provision of high-quality safe care. Indeed in countries where both audit and external inspection are carried out, the processes have been found to be broadly complementary: in clinical audits, a broader and deeper view of the clinical procedures is taken, while regulatory inspections mainly verify conformance to basic regulatory requirements (Hirvonen-Kari et al. 2010). Certainly audit data generated internally can be of great value in providing data for external regulatory bodies.

3 Models of Audit

The classical model of clinical audit is the audit cycle or spiral (Figs. 1 and 2).

A standard of performance is identified and agreed before the audit is carried out. The data to be collected and analysed (the indicator or outcome to be measured) are then agreed. The sample size then needs to be established. This has to be large enough to be indicative (although not necessarily statistically valid) while also taking into account the practicalities and time investment required. Once the data is collected and analysed, it will become apparent if the target performance has been achieved. If it has, and it is agreed that the target standard was appropriate (and not too low or 'easy' to achieve), the audit can be considered to be complete. If achieved, but in retrospect the target performance is considered to be too low, a higher standard can be set, turning the audit cycle into a spiral of ascending performance expectations.

If performance is suboptimal and the target is not met, the reasons for this must be explored. This includes an analysis of the steps in the process being audited, so that the cause/causes or source of underperformance be identified. With this knowledge, the question is then what can be done to ameliorate or improve the performance so that the target performance can be met. Following corrective action, reaudit is necessary to ensure that the change has indeed led to the expected improvement. Although over time the target performance can be raised to challenge the system to attempt to achieve better and better performance, perfection is rarely achieved, and performance cannot be improved ad infinitum, year on year.

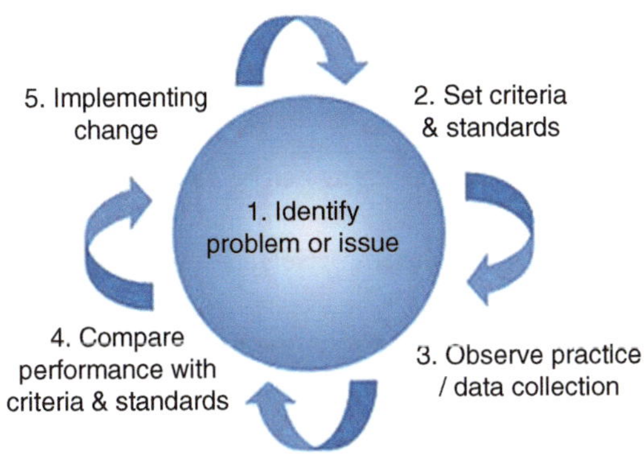

Fig. 1 Audit cycle

4 Internal vs. External Audit

If audit is regarded as a key professional activity, it should not be left to external bodies or inspections, but should be a continuous process taking

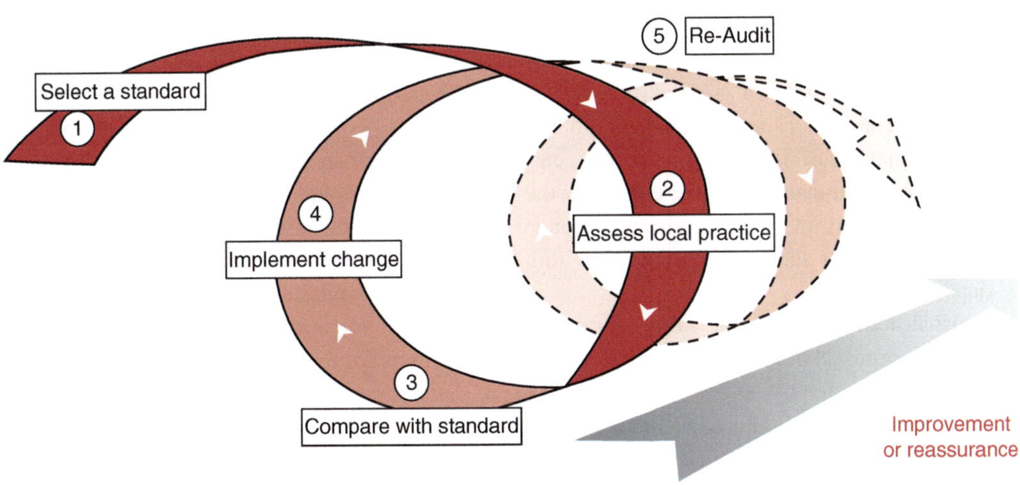

Fig. 2 Audit spiral

place in every department, that is, 'internal audit'. Many activities within radiology involve different professional groups including radiologists, technicians, radiographers, nursing and clerical staff. Medical physicists may also play an important role, especially in the field of radiation protection. European Commission and individual professional body guidelines on audit often emphasize the multidisciplinary aspect of audit, and encourage collaborative audits. Indeed the need for a multidisciplinary approach was the primary reason for renaming 'medical audit' as clinical audit in the 1990s. Within radiology, the patient journey involves multiple steps in the process, and a variety of staff members. All steps can be audited, and this can mean auditing work carried out by many different grades of staff. Some audits may also directly or indirectly audit the work of those outside the radiology department, e.g. referrers. Auditing others' work without their knowledge, and preferably co-operation, is not recommended because it can be viewed as potentially punitive rather than in the spirit of improvement. If improvement is the goal, then a no-blame, constructive approach is essential to obtain the co-operation and collaboration of all staff, and importantly wide acceptance of the validity of the results and any corrective actions suggested (Flottorp et al. 2010).

The ideal situation is where there is a rolling programme of key audits carried out regularly within a department, with additional ones carried out sporadically, or when it is perceived that an individual process or service needs to be improved. Analysis of disappointing results, carried out with a root-cause analysis, can allow the contributory factors of suboptimal performance to be identified and addressed internally within the department or unit.

External audits are also of value. European guidelines suggest that these are carried out by multidisciplinary teams every few years; 5 yearly is recommended. The additional value of external audit is the cross-fertilisation of ideas, and an objective view of the department. They also provide an opportunity for the pooling data from multiple sites, benchmarking and setting of standards. Unfortunately, external auditing processes may be very expensive because they are labour intensive, and many countries cannot devote the relevant resources (Vargha 2009). Here, professional bodies can be helpful by providing set audits that departments can carry out with predefined standards and self-reporting of results. In Europe, this work has been undertaken by the European Society of Radiology (European Society of Radiology 2010; European Society of Radiology, https://www.myesr.org/quality-safety/esr-basic-patient-safety-standards-and-audit-tool). Some countries also carry out national audits on specific topics, in some cases facilitated by national professional bodies, to achieve a snapshot of national performance in a specific area (Duncan et al. 2012).

5 Scope of Clinical Audit

Anything and everything can be audited. Broadly, audit is usually divided into audit of structure, process and outcome. Selected examples are given below:

5.1 Structure

1. Equipment available, e.g. per capita provision, age and specification of equipment, range of equipment available relative to clinical referral guidelines
2. Numbers of staff, e.g. numbers of radiologists relative to workload, numbers of radiographers per machine/workload, hours of operation of equipment
3. Provision of infrastructure, e.g. number of reporting workstations relative to reporters, image storage capacity relative to long-term storage recommendations, electronic alert systems for urgent findings
4. Safety, e.g. machine service contracts, provision of medical physics radiation protection oversight, provision of lead aprons relative to room staffing
5. Patient dignity/well-being, e.g. changing facilities, waiting rooms, translation and chaperone provision

5.2 Process

1. Referrer, e.g. documented referrer contact details, mechanisms for communicating urgent findings
2. Justification, e.g. documentation of roles and responsibilities, documentation of vetting, pregnancy status policies and documentation
3. Timeliness, e.g. waiting times for examinations, report turnaround times, machine time unoccupied, throughput per machine
4. Optimisation, e.g. documented specific imaging protocols for equipment, DRLs, recording of dose, monitoring and documentation of dose, documentation of contrast administered
5. Safety, e.g. process for checking renal function/contrast allergy, process for checking patient identity, process for recording radiation accidental or overexposure, procedure complication reporting, untoward incident reporting process and investigation pathways
6. Complaints, e.g. mechanism for investigation, turnaround times for response
7. Process for reporting of diagnostic discrepancy

5.3 Outcome

1. Number of incidents of accidental/overexposure
2. Numbers of complaints
3. Numbers of adverse incidents reported and their nature, e.g. contrast extravasation
4. Complication rates per interventional procedure
5. Technical success rates for interventional procedures
6. Discrepancy rates for interpretation on second review of imaging
7. Diagnostic accuracy rates
8. Patient satisfaction data
9. Referrer feedback

The success of medicine is ideally judged in terms of the patient outcome. In radiology, with the exception of interventional techniques, the patient health-related outcome which is directly attributable to diagnostic radiology is very difficult to measure. Surrogate measures are therefore often necessary, and these, such as discrepancy or accuracy rates for radiological reporting, are both challenging to collect and even more difficult to validate, which has to be accepted as a limitation of any attempted quality evaluation in this area.

Priorities for audit may include areas where national standards and guidelines exist, where problems have been encountered locally, or where there is a clear potential for improvement or increased efficiency.

6 Source of Target Standards

Ideally, target standards should be evidence based, from published and well-researched sources. One major issue in radiology is the paucity of data on which to base standards, both individual and institutional, particularly patient outcome data, and so target standards may be quite poorly validated. However, legal requirements are clear standards, and consensus guidelines from professional bodies are also a useful source of target standards for clinical audit. Sometimes, benchmarking derived from a range of institutions may form the basis of a target standard. In this case, the standard may not be a fixed number; instead it could be within a range, e.g. within a set number of standard deviations of the mean. This approach is based on the assumption that performance will inevitably fluctuate over time, but using an acceptable range avoids a league table approach whilst still detecting performance which is an 'outlier'. In addition, enough data has to be collected to make sure that the assessment is comprehensive, fair and robust. For radiologists, the ad hoc reporting of retrospectively discovered discrepancies or a sampling method of second review of a percentage of reports may be employed as part of quality assurance of radiologists' performance. However, sampling and reporting variability may be significant, the definition and proof of an error can be variable and the statistical reliability of some of these methods in respect of individual rather than group performance, particularly when relying on ad hoc reporting of retrospectively identified discrepancies, is questionable (The Royal College of Radiologists 2014). As evidence accrues however, it should be possible to update and revise standards across the speciality of radiology, and develop new ones where appropriate. Professional bodies have an important role here to avoid standards being set by those outside the profession or speciality which may be unrealistic or unachievable.

7 Ownership and Accuracy of Audit Data

If audit is considered to be a professional rather than regulatory activity, ownership of the data is local, but it is of management interest. There is a strong argument for personal anonymity in audit because of the risk of blame, and even intimidation or regulatory action which can lead to a fear of audit, concealment and disengagement from the process, but naturally patient protection issues may supersede anonymity in some circumstances. The accuracy of audit data must be realistically assessed, based on sample size and methods used, and not automatically assumed to be a robust enough basis on which to make major management decisions. Where these are intended, additional preplanning of the audit process is necessary in advance of data gathering to ensure that it is fit for purpose, and a sound basis for decision-making. In government-funded healthcare systems, there may be regulatory requirements to produce audit data for benchmarking and policy decisions, but the accuracy issues still pertain to their interpretation, and this needs to be taken into consideration where it may be used for reimbursement decisions. However, audit may reveal that underinvestment is the cause of a failure to reach the benchmark standard and here it can be a powerful tool to present in a case for increased investment in the service.

8 Education and Training

Clinical audit should be part of routine undergraduate and postgraduate training so that it is an expected part of professional life. Unfortunately, it is not generally a 'valued' professional activity amongst doctors, unlike research; and for older generations it may seem a waste of time. The perception that time and effort expended in carrying out audit is not rewarded by proportionate professional recognition has hampered the wider uptake of audit, and moves to make it compulsory, either for certification or reimbursement may be necessary to stimulate the engagement of doctors. The risk of non-engagement of radiologists, or doctors as a whole, is that the standards will be set by others, such as payers and governments, who will have less understanding of the processes than the professionals in that field. It is in the interests of doctors that the accuracy and relevance of any data collected are as robust and relevant as possible, and the engagement and voice of professional bodies are very important to support this.

References

Council Directive 2013/59/Euratom laying down basic safety standards for protection against the dangers arising from exposure to ionizing radiation (OJ L13, 17.01.2014, pp 1–73)

Department of Health (1989) Working for patients. The Stationery Office, London. (Cm 555)

Duncan KA, Drinkwater KJ, Frost C, Remedios D, Barter S (2012) Staging cancer of the uterus: a national audit of MRI accuracy. Clin Radiol 67:523–530

European Society of Radiology (2010) ESR Subcommittee on audit and standards clinical audit—ESR perspective. Insights Imaging 1(1):21–26

European Society of Radiology ESR Basic Patient Safety Standards and Audit Tool. https://www.myesr.org/quality-safety/esr-basic-patient-safety-standards-and-audit-tool

European Society of Radiology (ESR) (2011) European Commission guidelines on clinical audit. Statement by the European Society of Radiology. Insights Imaging 2(2):97–98. http://doi.org/10.1007/s13244-011-0065-8

Flottorp SA, Jamtvedt G, Gibis B, McKee M (2010) Using audit and feedback to health professionals to improve the quality and safety of health care Policy summary prepared for the Belgian EU Presidency Conference on Investing in Europe' health workforce of tomorrow: scope for innovation and collaboration (La Hulpe, 9–10 September 2010)

Hirvonen-Kari M, Salo S, Dean K, Kivisaari L (2009) Effect of clinical audits of radiation use in one hospital district in Finland. Acta Radiol 50(4):389–395.

doi:10.1080/02841850902755260. First published date: 1 May 2009

Hirvonen-Kari M, Järvinen H, Kivisaari L (2010) Clinical audits and regulatory inspections--double efforts and expenses for radiation protection? Acta Radiol 51(6):619–624. Accepted 10 Feb 2010, published online: 30 Apr 2010. https://www.ncbi.nlm.nih.gov/pubmed/20429768#

Johnston G, Crombie IK, Alder EM et al (2000) Reviewing audit: barriers and facilitating factors for effective clinical audit. Qual Health Care 9:23–36

Jutley RS, Mckinley A, Hobeldin M, Mohamed A, Youngson GG (2001) Use of clinical audit for revalidation: is it sufficiently accurate? J Qual Clin Pract 21:71–73. doi:10.1046/j.1440-1762.2001.00414.x

National Institute of Clinical Excellence (2002) Principles of best practice in clinical audit. NICE, London. (ISBN 1-85775-976-1)

The Royal College of Radiologists (2014) Quality assurance in radiology reporting: peer feedback. https://www.rcr.ac.uk/publication/quality-assurance-radiology-reporting-peer-feedback

Vargha A (2009) Harmonising clinical audit in European diagnostic radiology. What needs to be done to improve uptake? Imaging Manage 9:22. https://healthmanagement.org/c/imaging/issue/1590

Quality Metrics: Definition, Creation, Presentation, and Use

Romeo Laroya II and Ramin Khorasani

Contents

R. Laroya II, M.D. • R. Khorasani, M.D., M.P.H. (✉)
Department of Radiology, Center for Evidence-Based Imaging, Brigham and Women's Hospital, Harvard Medical School, Boston, MA, USA
e-mail: rkhorasani@bwh.harvard.edu

Abstract

Advances in diagnostic imaging have helped revolutionize the practice of medicine. These advances have enhanced physicians' understanding of diseases, improved diagnostic accuracy, and contributed tremendously to patient care. However, heterogeneity and on warranted variation in practice of radiology exists locally, regionally, nationally, and globally. Variations in diagnostic radiology practices are well-documented numerous. Even in a single radiology practice substantial unexplained variation exists in how imaging tests are requested, scheduled, performed, reported, communicated, and how frequently appropriate follow-up diagnostic and therapeutic tests and procedures are performed. Such unexplained words and variations in practice of diagnostic radiology can lead to some optimal quality of care, waste, and a diminished patient experience of care. Initiatives to close such performance gaps enhance the value of radiologists and diagnostic imaging to individual patients and to the healthcare system.

To improve quality, initiatives to define, measure, improve and monitor quality are critical. In this chapter, we define quality, describe the importance of measuring quality and characteristics of good quality metrics in radiology. We well describe examples of diagnostic radiology quality metrics in safety, timeliness, effectiveness, and patient centered domains. We will briefly describe the process for creation, presentation, and distribution of quality metrics to enable managing and leading the changes needed to improve the care of individual patients and the performance of the healthcare system.

Med Radiol Diagn Imaging (2018)
DOI 10.1007/174_2017_163, © Springer International Publishing AG
Published Online 05 April 2018

Key Points

- Diagnostic imaging has contributed substantially to patient care and the practice of medicine, but is accompanied by continuing gaps in quality of care and patient safety.
- The Institute of Medicine has defined six domains of healthcare quality—safe, timely, effective, efficient, equitable, and patient centered. Additional domains include measures of "value" as well as evaluations of patient experience and provider well-being.
- Quality measures serve to identify and quantify performance gaps, evaluate interventions to improve performance, monitor and sustain the gains achieved, and demonstrate accountability and value.
- Measures for accountability and value should optimally assess patient outcomes but process measures can serve as effective tools for performance improvement.
- Good quality metrics are clinically meaningful to good patient care, can be created and maintained with high quality using available data, are actionable, relate to a target for quality improvement, and have good validity and reproducibility.
- Exemplar measures for diagnostic radiology include percent of critical results communicated within appropriate predefined timeframes (safety domain), timeliness of examination and reporting completion, adherence to evidence-based clinical practice guidelines (effectiveness), and patient satisfaction with radiology services (patient-centeredness).
- Data from disparate database systems such as the picture archiving and communication system and electronic health record can be aggregated to form a radiology data warehouse from which quality measures can be constructed using visualization and analytics software tools to populate a performance dashboard or scorecards.
- Quality measures alone are insufficient to improve performance, which requires leading and managing change to address technology, processes, and behaviors (personnel).

1 Overview

Advances in diagnostic imaging have helped revolutionize the practice of medicine. These advances have enhanced physicians' understanding of diseases, improved diagnostic accuracy, and contributed tremendously to patient care. However, imaging studies are also associated with potential safety risks including kidney injury (Mitchell et al. 2012), allergic reactions from intravenous contrast, and exposure to radiation (Sodickson et al. 2009; Gee 2012). Despite benefits, significant performance gaps remain in diagnostic radiology relevant to quality of care. In their seminal report, *Crossing the Quality Chasm*, the Institute of Medicine (IOM) identified waste as a substantial feature of our healthcare delivery system (Institute of Medicine 2001). Heterogeneity and unwarranted practice variation contribute to this waste. Variations in diagnostic radiology practices are well documented and numerous. For example, in one large urban emergency department (ED), use of head CT for patients with trauma ranged by physician from 7.2 to 24.5% of patient encounters (with a single outlier of 41.7%) (Andruchow et al. 2012). Nationally, among 34 million Medicare fee-for-service beneficiaries in 2012, the average adjusted CT utilization intensity ranged from 330.4 studies per 1000 beneficiaries in the lowest decile hospital referral region (HRR) to 684.0 in the highest decile HRR; adjusted MR imaging utilization intensity varied from 105.7 studies per 1000 beneficiaries to 256.3 (Ip et al. 2015).

Even in a single radiology practice, substantial unexplained variation exists among radiologists in the frequency of follow-up recommendations in radiology reports, such as for pancreatic cysts—with a 2.8-fold difference in recommendation rates between readers (Ip et al. 2011), and in adherence to evidence-based guidelines for follow-up recommendations for pancreatic cysts (Bobbin et al. 2017), pulmonary nodules (Lu et al. 2016), and renal masses (Maehara et al. 2014).

Variations among radiologists in terminology used to convey diagnostic certainty (Khorasani et al. 2003; Hillman et al. 2004) can create ambiguity and confusion. Such unexplained and unwarranted variations in practice of diagnostic radiology can lead to suboptimal quality of care, waste, and a diminished patient experience. Initiatives to close such performance gaps will enhance the value of radiologists and diagnostic imaging in health care.

2 What Is Quality?

In 2001 as a part of *Crossing the Quality Chasm* (Institute of Medicine 2001), the IOM identified six domains of healthcare quality which have come to frame the definition of quality in the United States today:

- Safe: Avoiding harm to patients from the care that is intended to help them.
- Effective: Providing services based on scientific knowledge to all who could benefit and refraining from providing services to those not likely to benefit (avoiding underuse and misuse, respectively).
- Patient centered: Providing care that is respectful of and responsive to individual patient preferences, needs, and values and ensuring that patient values guide all clinical decisions.
- Timely: Reducing waits and sometimes harmful delays for both those who receive and those who give care.
- Efficient: Avoiding waste, including waste of equipment, supplies, ideas, and energy.
- Equitable: Providing care that does not vary in quality because of personal characteristics such as gender, ethnicity, geographic location, and socioeconomic status.

More recently, additional domains have been proposed, including those of value, as well as evaluations of patient experience and provider well-being. The IOM domains are not mutually exclusive; several are interrelated and interventions to improve quality in multiple domains have the most leverage to improve overall healthcare quality. For example, ensuring timely booking and conduct of appointments for imaging procedures will improve efficiency of the system (and potentially equitable distribution of care) in addition to timeliness. However, improvements in timeliness and efficiency should not come at the expense of patient safety or effectiveness, and an ability to perform more MRI and CT scans must be coupled with assurances that only appropriate orders are completed (i.e., be effective by refraining from providing services to those not likely to benefit), and that unnecessary radiation exposure and other patient safety risks are minimized.

3 Why Measure Quality?

"Quality" and "value" have become integral components of the US healthcare regulatory, compliance, and reimbursement systems. In order for radiology to successfully compete for resources in our rapidly changing healthcare system, we must be able to measure, demonstrate, and continually improve quality and value. However, measuring quality is necessary but not sufficient to change performance. "Insanity is doing the same thing over and over and expecting different results" (attributed to Albert Einstein). Therefore, to improve performance (quality, safety, and efficiency) and create value, we must successfully manage *change*, changes that address people, processes, and technology. Within this framework, quality measures serve multiple purposes, including to (1) identify and quantify performance gaps, (2) evaluate interventions to improve performance, (3) monitor and sustain the gains achieved, and (4) demonstrate value or accountability (Boland et al. 2017), such as adherence to regulatory or accreditation requirements. Measures for accountability or value should optimally assess patient outcomes; however, process measures can serve as effective tools for performance improvement.

4 Characteristics of Good Quality Metrics

"Not everything that counts is measurable, not everything that is measurable counts" (attributed to Albert Einstein). In other words, not all processes or desired outcomes can be measured, and while a process could be measured, not all processes can have meaningful effects to achieve the desired outcome(s). It is also important to distinguish metrics (e.g., radiology report turnaround time) from target performance (e.g., 80th percentile at 6 h). Characteristics of good quality metrics include the following:

- *Clinically meaningful*: The motivation behind a metric must be trusted by the people who will be using it and affected by it. Gaining user trust and support is significantly easier when a metric is sincerely clinically meaningful to the ultimate goal of good patient care. Aligning and demonstrating how a metric will affect patients as well as the interests of the clinician users will greatly improve impact. Metrics to address compliance requirements are critical to ensuring that necessary processes are in place. However, compliance metrics alone limit the opportunity to motivate clinically meaningful changes in practice to create value in healthcare delivery.
- *Relates directly to a defined target for quality improvement (QI)*: A metric must be clear and focused on an objective for QI. To optimize practice, measurement should be embedded in change management initiatives to address technology, people, and process gaps to enable the desired goals. Simply measuring performance may have short-term effects on performance of some, but any such gains are likely to be varied among users and unsustainable over time.
- *Distinguish metrics from target performance*: A good quality metric enables adjustment of

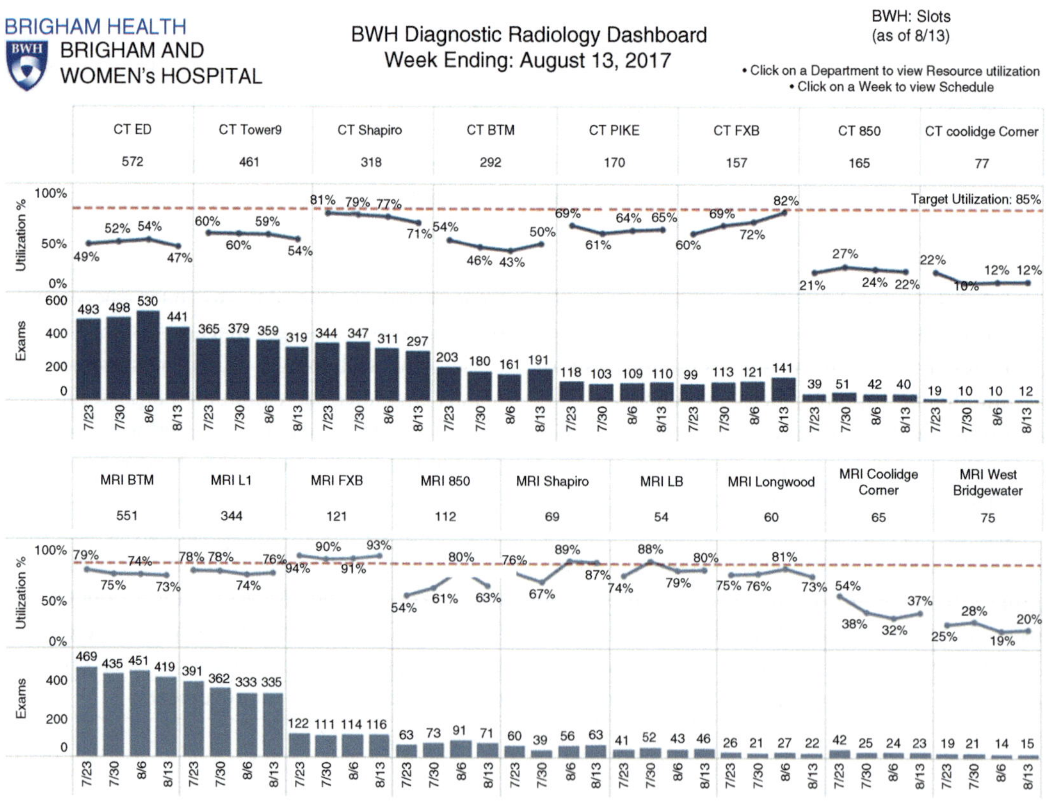

Fig. 1 Weekly scorecard of capacity utilization for CT and MRI slots (target = 85%)

the performance target, when clinically or operationally relevant, to ensure continuous QI.

- *Easy to measure*: This requirement seems simple, but numerous complexities may be encountered in accessing and comprehending the data necessary to create a quality metric. For example, if a metric is a proportion, the data in the numerator and denominator must be explicitly defined and measurable. There are several important caveats to consider. An important QI initiative in your practice may require data recording and capture by people who observe or participate in your current workflow. Such "manual" data collection strategies are often used in QI initiatives. However, to sustain any gains from such initiatives once the QI team has completed their work, easily measured, system-generated data will be needed to efficiently monitor the practice's performance over time to help avoid sliding back to prior behaviors, processes, or outcomes.

An asset utilization metric for an expensive capital asset such as MRI helps illustrate some of the complexities. If the metric is % of time the scanner is in clinical use, the numerator can be the number of minutes a patient was in the room (time stamp of patient entering the room subtracted from the timestamp of the patient leaving the room) for all the patients scanned each day, divided by the denominator of the total number of minutes the scanner was operational that day. This may seem simple enough, but it would require each timestamp for each patient be accurately and consistently documented, and available (easily extracted), and that expected and unexpected scanner downtime be accurately captured and available for calculation each day. Also, inefficient or unnecessarily long imaging protocols will not be apparent—a single patient scanned all day in the scanner will result in a 100% capacity utilization, utterly underrepresenting the performance gap. Thus a second metric may need to be added to measure the length of each exam—which is by necessity varied across different body parts and indications for the study. Figure 1 illustrates a weekly scorecard of a capacity utilization metric for CT and MRI, based on the proportion of predetermined appointment slots used at each imaging location at a large, urban, academic medical center radiology practice, Brigham and Women's Hospital (BWH), in Boston, MA.

- *"Easily" obtained*: This attribute is particularly important to the sustainability of a metric and related QI efforts. The data needed to create the metric should optimally reside in systems used in your practice, and the data should optimally be extractable from your operational systems for reporting using commercially available, off-the-shelf data visualization tools. The more that data to construct a metric can be automated, the more sustainable it is. An important caveat is the limitation of most systems used in clinical operations to visualize and present data in meaningful forms suitable for QI initiatives. Practices focused on QI will thus need to invest in data visualization and analytics tools, and human resources capable of extracting the needed data from operational systems. The advent of machine learning techniques such as natural language processing (NLP) is helping certain metrics, previously unsustainable over time, become more feasible. For example, NLP can replace manual chart review for indications when assessing the appropriateness of MRI lumbar spine examinations performed in the ED for back pain. It is likely that artificial intelligence will help further automate the creation of useful metrics.
- *Reproducible*: A foundation of the scientific process, a metric must be calibrated and reproducible, measuring the same thing consistently.
- *Valid*: Credibly measures the desired attribute. For example, if a technologist enters the timestamp manually for each patient entering and leaving a scanner, errors may occur by delays in data entry or erroneous data entry into systems. The proportion of such erroneous data can make a metric for patient exam time invalid for QI or performance monitoring purposes.
- *Easy to explain*: A metric's ultimate purpose is to be consumed by a user. If a metric is too

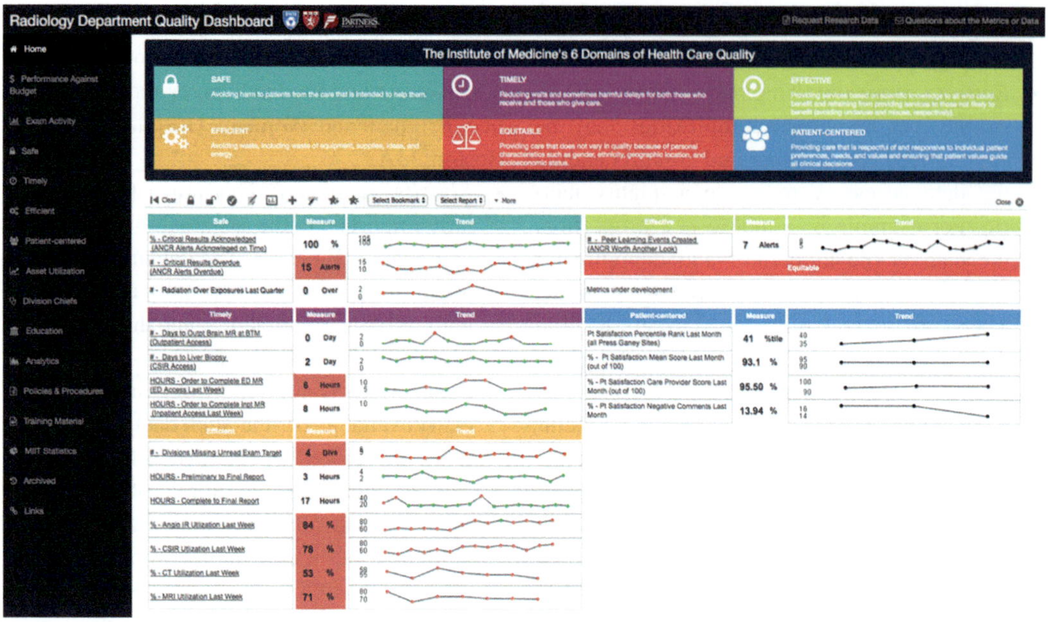

Fig. 2 Radiology Department Quality Dashboard at Brigham and Women's Hospital

convoluted, despite how ideologically accurate it may be, its message cannot be conveyed in a meaningful manner so as to affect behavior and, ultimately, meaningful change and improvement.

- *Actionable*: A metric whose results cannot be acted upon is useless as it will not produce the desired change or improvement.
- A good quality metric *enables identification of performance gaps and opportunities for improvement*. If the ideal target performance of a quality metric is achieved by all in your practice, the metric is no longer a tool for QI. Rather it may become a useful tool for marketing your practice's services. Thus a useful metric should help identify processes, behaviors, or outcomes that should be improved.

5 Examples of Imaging Quality Metrics

Quality measures for diagnostic radiology can be defined in each of the six IOM domains of quality. A recent report of the American College of Radiology's Economics Committee on value-based payment models also provides a very useful framework for developing clinically meaningful metrics for your practice (Boland et al. 2017). As one example, Fig. 2 displays a "dashboard" of key quality, safety, and performance metrics for the Radiology Department at BWH, arrayed by IOM quality domain. The subsections that follow review exemplar imaging quality metrics in several domains.

5.1 Safety

Failure to promptly communicate critical imaging test results is not uncommon and such delays are a major source of malpractice claims in radiology and a potential source of patient harm. Therefore, communication of critical results from diagnostic procedures between caregivers was named a 2011 Joint Commission national patient safety goal. BWH established an enterprise-wide communication of Critical Test Results policy for communication of critical imaging results (Khorasani 2009), and developed an automated system, Alert Notification of Critical Results (ANCR), designed to facilitate such communication (Lacson et al. 2014a, b, 2016; O'Connor et al. 2016). Nearly 50,000 critical result alerts are generated annually; >98% have closed loop acknowl-

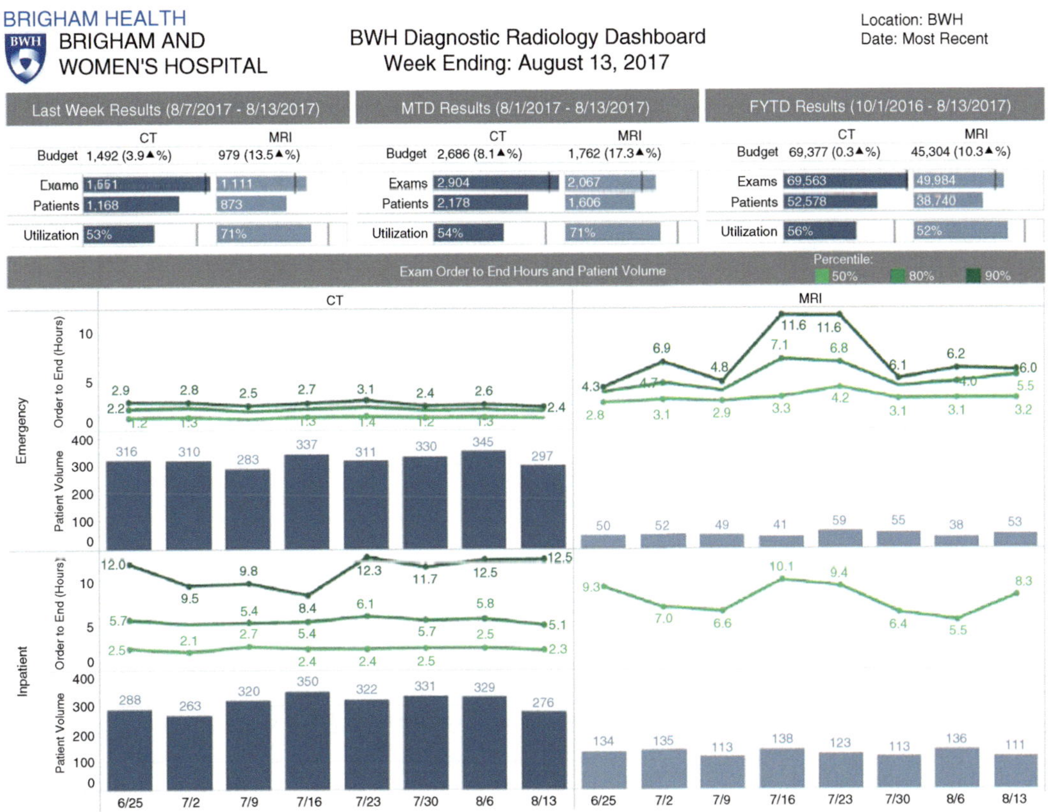

Fig. 3 Weekly scorecard of performance indications for CT and MRI for emergency department and inpatients

edgement within the timeframe stipulated by BWH policy. The BWH dashboard tracks the daily percentage of critical results with closed loop acknowledgment within BWH policy parameters, critical results ('alerts') acknowledged over time, as well as the number of alerts that are overdue (unacknowledged beyond the timeframe stipulated by BWH policy parameters). Target performance is >95% of critical results acknowledged within policy timeframe (1 h for Level 1 or red alerts; 3 h for Level 2 or orange alerts; 15 days for Level 3 or yellow alerts) (Lacson et al. 2014b).

5.2 Timeliness

These metrics should be created and measured for various modalities and care settings. At BWH, timely ambulatory MRI access is defined as the third available outpatient appointment. The third appointment is used because using the next available appointment invariably overstates capacity, as one or two cancellations occur daily. This is also congruent with how the healthcare delivery system reports outpatient access to other specialists. Inpatient and ED MRI access is defined by the time it takes from an examination request until it is performed (target performance: 90% of exams performed within 5 and 12 h, respectively). Clicking on the summary measure for ED or inpatient access on the dashboard's home page (Fig. 2) links to a more detailed weekly scorecard of performance for CT and MRI for ED and inpatients (Fig. 3) that depicts performance for these metrics. At most practices, this information resides in the Radiology Information System (RIS). At BWH, because of the full adoption of an electronic health record (EHR) and embedded computerized provider order entry (CPOE) system for all imaging studies, the request time is taken from the CPOE database, and the examination completion is taken from the RIS module of the EHR.

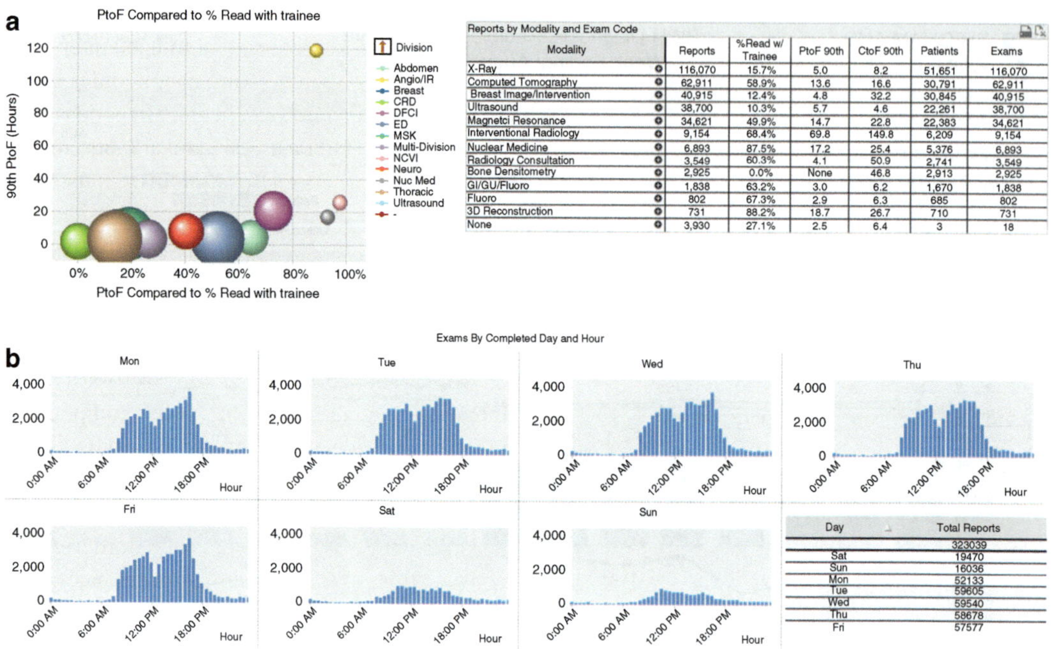

Reports by Modality and Exam Code

Modality	Reports	%Read w/ Trainee	PtoF 90th	CtoF 90th	Patients	Exams
X-Ray	116,070	15.7%	5.0	8.2	51,651	116,070
Computed Tomography	62,911	58.9%	13.6	16.6	30,791	62,911
Breast Image/Intervention	40,915	12.4%	4.8	32.2	30,845	40,915
Ultrasound	38,700	10.3%	5.7	4.6	22,261	38,700
Magnetci Resonance	34,621	49.9%	14.7	22.8	22,383	34,621
Interventional Radiology	9,154	68.4%	69.8	149.8	6,209	9,154
Nuclear Medicine	6,893	87.5%	17.2	25.4	5,376	6,893
Radiology Consultation	3,549	60.3%	4.1	50.9	2,741	3,549
Bone Densitometry	2,925	0.0%	None	46.8	2,913	2,925
GI/GU/Fluoro	1,838	63.2%	3.0	6.2	1,670	1,838
Fluoro	802	67.3%	2.9	6.3	685	802
3D Reconstruction	731	88.2%	18.7	26.7	710	731
None	3,930	27.1%	2.5	6.4	3	18

Day	Total Reports
	323039
Sat	19470
Sun	16036
Mon	52133
Tue	59605
Wed	59540
Thu	58678
Fri	57577

Fig. 4 (**a**) Scorecard of hours from preliminary to final (PtoF) report vs. %trainee-generated reports by subspecialty division, January–June, 2017. (**b**) Scorecard of the number of imaging studies completed each hour of each day (averaged over January–June, 2017)

Various timeliness of interpretation metrics can be constructed with data obtained from the RIS or report generation databases (e.g., speech recognition solutions), depending on the practice setting. These measures span the timeliness and efficiency domains of quality. Examination and report milestones can be designated as follows: (1) examination complete (all images obtained), (2) examination dictated by the radiologist, (3) report transcribed and ready for the radiologist's signature, and (4) report signed and finalized by the radiologist. The time interval between each milestone describes practice or individual radiologist performance for the timeliness of reporting. For example, the time from completion to finalization depicts report turnaround time, while the time from transcription (a report in preliminary status created by a trainee, or in a small and diminishing number of practices where a transcriptionist translated the voice file into text for edit and signature by the radiologist) to finalization refers to radiologist signature time. With the use of speech recognition technology, the time from dictation to transcription may be irrelevant at many practices.

The BWH Radiology Dashboard tracks the hours from preliminary to final report (preliminary reports are generated by a trainee), as well as the hours from examination completion to final report. Target performance for signature time is 90% of reports within 6 h, 7 × 24 × 365 inclusive of all care settings—ED, inpatients, and outpatients. Clicking on the summary measure on the dashboard's home page (Fig. 2) links to a more detailed analytics module displaying various additional complementing metrics such as proportion of reports generated by trainees in different radiology subspecialty divisions (Fig. 4a) or the number of imaging studies completed each hour of each day (averaged over a predefined time period) to enable optimization of the radiologist workforce for timely delivery of needed clinical care (Fig. 4b).

	OVERALL	BWH IMG CT 850	BWH IMG CT BTM	BWH IMG CT FXB	BWH IMG CT PIKE	BWH IMG CT SH	BSH IMG CT CCI	BWH IMG FL GI DIAG	BWH IMG IR ANGIO	BWH IMG IR CSIR	BWH IMG MSK IR XRAY BTM	BWP RAD VEIN CTR FXB	BWP RAD VEIN
Overall	10%	0%	38%	33%	24%	13%	25%	10%	13%	19%	15%	56%	0%
Category													
Registration	13%	0%	0%	0%	20%	13%	NA	6%	0%	20%	17%	67%	0%
Test or Treatment	9%	0%	100%	NA	50%	10%	100%	0%	50%	11%	18%	33%	0%
Personal Issue	15%	0%	100%	100%	0%	21%	0%	0%	0%	9%	33%	0%	0%
Care Provider	11%	NA	NA	NA	20%	NA	NA	NA	NA	NA	NA	NA	NA
Facility	21%	0%	100%	NA	0%	11%	NA	40%	NA	44%	13%	NA	0%
Overall assessment	10%	0%	0%	0%	33%	12%	0%	0%	0%	14%	0%	100%	0%

Fig. 5 Brigham and Women's Hospital (BWH) patient experience heat map. % of patient comments that are negative; by category and by imaging center

5.3 Effectiveness

Measures in the domain of effectiveness assess whether services are provided based on scientific knowledge to those who could benefit and not provided to those not likely to benefit (avoiding overuse and waste). Numerous measures are possible to assess the appropriateness of the radiology examination ordered ("the right procedure"), e.g., the % of appropriate head CT orders among ED patients with head trauma. For most radiology practices, the determination of appropriateness can typically be made by comparing the order indications to appropriate use criteria, such as the American College of Radiology (ACR) Appropriateness Criteria® (American College of Radiology 2017), or to published evidence-based or local best practice guidelines. Such metrics for adherence to evidence can be constructed and used in QI initiatives. Multifaceted health information technology-enabled QI initiatives can improve adherence to evidence-based guidelines during the radiology test ordering process (Gupta et al. 2014; Raja et al. 2014; Ip et al. 2014), reaching 85% adherence to Wells criteria when ordering chest CT for pulmonary embolism in the ED and 96% adherence to American College of Physicians guidelines for use of MRI in primary care patients with low back pain. Similar multifaceted interventions have been shown to improve report signature time (Andriole et al. 2010), quality of multiparametric prostate MRIs (Silveira et al. 2015), and quality of rectal cancer staging MRI reports (Sahni et al. 2015). Tracking and improving appropriate use of imaging will be an important focus of QI initiatives and potential target of federal regulations (Protecting Access to Medicare Act of 2014) as we transition from transactional healthcare financing to value-based payment systems.

Most practices have some program for interpretation accuracy as part of their quality assurance programs. More recently, information technology (IT) solutions have been developed and implemented at some practices. The ACR's RADPEER® system is an example of such a program and can be integrated into a picture archiving and communication system (PACS). While interpreting a current examination, a radiologist can review the report of a prior examination and agree or disagree with the prior interpretation. The substance of the disagreement can also be graded. Using such software, one can create metrics at the practice or individual radiologist level, using peer-reviewed agreement or disagreement as a proxy for accuracy of interpretation.

5.4 Patient Centered

Although debate persists regarding survey content, timing of survey administration, and relevant risk adjustment methodologies, there is evidence that self-reported measures of patient experience are distinctive indicators of healthcare quality (Manary et al. 2013). Thus engaging patients and eliciting their feedback to motivate improvements have become major initiatives across the nation's healthcare delivery systems. However, there are few reports of such initiatives in radiology. Surveys are typically delivered to patients on paper or electronically, using standard survey content to enable comparison between peer institutions. Results of surveys are presented as mean patient satisfaction scores and percentile rankings when compared to peer institutions. Free text comments from patient respondents can be categorized as negative, positive, or mixed. Given the multitude of imaging locations within some practices (distributed by physical location and modality for example) it is possible to create a heat map based on the percentage of surveys with negative patient comments to identify targets for performance improvement (Fig. 5). Though it remains to be seen if such an approach can help improve patient satisfaction performance, experiments with various strategies to engage and train the workforce to improve patient interactions will be needed to shape optimal intervention to address this import quality domain.

6 Creation, Presentation, and Distribution of Quality Metrics

In a typical practice, multiple health IT systems are used in clinical operations. In radiology, such systems include the EHR, RIS module, report generation system (e.g., speech recognition system), and PACS, among others. Each system has its own database, often with different definitions for similar data/milestones. Combining the data from these various databases can provide a very useful infrastructure for developing metrics. However, in reality, informatics challenges as well as needed human resources with appropriate skills hamper such an approach in many organizations. Still, the most practical approach for quality metrics creation and reporting requires creating a new database (a data warehouse), populated by data from the disparate systems in use (Prevedello et al. 2008). Business intelligence refers to the set of tools needed to integrate, store, analyze, and present data from nonintegrated sources. Integration is a key process step to ensure that data from different sources are checked for consistency and subsequently converted into a unified format. This integration is referred to as Extract Transform Load (ETL) process and can be used to extract data from each database to populate the data warehouse. This process can be enhanced to normalize data across the varied operational databases to help automate the near-real-time population of the data warehouse.

The normalization of data is needed to minimize heterogeneous encoding of data across various databases. A simple example is to validate and ensure that a milestone called "exam begin" in one system is or is not the same as "exam start" in another operational system. Such attention to detail is critical when creating the data warehouse to help ensure that metrics can ultimately be clinically relevant, accurate, and reproducible. Relational databases, where data are represented in numerous related tables, are very common but are not ideal for ad hoc analysis because of additional needed data processing to easily understand the results of queries. Another method of organizing the data is using multidimensional data cubes using On-Line Analytical Process (OLAP) tools to enable the user to better understand the results during ad hoc queries. Relational databases can thus be enhanced by connecting to OLAP tools to enable easily understood real-time queries to the data warehouse (Prevedello et al. 2010). Once the data warehouse is created, analytic and visualization tools can thus leverage the normalized data in the warehouse to create near-real-time views of desired metrics. Although definitions are somewhat arbitrary, a dashboard often refers to near-real-time, online view of performance measures, analogous to a speedometer in an automobile. A scorecard, in distinction, will refer to a static view of performance updated at some predetermined interval (e.g., weekly, monthly). Analytics tools in contrast enable a user to create numerous custom queries of the data warehouse as needed. Figure 1 represents the current BWH quality "dashboard" with key quality, safety, and performance indicators on the home page with some updated daily, others weekly or monthly.

7 Managing Change

Creating and publishing the results of quality metrics alone is highly unlikely to result in sustainable meaningful improvement in your practice. Rather, performance improvement requires managing change in your practice, including leaders who can address technology, process, and people issues to create and sustain gains. Within such a change framework, quality measures are a necessary, but not sufficient, tool. Successful change management is a discipline to its own and requires dedicated skills and resources (Khorasani 2004; Kotter 1995), a topic beyond the scope of this chapter.

Conclusion

National initiatives (Choosing Wisely—An Initiative of the ABIM Foundation [Internet] 2015; Medicare Access and CHIP Reauthorization Act of 2015 (MACRA) [Internet] 2015) are under way to improve quality, reduce waste, and transform the healthcare system from its current transactional payment model to one based on quality and value. Measuring, monitoring, and reporting radiology quality measures, combined with multifaceted change management initiatives to address information technology, care processes, and behaviors (people) of providers who order radiology studies, and those who perform and interpret them, can encourage and enable evidence-based practice, improve quality and patient experience of care, and reduce waste. Additional research will continue to inform best practices to develop, measure, and employ quality measures as part of meaningful interventions to improve the healthcare delivery system.

References

American College of Radiology (2017) ACR Appropriateness Criteria® [Internet]. [cited 2017 Aug 24]. https://www.acr.org/Quality-Safety/Appropriateness-Criteria

Andriole KP, Prevedello LM, Dufault A, Pezeshk P, Bransfield R, Hanson R et al (2010) Augmenting the impact of technology adoption with financial incentive to improve radiology report signature times. J Am Coll Radiol 7(3):198–204

Andruchow JE, Raja AS, Prevedello LM, Zane RD, Khorasani R (2012) Variation in head computed tomography use for emergency department trauma patients and physician risk tolerance. Arch Intern Med 172(8):660–661

Bobbin MD, Ip IK, Sahni VA, Shinagare AB, Khorasani R (2017) Focal cystic pancreatic lesion follow-up recommendations after publication of ACR White Paper on managing incidental findings. J Am Coll Radiol 14(6):757–764

Boland GW, Glenn L, Goldberg-Stein S, Jha S, Mangano M, Patel S et al (2017) Report of the ACR's economics committee on value-based payment models. J Am Coll Radiol 14(1):6–14

Choosing Wisely - An Initiative of the ABIM Foundation [Internet] (2015) [cited 2017 Aug 25]. http://choosingwisely.org/

Gee A (2012) Radiation Concerns Rise with Patients' Exposure. The New York Times [Internet]. http://www.nytimes.com/2012/06/13/health/as-medical-imaging-rises-radiation-concerns-follow.html?_r=0

Gupta A, Ip IK, Raja AS, Andruchow JE, Sodickson A, Khorasani R (2014) Effect of clinical decision support on documented guideline adherence for head CT in emergency department patients with mild traumatic brain injury. J Am Med Inform Assoc 21(e2):e347–e351

Hillman BJ, Amis ES, Neiman HL, FORUM Participants (2004) The future quality and safety of medical imaging: proceedings of the third annual ACR FORUM. J Am Coll Radiol 1(1):33–39

Institute of Medicine (2001) Crossing the quality chasm: a new health system for the 21st century. National Academy Press, Washington, DC

Ip IK, Mortele KJ, Prevedello LM, Khorasani R (2011) Focal cystic pancreatic lesions: assessing variation in radiologists' management recommendations. Radiology 259(1):136–141

Ip IK, Gershanik EF, Schneider LI, Raja AS, Mar W, Seltzer S et al (2014) Impact of IT-enabled intervention on MRI use for back pain. Am J Med 127(6):512–518.e1

Ip IK, Raja AS, Seltzer SE, Gawande AA, Joynt KE, Khorasani R (2015) Use of public data to target variation in providers' use of CT and MR imaging among Medicare beneficiaries. Radiology 275(3):718–724

Khorasani R (2004) Leading your organization through a successful software implementation has little to do with the technology. J Am Coll Radiol 1(6):430–431

Khorasani R (2009) Optimizing communication of critical test results. J Am Coll Radiol 6(10):721–723

Khorasani R, Bates DW, Teeger S, Rothschild JM, Adams DF, Seltzer SE (2003) Is terminology used effectively to convey diagnostic certainty in radiology reports? Acad Radiol 10(6):685–688

Kotter J (1995) Leading change: why transformation efforts fail. Harv Bus Rev

Lacson R, O'Connor SD, Andriole KP, Prevedello LM, Khorasani R (2014a) Automated critical test result notification system: architecture, design, and assessment of provider satisfaction. AJR Am J Roentgenol 203(5):W491–W496

Lacson R, Prevedello LM, Andriole KP, O'Connor SD, Roy C, Gandhi T et al (2014b) Four-year impact of an alert notification system on closed-loop communication of critical test results. AJR Am J Roentgenol 203(5):933–938

Lacson R, O'Connor SD, Sahni VA, Roy C, Dalal A, Desai S et al (2016) Impact of an electronic alert notification system embedded in radiologists' workflow on closed-loop communication of critical results: a time series analysis. BMJ Qual Saf 25(7):518–524

Lu MT, Rosman DA, Wu CC, Gilman MD, Harvey HB, Gervais DA et al (2016) Radiologist point-of-care clinical decision support and adherence to guidelines for incidental lung nodules. J Am Coll Radiol 13(2):156–162

Maehara CK, Silverman SG, Lacson R, Khorasani R (2014) JOURNAL CLUB: renal masses detected at abdominal CT: radiologists' adherence to guidelines regarding management recommendations and communication of critical results. AJR Am J Roentgenol 203(4):828–834

Manary MP, Boulding W, Staelin R, Glickman SW (2013) The patient experience and health outcomes. N Engl J Med 368(3):201–203

Medicare Access and CHIP Reauthorization Act of 2015 (MACRA) [Internet] (2015) [cited 2017 Aug 25]. https://www.cms.gov/Medicare/Quality-Initiatives-Patient-Assessment-Instruments/Value-Based-Programs/MACRA-MIPS-and-APMs/MACRA-MIPS-and-APMs.html

Mitchell AM, Jones AE, Tumlin JA, Kline JA (2012) Prospective study of the incidence of contrast-induced nephropathy among patients evaluated for pulmonary embolism by contrast-enhanced computed tomography. Acad Emerg Med 19(6):618–625

O'Connor SD, Dalal AK, Sahni VA, Lacson R, Khorasani R (2016) Does integrating nonurgent, clinically significant radiology alerts within the electronic health record impact closed-loop communication and follow-up? J Am Med Inform Assoc 23(2):333–338

Prevedello LM, Andriole KP, Khorasani R (2008) Business intelligence tools and performance improvement in your practice. J Am Coll Radiol 5(12):1210–1211

Prevedello LM, Andriole KP, Hanson R, Kelly P, Khorasani R (2010) Business intelligence tools for radiology: creating a prototype model using open-source tools. J Digit Imaging 23(2):133–141

Protecting Access to Medicare Act of (2014) Public Law 113-93 Apr 1, 2014 p. Congressional Record Vol 160

Raja AS, Gupta A, Ip IK, Mills AM, Khorasani R (2014) The use of decision support to measure documented adherence to a national imaging quality measure. Acad Radiol 21(3):378–383

Sahni VA, Silveira PC, Sainani NI, Khorasani R (2015) Impact of a structured report template on the quality of MRI reports for rectal cancer staging. Am J Roentgenol 205(3):584–588

Silveira PC, Dunne R, Sainani NI, Lacson R, Silverman SG, Tempany CM et al (2015) Impact of an information technology-enabled initiative on the quality of prostate multiparametric MRI reports. Acad Radiol 22(7):827–833

Sodickson A, Baeyens PF, Andriole KP, Prevedello LM, Nawfel RD, Hanson R et al (2009) Recurrent CT, cumulative radiation exposure, and associated radiation-induced cancer risks from CT of adults. Radiology 251(1):175–184

Part V

Reporting

Reporting: Recommendations/ Guidelines

Jessica G. Zarzour and Lincoln L. Berland

Contents

J.G. Zarzour, M.D.
Department of Radiology, University of Alabama at Birmingham, 619 19th Street South, JTN 357, Birmingham, AL 35249, USA

L.L. Berland, M.D., F.A.C.R. (✉)
Chair, ACR Body Imaging Commission Professor Emeritus, Department of Radiology, University of Alabama at Birmingham, 619 19th Street South, JT N455D, Birmingham, AL 35249, USA
e-mail: lberland@uabmc.edu

Abstract

A core principle of quality improvement for better outcomes is consistency. With the increased use of medical imaging, incidental findings are more commonly being discovered. There is significant variability in the reporting and follow-up regarding incidental findings. This can lead to confusion for the referring physician unless specific guidance is offered by the radiologist. Other guidelines have also been developed for specific conditions and to help guide the management of the patient. The development, implementation, and use of guidelines can help foster consistency and lead to quality improvement.

In this chapter, the scope of the problem and process for development of guidelines will be addressed. Medicolegal and ethical implications of using guidelines are also discussed. Quality is enhanced by decreasing variation in practice and guidelines are an important tool. Guidelines should be broadly acceptable, easy to access, and straightforward to understand and apply. Development of guidelines under the auspices of established professional societies allows for endorsement and dissemination of recommendations. Radiologist adherence to guidelines can enhance informed decision-making, decrease variations in recommendations, decrease cost, and limit medical liability. This has potential to provide standardization, to improve patient care, and to improve confidence of the referring physicians.

Med Radiol Diagn Imaging (2017)
DOI 10.1007/174_2017_87, © Springer International Publishing AG
Published Online 23 June 2017

1 Scope of the Problem

The use of medical imaging has increased rapidly in the past several decades, although that trend has recently flattened (Baker et al. 2008; Smith-Bindman et al. 2008). That increase has been accompanied by an improvement in image quality and a substantial expansion of the knowledge about the implications of both primary findings and incidental findings. This expansion of knowledge has led to efforts to analyze, systematize, and operationalize complex knowledge to make it more easily consumable. This includes multiple criteria used to manage specific conditions, such as indications for liver and cardiac transplantation and placement on transplant waiting lists.

To address these issues, there has been a proliferation of guidelines and recommendations because one of the core principles of quality improvement to improve outcomes is consistency, which guidelines can foster. Such guidelines are most often created under the auspices of established professional societies. Without clear, acceptable, accessible, easily applicable guidelines at least partly integrated into the physicians' workflow, independent radiologists tend to develop their own subjective and inconsistent criteria for managing them (Berland et al. 2014). Given these challenges, the process of developing and applying guidelines is still rapidly evolving.

2 Guidelines for Incidental Findings

Incidental findings, defined as findings that are unrelated to the patients presenting symptom or diagnosis (Berland 2011; Berland et al. 2010), are one source of inconsistent practice and are increasingly being discovered on CT and MRI scans. These incidental findings are an inevitable product of radiologists being taught to carefully scrutinize each examination during their training (Brown 2013).

The remarkable detail provided in modern imaging has led to a reassessment of the natural history of many diseases. For example, the recognized incidence of thyroid cancer has more than doubled over the last 30 years, which is thought to be because of increasing use of thyroid ultrasound (Davies and Welch 2006; Cronan 2008). Similarly, a 61% increase in renal cell cancer diagnosis is attributed to their incidental discovery on CT scans performed for other reasons (Berland 2011). While some incidental findings are clinically important and can lead to interventions that may change the course of the disease, many such findings would never affect the patient's health if not recognized and no intervention was performed (Berland 2011; Berland et al. 2010).

Regarding CT colonography, several studies have reported detection of incidental findings in 41–98% of cases, with clinically significant findings in 5–18% of the cases (Pickhardt et al. 2008; Yee et al. 2010; Berland 2009a; Hara et al. 2000; Xiong et al. 2005, 2006; Hellstrom et al. 2004; Hassan et al. 2008a; Liu et al. 2005; Song et al. 2012; Flicker et al. 2008; Gluecker et al. 2003; Veerappan et al. 2010; Kimberly et al. 2009), but with a higher frequency of clinically significant findings in symptomatic patients (Berland 2009a; Hara et al. 2000; Xiong et al. 2005, 2006; Hellstrom et al. 2004). The detection of incidental findings increases with the patient's age (Furtado et al. 2005), being found in nearly everyone over the age of 70. The percentage of patients subjected to procedures for managing incidental findings ranges from 2 to 11% (Pickhardt et al. 2008; Xiong et al. 2005). In a retrospective review of 2195 patients who underwent screening CT colonography, further workup was required in 6.1% of the patients for incidental findings including additional imaging, noninvasive and invasive procedures (Pickhardt et al. 2008). Benign, insignificant findings were confirmed in most patients and only 2.5% had relevant new diagnoses (Pickhardt et al. 2008).

In abdominal CTs other than CT colonography, clinically significant incidental findings were found in 18% of patients undergoing CT urography for evaluating hematuria (Liu et al. 2005) and in 10.3% of patients undergoing a CT angiography for renal donor candidates

(Maizlin et al. 2007). In a review of 1295 patients who underwent CT for hematuria, 214 (16.5%) important incidental findings were found in 143 (11.0%) of the patients leading to invasive procedures in 30 patients and further evaluation without invasive procedures in 63 patients, which lead to a therapeutic benefit in 25 patients and serious complications in 6 patients (Morgan et al. 2015). In another study of 1192 patients undergoing whole body CT screening, 37% of the patients had recommendations for further testing (Furtado et al. 2005).

Regarding chest CT examinations, the detection of lung nodules, emphysema, coronary artery disease, and thyroid nodules are the most commonly reported incidental findings (MacRedmond et al. 2004). In patients undergoing screening chest CT, the rate of detecting incidental findings varies from 19.2 to 62% (MacRedmond et al. 2004; Kucharczyk et al. 2011). Extracardiac incidental findings at coronary CT angiography are discovered in 25–61% of patients (Lee et al. 2010; Sosnouski et al. 2007; Machaalany et al. 2009).

3 Inconsistencies in Managing Incidental Findings

Determining how to handle incidental findings can be confusing for the treating physician unless specific guidance is offered by the radiologist (Berland 2011). The reporting and follow-up of incidental findings is inconsistent (Obuchowski et al. 2007). In a report describing how 27 academic radiologists at 3 major academic centers manage incidental findings, the rate of agreement ranged from 30 to 85% (Johnson et al. 2011). Another study of 5.9 million radiology reports showed significant variation in the recommendation rates for additional imaging within a single department (Sistrom et al. 2009). After publication of the Society of Radiologists in Ultrasound (SRU) Consensus guidelines regarding adnexal cystic lesions, recommendations for additional imaging dramatically decreased (Ghosh and Levine 2013; Levine et al. 2010). Inconsistencies in how radiologists handle incidental findings are problematic and may diminish radiologists' credibility and perceived value (Brown 2013; Johnson et al. 2011; Eisenberg et al. 2010; Megibow 2011). Problems arise due to varying reporting patterns that lead to inconsistencies in documentation and clinical care (Johnson et al. 2011; Eisenberg et al. 2010). The variation frustrates referrers who may choose to ignore the recommendations (Boland et al. 2011). Referring physicians may regard recommendations for additional imaging as a form of "self-referral" (Kilani et al. 2011). Recommendations made by the radiologist acting in his or her role as a consultant can offer helpful information and guidance to the patient and treating physician (Silverman et al. 2008). Guidelines can help decrease variations in follow-up recommendations.

So, applying recommendations as inconsistently as is currently practiced cannot generate the highest quality care and may not continue to be tolerated by government and other regulatory organizations. The passage of MACRA (2016), mandating merit-based incentive payment systems or alternative payment models, imposes quality requirements that include metrics that are regularly updated, and include adherence to some ACR incidental findings recommendations (PQRS measures #405, and #406, which can be accessed online from CMS.gov).

Sparse data are present to suggest what drives how a radiologist handles incidental findings. While younger radiologists are more likely to recommend additional imaging examinations than their more experienced colleagues (Sistrom et al. 2009), less experienced radiologists are more likely to follow guidelines (Eisenberg et al. 2010). Perhaps the greater compliance in following guidelines is because of their greater familiarity with them (Eisenberg et al. 2010). One study showed that radiologists who were abdominal specialists complied with reporting renal critical results 93% of the time versus only 57% for non-abdominal specialists (Maehara et al. 2014). Variation in recommendations for additional imaging is multifactorial, including the radiologist's diagnostic confidence, experience, subspecialty expertise, perception, and fear of litigation (Boland et al. 2011).

4 Guidelines for Other Conditions

Numerous guidelines have been developed to help diagnose and manage specific conditions other than incidental findings, including (1) pregnancies of unknown location or viability (Doubilet et al. 2014), (2) low-radiation-exposure CT for lung cancer screening using the Lung-RADS guidelines (American College of Radiation 2016), (3) Li-RADS for hepatocellular carcinoma in patients with cirrhosis (American College of Radiology 2014), (4) thyroid nodules regarding whether they should undergo fine needle aspiration (Ghosh and Levine 2013), (5) image-based cancer staging, and (6) categorization to assist management, such as the American Association for the Surgery of Trauma (AAST) system for grading organ trauma.

The purposes of these guidelines are strikingly varied, although all attempt to organize disparate and controversial data and opinions. The guideline on pregnancy of unknown location or viability reflects the results of an SRU consensus conference reviewing a complex set of findings where recommendations had been fragmented into a large number of papers with conflicting information (Doubilet et al. 2014). The guideline on lung cancer screening is based on Lung-RADS and reflects the need to collect a large set of data in high-risk patients to determine the patient's specific risk of having a lung cancer (American College of Radiation 2016). This data also is required to populate a registry. The Li-RADS guideline provides a lexicon and describes a number of criteria that rate the probability that a patient with cirrhosis and liver lesions has hepatocellular carcinoma, helps determine therapy and helps place patients in the appropriate positioning on liver transplant lists (American College of Radiology 2014).

Guidelines for determining the need for fine needle aspiration of thyroid nodules are among the most controversial because there are strong disagreements regarding the need to aggressively pursue a condition with such a high rate of curability. Therefore, existing guidelines vary considerably and lead to confusing guidance for radiologists performing neck ultrasound. Cancer staging has been performed for decades, but the radiologist's role in staging has been expanding, mostly because cross-sectional imaging provides so much valuable information that affects staging and treatment. Categorizations systems such as the AAST organ trauma grading system help triage the severity of injuries and help determine whether surgical intervention is appropriate. Additionally, grading is required for accredited trauma institutions.

What all of these scenarios have in common is that they represent complex sets of multiple imaging and clinical features that must be evaluated in combination to arrive at a potential action. The need for having these guidelines in a form that is easy to refer to reflects that these guidelines can rarely be memorized by radiologists of varying experience and even if they can be remembered, following defined pathways would be a very challenging mental exercise without visually referring to the algorithms.

5 Medicolegal Implications of Using Guidelines

Managing incidental findings is a dilemma for the radiologist, treating physician, patient, and patient's family. The chance that an incidental finding could represent a lethal carcinoma is <1% (Welch 2011). Evaluating incidental findings is of uncertain benefit as the findings vary in clinical importance, but can lead to a series of tests with increased cost, patient anxiety, decreased productivity, and morbidity (Berland et al. 2010; Berland 2009a; Morgan et al. 2015; Casarella 2002; Ding et al. 2011). On the other hand, if an incidental finding is not mentioned in the radiological report and in the unlikely event that the finding turns out to represent a significant disease, then the patient's health has been jeopardized and medical malpractice litigation could ensue (Berlin 2011). In the New York Appeals Court decision declared over a century ago that has served as the foundation for informed consent between a patient and doctor, Justice Benjamin Cardozo stated, "Any human being of adult years and sound mind has a right to determine what shall be done with his own body (Court of Appeals of New York 1914)." The Code of Ethics of the American Medical Association says, "The physician's obligation is to present the medical facts accurately to the patient… Physicians should disclose all relevant medical information to patients (AMA's Council on Ethical and Judicial Affairs 2006)." The fear of medicolegal consequences may be the reason for pursuing incidental findings (Berland 2011; Berlin 2011). Radiologists do not want to get sued or harm the patient and the tendency is to report all incidental findings. This may result in overdiagnosis, which is the diagnosis of a disease that will not cause the patient's symptoms or death (Esserman et al. 2013).

The most common reason to pursue an incidental finding is to differentiate benign from potentially serious conditions (Berland et al. 2010). While most incidental findings prove to be benign, there is an unwillingness of many physicians to accept uncertainty even when the chance of a serious diagnosis is extremely unlikely (Berland et al. 2010; Hillman 2015). However, it should also be appreciated that not all clinically important incidental findings are suspicious for malignancy, such as abdominal aortic aneurysms. One study representing a Monte Carlo simulation suggested that in a theoretical group of 100,000 patients there would be a 2292 life years gained, but only 13% of them from early identification of cancers, with much of the remainder from early detection of abdominal aortic aneurysms (Hassan et al. 2008b).

The unwillingness to accept uncertainty is driven in part by paucity of data and lack of algorithms for diagnostic and treatment strategies (Berland et al. 2010). Despite our best intentions, the anxiety provoked by the fear of a missed cancer may lead to overtreatment (Heath 2014; Gawande 2015). However, it is important to consider anxiety that may be caused to a patient by forgoing the workup of a lesion with very low, but greater than no, chance of malignancy (Ding et al. 2011). What has the greater risk—not to biopsy and potentially miss a cancer or to continue on the path to feel compelled to know the diagnosis of every lesion with absolute certainty (Esserman and Thompson 2010)? Is there a reasonable threshold of risk below which reporting a finding has a substantial risk of doing more harm than good? The dilemma of overdiagnosis has been asked as, "What is responsible use of information that nobody asked for but once found is difficult to ignore? (Fletcher and Pignone 2008)."

Patients may opt to test for low-probability conditions despite costs, anxiety, and risks, a decision that is often supported by their physician (Brown 2013). Some authors suggest, "Patients would be better served if physicians limited their access to unsolicited diagnostic information (Volk and Ubel 2011)." The decision to pursue incidental findings are framed by the individual patient's values, perceived severity and significance of the consequences, and unique life experiences (Brown 2013). There has been a shift from autocratic physician ownership of medical decisions to enhanced autonomy of the patient with shared decision-making (Barry and Edgman-Levitan 2012; Epstein and Peters 2009; Truog 2012). Physicians are obligated to discuss risks with patients; however, there could be potential harms in divulging extraneous information (Brown 2013). This information may be confusing and distressing to the patient as well as to their physician (Brown 2013), and carries the risk of unnecessary medical testing and of distracting attention and time from considering more important findings.

It has been recently suggested that radiologists should consider "rethinking normal," perhaps refraining from reporting some findings that have virtually no chance of being clinically important (Pandharipande et al. 2016). The ACR white paper on thyroid incidental findings also suggested that some incidentally discovered thyroid nodules should not be referred for examination with a complete diagnostic ultrasound (Hoang et al. 2015). Also, the SRU consensus paper on adnexal US recommends not reporting small physiologic cysts. Such proposals have sometimes been met with determined opposition. For example, Dr. Leonard Berlin stated in his letter to the editor of JACR regarding the suggestion to not, for example, report small benign-appearing renal cysts: " …'do not report' means to ignore, a word defined in the dictionary as 'to refuse to take notice…to neglect.' The noun neglect is synonymous with negligence, which in the courtroom is equivalent to malpractice" (Berlin 2016). Drs. Turano and Cummings pointedly stated in their comment on the incidental findings paper in JACR in the journal *Thyroid*: "Withholding this information, because it is believed that it may cause the patient more harm to know about their condition, reeks of paternalism and leaves out the patient and treating physician – both key stakeholders in the process of informed decision-making."

(Tufano et al. 2015). The ACR has also recently initiated "ACR Engage" [<engage.acr.org>], which is an online forum for ACR members, and there has been a lively, often polarized, discussion of this topic. We disagree with these objections, but a change in mindset and further evidence may be required to alter the ingrained practice that everything seen should be reported.

Radiologists should attempt to adhere to a standard of care that is "usual and customary in the local or national community, under the same or similar circumstances" (Berlin 2011). This can be done by consulting the published scientific literature to determine if there is a "usual and customary manner" in which other radiologists deal with an incidental finding (Berlin 2011). Guidelines can help the patient, radiologist, and treating physician navigate through the management of incidental findings. The radiologist has a crucial role in determining how incidental findings are handled as well as educating the patient and treating physicians (Brown 2013).

One commonly cited concern is that if a patient is managed for a condition for which a guideline exists, but is not followed, that there is an increased medicolegal risk to the diagnosing and treating physicians if there is a bad outcome. While this is a sensible fear, there are a number of mitigating factors limiting such risk. Healthcare providers are expected to adhere to a standard of care (SOC), not specifically to published guidelines for specific conditions. Indeed, statements that they should not be used to establish the legal standard of care in any particular situation accompany most guidelines. They may also be sometimes ruled to be inadmissible as evidence. In many cases, it can be argued that adhering to such guidelines is not (at least yet) the SOC. Guidelines for similar conditions issued by various specialty societies sometimes conflict and so guidelines for such conditions may not be definitive. Many guidelines are based on relatively weak evidence and their validity can be called into question. Guidelines cannot specify all of the complicating factors and comorbidities that exist in individual patients and may not apply. Furthermore, aspects of some guidelines are often outdated relatively soon after they are issued. The purpose of guidelines is to improve consistency of practice with reasonably well-founded medical principles, not to be used to establish legal precedent.

Guidelines should be perceived as just that—guides, rather than rules to which physicians are required to adhere. If guidelines are not followed in any particular instance, it is helpful for the radiologist or treating physician to indicate that they are aware of such guidelines, but diverged from them for a particular reason.

Regardless of the arguments as to whether the existence of guidelines places radiologists or referring physicians at risk, they do exist and the number of them is even increasing, so physicians should take an interest in becoming more aware of ones that are relevant to their practice. Finally, up to the present, the number of legal actions that have been brought that could be attributed to failure to follow published guidelines is very limited.

6 Costs Associated with Managing Incidental Findings

Given the current climate of rising healthcare costs and efforts for cost containment, we must be aware of the costs associated with managing incidental findings. The balance of additional workup and the associated costs and potential patient morbidity must be handled judiciously. Several studies have attempted to assess the burden of extra costs generated with management of incidental findings. Most of the published literature regarding the economic burden of managing incidental findings is centered on the CT of the chest, abdomen, and pelvis. Regarding CT colonography, multiple studies reported additional costs associated with the incidental finding of \$13 to \$248 per scan (Pickhardt et al. 2008; Yee et al. 2010; Hara et al. 2000; Xiong et al. 2005; Flicker et al. 2008; Gluecker et al. 2003; Veerappan et al. 2010; Kimberly et al. 2009). In abdominal CT (non-CT colonography) examinations, the costs associated with incidental findings range from \$35 to \$385 per patient (Liu et al. 2005; Maizlin et al. 2007; Morgan et al. 2015). Costs for investigating incidental findings discovered on chest CT ranges from \$17 to \$86 (Lee et al. 2010; Machaalany et al. 2009). Most authors indicated they believed they were underestimating costs as they were focused on costs generated by additional imaging studies rather than the surgical procedures, hospitalizations, and other non-imaging diagnostic procedures that were the result of the incidental findings (Morgan et al. 2015). The vast majority of the costs are related to invasive procedures in a small percentage of patients (Morgan et al. 2015). Reporting recommendations for management of incidental findings can direct cost-efficient and -effective care (Morgan et al. 2015).

7 Processes for Developing Guidelines

Practice guidelines provide a framework that, if widely accepted and utilized, can disseminate best practice among peers. Ideally, practice guidelines should be built on high quality medical evidence, with randomized control trials of patient outcomes generally being considered the highest level of evidence (National Institute for Health and Clinical Excellence 2012; Schunemann et al. 2008). The United States Institute of Medicine defines clinical practice guidelines as "statements that include recommendations intended to optimize patient care that are informed by a systematic review of evidence and an assessment of the benefits and harms of alternative care options" (Institute of Medicine 2011). Clinical practice guidelines have also been described as "systematically developed statements to assist practitioner and patient decisions about appropriate health care for specific clinical circumstances" (Woolf et al. 1999). Thorough and systematic review of evidentiary research studies should be well documented as pillars of guidelines. The quality of the evidence should also be taken into consideration.

The degree to which medical evidence may drive development of guidelines depends on the nature of the intended guideline (Brink 2010). Guidelines for specific disease processes are more likely to be based on evidence than are guidelines for medical imaging (Brink 2010). In diagnostic imaging, randomized control trials are not always the most appropriate type of evidence (Zuiderent-Jerak et al. 2012; Reed 2015). Historically, advances in radiology have been made through descriptive studies rather than randomized controlled clinical trials. Practice guidelines for medical imaging relies more on the consensus opinion of a panel of experts to fill in the gaps of medical evidence (Brink 2010). Unfortunately, for topics such as incidental findings, there is a scarcity of high quality medical evidence, or often even any evidence at all. This leads to the necessity to develop recommendations that are based on expert consensus opinions. These may not be as highly regarded as formal guidelines, but they can improve uniformity in clinical practice.

Various techniques have been used to strengthen the value of expert opinion. The American College of Radiology uses the modified Delphi procedure for establishing appropriateness criteria for imaging procedures. In this technique, expert panel members are presented with an evidence table and narrative that relates to the clinical condition. Each expert individually answers questionnaires in two or more rounds with an anonymous summary of the results between each round. This method allows for each panelist to articulate his or her voice without the peer pressure of in-person meetings and discussions (Brink 2010).

The ACR Incidental Findings Committee determined the most efficient way to codify and disseminate guidelines for management of incidental findings was a consensus-based process leading to developing white papers (Berland 2011; Pandharipande et al. 2016; Patel et al. 2013; Khosa et al. 2013; Heller et al. 2013; Sebastian et al. 2013), which are defined as authoritative reports issued by organizations. The committee used a consensus method based on repeated reviews and revisions by a panel of experts utilizing the best scientific evidence available. Expert radiologists in the relevant organ systems were recruited to take part in creating, reviewing, and revising the recommendations, supported by the available literature. The white papers are meant to serve as general guidance for managing incidentally discovered conditions and will require revision on the basis of new research. While non-radiology expert physicians in relevant domains were not involved in the initial ACR white papers, they may be enrolled in revising them (Berland 2011). While the choice to include only radiologists in developing the incidental findings recommendations has been controversial, we took this approach because: (1) our goals were to focus on the radiologic aspects of the conditions being evaluated, (2) inconsistency in guidelines is common among different non-radiology groups, so reconciling these would be difficult, and (3) we believe that many guidelines developed by non-radiologists have been too aggressive in recommending additional imaging and other testing for incidental findings and we wanted to initially limit the influence of strongly held opinions by specialty groups and generate our own independent evaluation prior to involving non-radiology specialists.

Although the ACR Appropriateness Criteria® have been developed for over 20 years using a modified Delphi consensus approach, such a formal process has not been applied within the Incidental Findings Committee. A less formal process of informal consensus building, with the endorsement of the ACR, has led to the current white paper recommendations (Berland 2011). The Incidental Findings Committee white papers and other guidelines can direct radiologists towards best practices and serve as a baseline on which evidence-based clinical trials could be developed to confirm or modify the baseline (Boland et al. 2011; Brink 2010).

8 Nature and Form of Guidelines

Guidelines take many forms, but are commonly displayed in the form of algorithmic flowcharts or tables. Incidental findings recommendations are mostly shown as colored flowcharts, with boxes differentiated by color between information gathering, recommending an action or indicating that evaluation should be ended (as shown in Fig. 1).

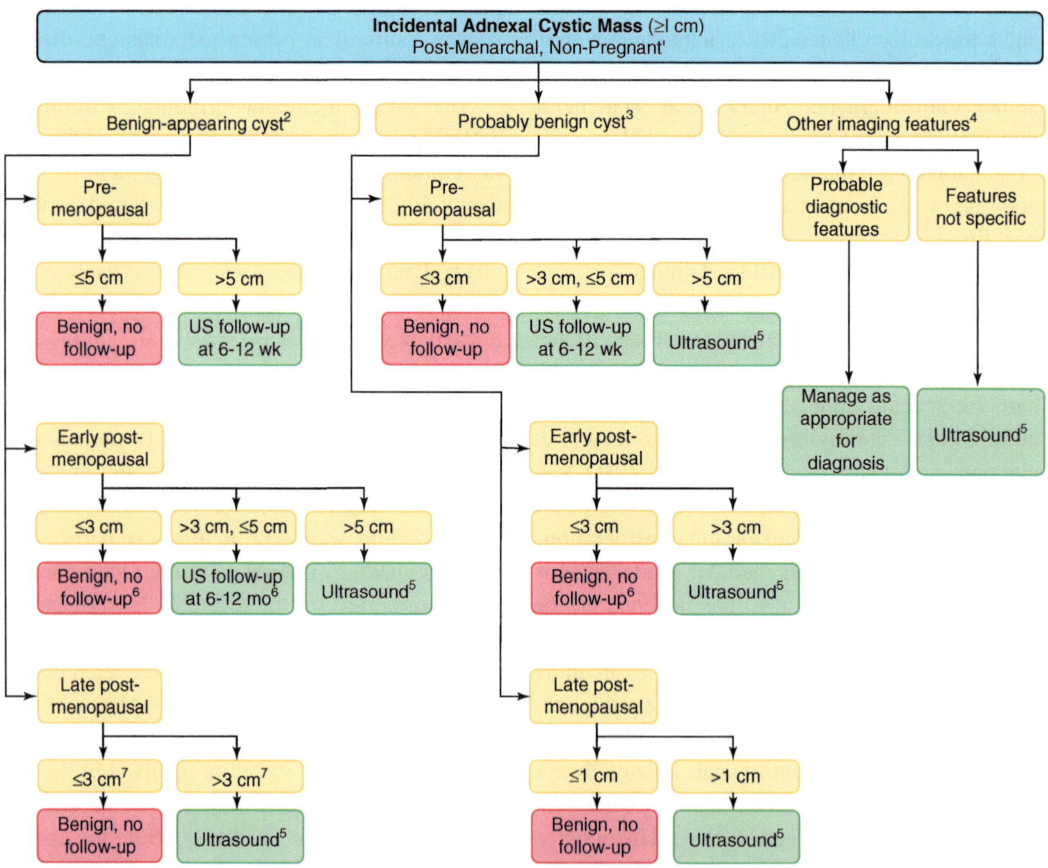

Fig. 1 Figure shows a typical flowchart created by the Incidental Findings Committee. Reprinted with permission (Patel 2013)

9 Integrating Guidelines into Reports

We are not aware of any radiology group that successfully applies guidelines universally. There are a number of challenges to achieving this. One issue is that the guidelines themselves have limitations, including that they may be outdated or have some details that are controversial or be inaccurate because of limitations of available evidence. The display of recommendations may be confusing or only cover a limited set of alternatives. It is also very difficult to stratify for risk and specify different recommendations for variations in age, gender, and comorbidities. Confusion may also be caused by differences among guidelines promulgated by different organizations.

Limited use of guidelines also has multiple other obstacles to broad use. The radiologist may consider himself or herself too busy to take the time to look them up if they are not immediately at hand. They may believe that referring physician is more responsible for providing the level of detail found in such guidelines than the radiologist. Radiologists may reject guidelines that don't reflect their traditional approach and believe that they are not at significant risk for a malpractice suit by not including references to guidelines. The individual radiologist's underlying level of both medical and legal risk tolerance may influence all these factors. In the absence of strong incentives for using guidelines or penalties for not doing so, there are no substantial pressures to modify workflow and practices, especially given the pressures of productivity.

To optimize their use, guidelines should be broadly acceptable, easy to access, and straightforward to understand and apply (Berland 2011). Consensus recommendations can help make patient care more consistent and can optimize management, but the recommendations cannot be adopted and implemented without education of radiologists. A 2014 survey of the ACR membership revealed that 38% of the members had read the white papers regarding incidental findings and 89% of those reported use of the guidelines in clinical practice (Berland et al. 2014). A survey in 2010 indicated that 77.8% of the respondents were aware of the Fleischner Society guidelines and 35–61% used them appropriately in clinical practice (Eisenberg et al. 2010). Variations in guideline adherence is multifactorial including difficulty staying current with all guidelines, the time-consuming nature of looking up specific guidelines, medicolegal concerns, or the decision to ignore them (Boland et al. 2011).

The ACR Incidental Finding Committee created flowcharts to illustrate recommendations to attempt to make them easy to access and follow (Fig. 1) (Berland 2011). Institutions have shown increased adherence to guidelines by printing the guidelines and posting them to the dictating machine or displayed at the PACS station (Eisenberg and Fleischner 2013; Masciocchi et al. 2012). A similar method could be used to make the incidental findings flowcharts easy to access and could increase their use. Guidelines could be printed, tabulated, and placed in binders at each PACS station. Alternatively, they could be made electronically available on each workstation. Utilizing the voice recognition reporting system, "macros" and templates could be used to prompt the radiologist to report the recommendations in a standard way. One study emphasized the value of integration of decision support tools with PACS workflow. Forty-eight radiology residents were provided a decision support tool from the web or through direct PACS access. Those that had integrated access had higher usage by a factor of 3 and when removed, their use of the system decreased by 52% (Morgan et al. 2011).

Clinical decision support between a computer and a user has been utilized to help determine the need for imaging and to assist in selecting the most optimal diagnostic exam (Bates et al. 2003). Electronic decision support is also promising as a means to delivering guidelines to a radiologist in making recommendations for further imaging (Boland et al. 2011). One point of care decision support tool has the radiologist enter specific observations about the finding and relevant patient parameters into the voice reporting system and then automatically generates text that includes the findings, impression and recommendations (see Chap. 10 by Alkasab and Harvey). This has been shown to increase adherence to incidental pulmonary nodule guidelines from less than 50% when not using the DS system to greater than 95% when they do (Boland et al. 2011, 2014; Lu et al. 2016). However, the quality and flexibility of the computer user interface can strongly affect the willingness of radiologists to use such systems. Nevertheless, decision support systems could decrease the bias of personal preference or experience and can direct to recognized best practices (Boland et al. 2011).

The capabilities of artificial intelligence (AI) (e.g., machine learning and deep learning) are evolving rapidly and promise to further improve compliance with guidelines, although sophisticated AI systems have not yet been applied to this area. One concept of how such a system would work is for it to learn to recognize and parse dictated data and automatically populate the report with the text of the findings and recommendations. Improved interfaces with electronic health records are also likely to allow tracking of how often such recommendations are followed and the outcomes of following versus not complying with guidelines.

With the exception of the ACR's Breast Imaging Reporting and Data System® (BI-RADS®), there are no mandates for radiologists to follow guidelines once they are developed (Boland et al. 2011). Incentives and audit processes could be developed to measure performance and increase adherence to guidelines. Formal policies could require their adoption to decrease the degree of variability in following guidelines. Follow-up analysis of compliance could confirm effects on adherence to the guidelines (Rosenkrantz and Kierans 2014). Measures published in the Physician Quality Reporting System (PQRS) include recommendations for managing incidentally discovered liver lesions and thyroid nodules (PQRS 2015, 2016), but these measures can be difficult to apply and may not be the most relevant measures of quality.

Guidance to change practice and behavior is more likely to be accepted when it comes from professional medical groups including both those who interpret and request imaging (Remedios et al. 2015). Involvement of many organizations and societies allows for endorsement and dissemination of the recommendations. Newly accepted guidelines can be disseminated to members of the organizations through mailings and can be posted on their websites. This has the potential to improve patient care, improve confidence of referring physicians, and provide standardization (Boland et al. 2011).

Conclusion

Guidelines are not intended to be final documents, as they continuously need updating, revision, and review as processes evolve. The ultimate decision on how to manage an incidental finding will be multifactorial including patient specific factors, disease prevalence, and availability of equipment. Quality is enhanced by decreasing variations in practice (Berland 2011). Radiologist's adherence to guidelines and recommendations regarding incidental radiologic findings can enhance informed decision-making, decrease variations in recommendations, decrease cost, limit medical liability, and improve consistency in patient care (Brown 2013; Berland 2009b).

References

AMA's Council on Ethical and Judicial Affairs (2006) Opinion 8.08—Informed Consent, in Code of Medical Ethics. AMA, Chicago, IL

American College of Radiology (2014) Liver Imaging Reporting and Data System ACR.org: American College of Radiology [cited 29 Jul 2016]. Quality & Safety | Additional Resources | LI-RADS. http://www.acr.org/Quality-Safety/Resources/LIRADS

American College of Radiology (2016) Lung CT Screening Reporting and Data System (Lung-RADS™). ACR.org: American College of Radiology [cited 29 Jul 2016]. Quality Safety | Additional Resources | Lung-RADS™. http://www.acr.org/Quality-Safety/Resources/LungRADS

Baker LC, Atlas SW, Afendulis CC (2008) Expanded use of imaging technology and the challenge of measuring value. Health Aff (Millwood) 27(6):1467–1478

Barry MJ, Edgman-Levitan S (2012) Shared decision making—pinnacle of patient-centered care. N Engl J Med 366(9):780–781

Bates DW et al (2003) Ten commandments for effective clinical decision support: making the practice of evidence-based medicine a reality. J Am Med Inform Assoc 10(6):523–530

Berland LL (2009a) Incidental extracolonic findings on CT colonography: the impending deluge and its implications. J Am Coll Radiol 6(1):14–20
Berland LL (2009b) Author's reply. J Am Coll Radiol 6(8):599–600
Berland LL (2011) The American College of Radiology strategy for managing incidental findings on abdominal computed tomography. Radiol Clin N Am 49(2):237–243
Berland LL et al (2010) Managing incidental findings on abdominal CT: white paper of the ACR incidental findings committee. J Am Coll Radiol 7(10):754–773
Berland LL et al (2014) ACR members' response to JACR white paper on the management of incidental abdominal CT findings. J Am Coll Radiol 11(1):30–35
Berlin L (2011) The incidentaloma: a medicolegal dilemma. Radiol Clin N Am 49(2):245–255
Berlin L (2016) Rethinking normal: benefits and risks of not reporting harmless incidental findings. J Am Coll Radiol 13(9):1025
Boland GW et al (2011) Decision support for radiologist report recommendations. J Am Coll Radiol 8(12):819–823
Boland GW, Enzmann DR, Duszak R Jr (2014) Actionable reporting. J Am Coll Radiol 11(9):844–845
Brink JA (2010) The art and science of medical guidelines: what we know and what we believe. Radiology 254(1):20–21
Brown SD (2013) Professional norms regarding how radiologists handle incidental findings. J Am Coll Radiol 10(4):253–257
Casarella WJ (2002) A patient's viewpoint on a current controversy. Radiology 224(3):927
Court of Appeals of New York (1914) Mary E. Schloendorff v. The Society of the New York Hospital in New York; New England. Court of Appeals of New York p 125; 92
Cronan JJ (2008) Thyroid nodules: is it time to turn off the US machines? Radiology 247(3):602–604
Davies L, Welch HG (2006) Increasing incidence of thyroid cancer in the United States, 1973–2002. JAMA 295(18):2164–2167
Ding A, Eisenberg JD, Pandharipande PV (2011) The economic burden of incidentally detected findings. Radiol Clin N Am 49(2):257–265
Doubilet PM, Benson CB, Bourne T, Blaivas M (2014) Pregnancy SoRiUMPoEFTDoMaEoaVI. Diagnostic criteria for nonviable pregnancy early in the first trimester. Ultrasound Q 30(1):3–9
Eisenberg RL, Fleischner S (2013) Ways to improve radiologists' adherence to Fleischner Society guidelines for management of pulmonary nodules. J Am Coll Radiol 10(6):439–441
Eisenberg RL, Bankier AA, Boiselle PM (2010) Compliance with Fleischner Society guidelines for management of small lung nodules: a survey of 834 radiologists. Radiology 255(1):218–224
Epstein RM, Peters E (2009) Beyond information: exploring patients' preferences. JAMA 302(2):195–197
Esserman L, Thompson I (2010) Solving the overdiagnosis dilemma. J Natl Cancer Inst 102(9):582–583
Esserman LJ, Thompson IM Jr, Reid B (2013) Overdiagnosis and overtreatment in cancer: an opportunity for improvement. JAMA 310(8):797–798
Fletcher RH, Pignone M (2008) Extracolonic findings with computed tomographic colonography: asset or liability? Arch Intern Med 168(7):685–686
Flicker MS et al (2008) Economic impact of extracolonic findings at computed tomographic colonography. J Comput Assist Tomogr 32(4):497–503
Furtado CD et al (2005) Whole-body CT screening: spectrum of findings and recommendations in 1192 patients. Radiology 237(2):385–394
Gawande A (2015) Overkill. In: The New Yorker. Conde Nast, New York
Ghosh E, Levine D (2013) Recommendations for adnexal cysts: have the Society of Radiologists in Ultrasound consensus conference guidelines affected utilization of ultrasound? Ultrasound Q 29(1):21–24
Gluecker TM et al (2003) Extracolonic findings at CT colonography: evaluation of prevalence and cost in a screening population. Gastroenterology 124(4):911–916
Hara AK et al (2000) Incidental extracolonic findings at CT colonography. Radiology 215(2):353–357
Hassan C et al (2008a) Computed tomographic colonography to screen for colorectal cancer, extracolonic cancer, and aortic aneurysm: model simulation with cost-effectiveness analysis. Arch Intern Med 168(7):696–705
Heath I (2014) Role of fear in overdiagnosis and overtreatment—an essay by Iona Heath. BMJ 349:g6123
Heller MT et al (2013) Managing incidental findings on abdominal and pelvic CT and MRI, part 3: white paper of the ACR Incidental Findings Committee II on splenic and nodal findings. J Am Coll Radiol 10(11):833–839
Hellstrom M, Svensson MH, Lasson A (2004) Extracolonic and incidental findings on CT colonography (virtual colonoscopy). Am J Roentgenol 182(3):631–638
Hillman BJ (2015) Certainty. J Am Coll Radiol 12(4):321
Hoang JK et al (2015) Managing incidental thyroid nodules detected on imaging: white paper of the ACR Incidental Thyroid Findings Committee. J Am Coll Radiol 12(2):143–150
Institute of Medicine (2011) Clinical practice guidelines we can trust. National Academic Press, Washington, DC
Johnson PT et al (2011) Common incidental findings on MDCT: survey of radiologist recommendations for patient management. J Am Coll Radiol 8(11):762–767
Khosa F et al (2013) Managing incidental findings on abdominal and pelvic CT and MRI, part 2: white paper of the ACR Incidental Findings Committee II on vascular findings. J Am Coll Radiol 10(10):789–794
Kilani RK et al (2011) Self-referral in medical imaging: a meta-analysis of the literature. J Am Coll Radiol 8(7):469–476
Kimberly JR et al (2009) Extracolonic findings at virtual colonoscopy: an important consideration in asymptomatic colorectal cancer screening. J Gen Intern Med 24(1):69–73

Kucharczyk MJ et al (2011) Assessing the impact of incidental findings in a lung cancer screening study by using low-dose computed tomography. Can Assoc Radiol J 62(2):141–145

Lee CI et al (2010) Incidental extracardiac findings at coronary CT: clinical and economic impact. Am J Roentgenol 194(6):1531–1538

Levine D et al (2010) Management of asymptomatic ovarian and other adnexal cysts imaged at US: Society of Radiologists in Ultrasound Consensus Conference Statement. Radiology 256(3):943–954

Liu W, Mortele KJ, Silverman SG (2005) Incidental extraurinary findings at MDCT urography in patients with hematuria: prevalence and impact on imaging costs. Am J Roentgenol 185(4):1051–1056

Lu MT et al (2016) Radiologist point-of-care clinical decision support and adherence to guidelines for incidental lung nodules. J Am Coll Radiol 13(2):156–162

Machaalany J et al (2009) Potential clinical and economic consequences of noncardiac incidental findings on cardiac computed tomography. J Am Coll Cardiol 54(16):1533–1541

MACRA (2016) The Merit-Based Incentive Payment System (MIPS) and Alternative Payment Models (APMs). CMS.gov: Centers for Medicare & Medicaid Services. https://www.cms.gov/Medicare/Quality-Initiatives-Patient-Assessment-Instruments/Value-Based-Programs/MACRA-MIPS-and-APMs/MACRA-MIPS-and-APMs.html

MacRedmond R et al (2004) Screening for lung cancer using low dose CT scanning. Thorax 59(3):237–241

Maehara CK, Silverman SG, Lacson R, Khorasani R (2014) Journal club: renal masses detected at abdominal CT: radiologists' adherence to guidelines regarding management recommendations and communication of critical results. Am J Roentgenol 203(4):828–834

Maizlin ZV et al (2007) Economic and ethical impact of extrarenal findings on potential living kidney donor assessment with computed tomography angiography. Transpl Int 20(4):338–342

Masciocchi M, Wagner B, Lloyd B (2012) Quality review: Fleischner criteria adherence by radiologists in a large community hospital. J Am Coll Radiol 9(5):336–339

Megibow AJ (2011) Preface imaging of incidentalomas. Radiol Clin N Am 49(2):xi–xii

Morgan MB, Branstetter BF, Clark C, House J, Baker D, Harnsberger HR (2011) Just-in-time radiologist decision support: the importance of PACS-integrated workflow. J Am Coll Radiol 8(7):497–500

Morgan AE et al (2015) Extraurinary incidental findings on CT for hematuria: the radiologist's role and downstream cost analysis. Am J Roentgenol 204(6):1160–1167

National Institute for Health and Clinical Excellence (2012) The guidelines manual. NICE, London

Obuchowski NA et al (2007) Total-body screening: preliminary results of a pilot randomized controlled trial. J Am Coll Radiol 4(9):604–611

Pandharipande PV, Herts BR, Gore RM et al (2016) Rethinking normal: benefits and risks of not reporting harmless incidental findings. J Am Coll Radiol 13(7):764–767

Patel MD et al (2013) Managing incidental findings on abdominal and pelvic CT and MRI, part 1: white paper of the ACR Incidental Findings Committee II on adnexal findings. J Am Coll Radiol 10(9):675–681

Pickhardt PJ et al (2008) Unsuspected extracolonic findings at screening CT colonography: clinical and economic impact. Radiology 249(1):151–159

PQRS (2015) Measure #405: appropriate follow-up imaging for incidental abdominal lesions—national quality strategy domain: effective clinical care 2016 PQRS options for individual measures [serial online]. vol Version 10.0. http://www.acr.org/%20~/media/ACR/Documents/P4P/2016%20PQRS/DX/2016_PQRS_Measure_405_11_17_2015.pdf. Accessed 24 Aug 2016

PQRSPRO (2016) PQRS Measure #406: appropriate follow-up imaging for incidental thyroid nodules in patients. pqrspro.com: Healthmonix [cited 24 Aug 2016]. https://www.pqrspro.com/cmsmeasures//appropriate_follow-up_imaging_for_incidental_thyroid_nodules_in_patients

Reed MH (2015) Evidence for diagnostic imaging guidelines. J Am Coll Radiol 12(4):325–326

Remedios D et al (2015) Clinical imaging guidelines part 1: a proposal for uniform methodology. J Am Coll Radiol 12(1):45–50

Rosenkrantz AB, Kierans AS (2014) US of incidental adnexal cysts: adherence of radiologists to the 2010 Society of Radiologists in Ultrasound guidelines. Radiology 271(1):262–271

Schunemann HJ et al (2008) Grading quality of evidence and strength of recommendations for diagnostic tests and strategies. BMJ 336(7653):1106–1110

Sebastian S et al (2013) Managing incidental findings on abdominal and pelvic CT and MRI, part 4: white paper of the ACR Incidental Findings Committee II on gallbladder and biliary findings. J Am Coll Radiol 10(12):953–956

Silverman SG et al (2008) Management of the incidental renal mass. Radiology 249(1):16–31

Sistrom CL et al (2009) Recommendations for additional imaging in radiology reports: multifactorial analysis of 5.9 million examinations. Radiology 253(2):453–461

Smith-Bindman R, Miglioretti DL, Larson EB (2008) Rising use of diagnostic medical imaging in a large integrated health system. Health Aff (Millwood) 27(6):1491–1502

Song JH, Beland MD, Mayo-Smith WW (2012) Incidental clinically important extraurinary findings at MDCT urography for hematuria evaluation: prevalence in 1209 consecutive examinations. Am J Roentgenol 199(3):616–622

Sosnouski D et al (2007) Extracardiac findings at cardiac CT: a practical approach. J Thorac Imaging 22(1):77–85

Truog RD (2012) Patients and doctors—evolution of a relationship. N Engl J Med 366(7):581–585

Tufano RP, Noureldine SI, Angelos P (2015) Ethical responsibilities of caring for patients with incidental thyroid nodules. Thyroid 25(5):467–468

Veerappan GR et al (2010) Extracolonic findings on CT colonography increases yield of colorectal cancer screening. Am J Roentgenol 195(3):677–686

Volk ML, Ubel PA (2011) Better off not knowing: improving clinical care by limiting physician access to unsolicited diagnostic information. Arch Intern Med 171(6):487–488

Welch HG (2011) We stumble onto incidentalomas that might be cancer, in overdiagnosed: making people sick in the pursuit of health. Beacon Press, Boston, MA, pp 90–101

Woolf SH et al (1999) Clinical guidelines: potential benefits, limitations, and harms of clinical guidelines. BMJ 318(7182):527–530

Xiong T et al (2005) Incidental lesions found on CT colonography: their nature and frequency. Br J Radiol 78(925):22–29

Xiong T et al (2006) Resources and costs associated with incidental extracolonic findings from CT colonogaphy: a study in a symptomatic population. Br J Radiol 79(948):948–961

Yee J et al (2010) Extracolonic findings at CT colonography. Gastrointest Endosc Clin N Am 20(2):305–322

Zuiderent-Jerak T, Forland F, Macbeth F (2012) Guidelines should reflect all knowledge, not just clinical trials. BMJ 345:e6702

Structured Reporting: The Value Concept for Radiologists

Marta E. Heilbrun, Justin Cramer, and Brian E. Chapman

Contents

M.E. Heilbrun, M.D. (✉)
Department of Radiology and Imaging Sciences, Emory University School of Medicine, Atlanta, GA, USA
e-mail: marta.heilbrun@emory.edu

J. Cramer, M.D.
Department of Radiology, University of Nebraska Medical Center, Omaha, NE, USA
e-mail: jcramer@unmc.edu

B.E. Chapman, Ph.D.
Department of Radiology and Imaging Sciences, University of Utah School of Medicine, Salt Lake City, UT, USA
e-mail: Brian.Chapman@utah.edu

Abstract

Narrative reporting has been the mainstay of the radiologist's work for as long as the domain of radiology has been in existence. Structured radiology reporting, containing coded and consistent information, will facilitate information exchange in the digital health record. This chapter will define structured reporting, review recent legislation that incentivizes structured reporting, and discuss the quality and value propositions that are supported by structured reporting. Constrained vocabularies and coded terminologies, including the American College of Radiology's disease-specific Imaging Reporting and Data Systems (IRADS) and the Radiological Society of North America's RadLex™, are described. Data exchange tools including the Management of Radiology Report Templates (MRRT) and Common Data Elements (CDEs) are discussed. Benefits of machine learning from report analysis are discussed. Limitations to implementation and realizing the full benefits of structured reporting are also acknowledged.

1 Introduction

Narrative reporting has been the mainstay of the radiologist's work for as long as the domain of radiology has been in existence (Langlotz 2015). The free-text narrative is a highly efficient

Med Radiol Diagn Imaging (2017)
DOI 10.1007/174_2017_167, © Springer International Publishing AG
Published Online 16 November 2017

method for the radiologist to record observations and interpretations when reviewing a patient's imaging and digital health record. Picture archiving and communication systems (PACS) and digital voice recognition transcription systems emerged in the end of the twentieth century. These disruptive technologies changed the radiologists' relationships and interactions with the providers who order imaging tests, but did not fundamentally change the radiologist's work product. As radiologists are challenged to demonstrate the value of their work product, it is becoming increasingly evident that the narrative report is limiting.

Overcoming the limitations of the narrative report requires a willingness on the part of the radiology community to embrace consistency as a core value. Structured and templated radiologist reporting is emerging as a tool to demonstrate the impact of the radiologist's work on patient outcomes. Structured and template report formats are being increasingly adopted by academic and community practice groups around the country (Powell and Silberzweig 2015). There is increasing literature demonstrating a preference for structured radiology reports by referring providers and radiologists (Bosmans et al. 2011; Schwartz et al. 2011). A structured report utilizing common vocabularies lays the groundwork for analysis including machine learning that will refine and improve understandings of disease processes and promotion of meaningful comparison of the work product of the radiologist. A clear report that contains consistent information will facilitate the interchange of information between systems and providers.

This chapter will define what is meant by structured reporting, review recent legislation that may incentivize radiologists to embrace structured reporting, and discuss the quality and value propositions that are supported by structured reporting. It will also address the process improvement and team building benefits of engaging your practice group in developing templates for structured reporting. Subsequent chapters in this section will review the benefits of specific content in radiology reports, from critical to incidental findings.

2 Definition of Structured Reporting

To varying degrees, all recorded data contains some inherent structure. It is helpful to clarify what is meant by the phrase "structured reporting" in radiology. Structured reporting may be thought of as three progressively structured tiers (Langlotz 2015). The first, simple, and well-accepted tier relates to having common headings for all reports such as "Indication" and "Impression" (Bosmans et al. 2012; Weiss and Langlotz 2008). The second tier involves subheadings such as organs and organ systems within the "Findings" or "Observations" section, which is sometimes called "itemized reporting" or "templated reporting." This is relatively easy to implement and is increasingly prevalent. These first two tiers represent organized reporting.

The third tier requires the use of standardized language in reports. To enforce such consistency, this tier uses pick lists, buttons, and other form elements. This last tier is orders of magnitude more difficult, both in development and in practice. When report components are subsequently represented as coded and searchable elements, the true definition of "structured reporting" is manifest.

The use of standardized and constrained language is the means by which the most benefits of structured reporting are realized. This type of structure is already prevalent in other areas of medicine, as it is required to satisfy various legislative and payment standards such as reviewing problem lists (Kahn et al. 2013). The Breast Imaging Reporting and Data System (BIRADS) is the most mature example within radiology (D'Orsi et al. 2013). However, there is increasing effort to standardize language and reporting in many disease processes and around many types of communications.

3 Constrained Vocabularies, Lexicons, and Common Data Elements

Constrained vocabularies and standard terminologies are critical components of achieving the consistency and reliability potential of structured reporting. Structure and meaning are facilitated by the consistent use of constrained vocabularies. In theory, radiologists are trained in and use a common vocabulary. However, in practice, both the radiologists and the care providers who receive radiology reports variably understand the meaning of specific phrases and words used in reports (Hobby et al. 2000; Reiner et al. 2007). Emerging constrained vocabularies are modeled after the success of the BIRADS and often lead by groups formed through the American College of Radiology (ACR). Examples include TIRADS for thyroid nodules (Tessler et al. 2017), LIRADS for liver lesions (Jha et al. 2014), and PIRADS for prostate MRI (Weinreb et al. 2015), among others. These are intended to mitigate differences in reporting that may hinder successful communication and subsequent management.

The benefits of constrained vocabularies are best demonstrated with examples. Consider a very typical free-text statement describing a thyroid nodule: "A1.7 cm mixed cystic and solid oval nodule is present on the left, consider biopsy." The ordering provider is left to wonder under what conditions should the biopsy be considered? What is the risk to the patient if the biopsy is not done? Will a cancer be diagnosed too late for a cure? Building on prior guidelines and emerging evidence, including those developed by the Society of Radiologists in Ultrasound in 2005 and the American Thyroid Association in 2015 (Frates et al. 2005; Haugen et al. 2016), TIRADS provides specific features that should be included in order to provide a definitive answer and recommendation (Tessler et al. 2017). The free-text description would be inadequate, as specific features including echogenicity, margin, shape, and orientation are not mentioned. A structured report that includes all these features as pick lists ensures that the radiologist generates a complete description of the nodule. Based on a summation of points for these different features, the radiologist provides very specific recommendations to the ordering provider and by extension to the patient.

Steps beyond constrained vocabularies are coded vocabularies. These facilitate digital information exchange. Lexicons originally developed outside of radiology to capture coded medical terminology and facilitate the electronic exchange of clinical health information include Systematized Nomenclature of Medicine-Clinical Terms (SNOMED-CT) and Logical Observation Identifiers Names and Codes (LOINC). While there is more current integration, in the early 2000s, these lexicons did not contain most of the terms used by radiologists or those related to imaging tests.

The gap was filled by the Radiological Society of North America (RSNA) and the creation of a radiology-specific lexicon, RadLex™ (Langlotz 2006). RadLex™ contains over 45,000 terms that are coded numerically and mapped for synonyms. Integration of these terms into templates will promote interoperability between institutions for patient care and research. To achieve this benefit, however, the codes must be portable between the systems where the reports are created and the final data repositories, whether an electronic health record (EHR) or a data warehouse. Post hoc mapping of reports or report templates to the RadLex™ lexicon is time-intensive and difficult.

Nonstandardized examination codes also limit interoperability. To overcome this limitation, the RadLex™ effort was extended to create the RadLex™ Playbook, a unifying resource of examination codes (Wang et al. 2017). For example, a patient might in one institution receive a "barium swallow," in another a "modified barium swallow," and in the third a "cookie swallow" or a "speech/swallowing evaluation." This variety of naming conventions could cause the patient to undergo unnecessary repeat examinations if there is no understanding that these exam descriptions are all synonyms for the preferred exam code "swallowing function assessment" (Radiology Lexicon (RADLEX) 2007). Apart from the content within a report, reducing variability in naming conventions for imaging exams reduces the potential for error.

4 Legislative Framework Promoting Structured Reporting

As a key component of the American Recovery and Reinvestment Act (ARRA) and the Health Information Technology for Economic and

Clinical Health (HITECH) Act of 2009, the US government has made a significant investment in growing EHR. The rationale for EHR adoption assumes that the information contained in EHR will be harnessed in order to improve medical decision-making with an associated improvement in patient outcomes (Blumenthal 2010). The motivation stems from the idea that by capturing every patient encounter within a healthcare system as unique and digital events, it will be possible to analyze, understand, and improve the quality of care that is delivered.

The intended goals and benefits of HITECH and ARRA were both streamlined and further legislated into action by the Medicare Access and CHIP Reauthorization Act (MACRA) passed in 2015 (Rosenkrantz et al. 2017). In addition to repealing the sustainable growth rate (SGR) formula that calculated annual physician payment cuts, MACRA replaced quality programs like the Physician Quality Reporting System and Meaningful Use Reporting Requirements with Quality Payment Programs (QPP).

Via QPP, MACRA proposes a framework for rewarding physicians to provide better care rather than merely more care, thus legislating the transition from volume to value. QPP physician payments will be based on participation in one of the two pathways, the Merit-based Incentive Payment System (MIPS) or alternative payment models (APMs). In order to participate in these new payment reward programs, physicians must submit performance data and be willing to be measured. MIPS assesses physicians in four performance categories, including Quality, Cost, Improvement Activities, and Advancing Care Information.

There are multiple MIPS quality measures for which structured reporting will facilitate reporting. For example, measure 406, "Appropriate Follow-up Imaging for Incidental Thyroid Nodules in Patients" is described as the:

> Percentage of final reports for computed tomography (CT), CT angiography (CTA) or magnetic resonance imaging (MRI) or magnetic resonance angiogram (MRA) studies of the chest or neck or ultrasound of the neck for patients aged 18 years and older with no known thyroid disease with a thyroid nodule <1.0 cm noted incidentally with follow-up imaging recommended. [https://www.acr.org/~/media/ACR/Documents/P4P/2017-MIPS/DX/2017_Measure_406_Registry.pdf]

The denominator for this measure is all CPT exam codes for cross-sectional imaging covering the thyroid gland. Ensuring that it is relatively simple to retrieve these reports and measure a denominator would be facilitated by a coded designation at the time of report generation and/or standardized language that could be easily found by a search engine after report generation (Langlotz 2015).

5 Development of Report Templates as a Team

The development of group-accepted report templates is an important task in team building. Because the report represents the radiologist's patient facing activity, there is a very strong emotional attachment to the form and content. The patterns and verbiage used by each radiologist are learned during training and reinforced over time. There is evidence that structured reports are preferred (Schwartz et al. 2011; Naik et al. 2001) and that there may be financial benefits for structured reporting (Pysarenko et al. 2017). The evidence is starting to emerge demonstrating that the imposition of such structure has the potential to impact patient outcomes (Kabadi and Krishnaraj 2017).

Coming together as a group to agree on unified reporting requires both skillful leadership and a willingness to negotiate and compromise. The organizational hurdles are likely to be as significant as technical hurdles. Larson et al. from Cincinnati Children's Hospital outline a rigorous and effective approach to implementing a department-wide structured reporting approach (Larson et al. 2013). This team explicitly acknowledged that merely writing the templates was only an initial step in the process. Gaining buy-in from all radiologists by considering their input and modifying templates when appropriate, "hounding" nonusers to use the templates, and basing modest bonuses on achieving usage goals all contributed to the ultimate success of the initiative.

Because of the challenge in overcoming individual reporting preferences, it may be useful to seek "independent" templates when beginning development in a radiology group. A resource is the RSNA template library that is hosted on radreport.org and open.radreport.org. Between the two sites, 350 reporting templates contributed by radiology societies, institutions, and individuals, with many translated into multiple languages, are represented. Additionally, subspecialty societies, including the Society of Interventional Radiology and the Society of Abdominal Radiology, are developing templates to be shared among society members.

6 The Value Proposition of Structured Reporting

The radiology work product has the potential to become relatively uniform through the imposition of structure and the use of constrained and coded vocabularies and elements. Consistency will facilitate the interchange of information with resultant improvements in patient care and associated patient outcomes. With structure, free-text reports can be more effectively analyzed. In addition there is a lower chance for error when translating information from a report into discrete data fields.

It is these ideas of benefit that are driving the adoption of EHR and the promotion of machine learning and artificial intelligence in medicine (Brink et al. 2017). There are many barriers to realizing the potential knowledge gain through widespread adoption of EHR. In health care, the attributes of Big Data are described by the terms silo, security, and variety (Jee and Kim 2013). Silo refers to the fact that data exists in incomplete, proprietary, and incompatible legacy systems, representing disparate clinical environments and sources (Bisbal and Berry 2011). Overcoming the silo is challenged by security concerns, the second attribute of health-care Big Data. Extracting information from a system with safeguards protecting patient privacy and maintaining those safeguards adds additional complexity to aggregating, organizing, and mining health-care Big Data.

Variety refers to the various types of structured and unstructured data available for consumption. When the discussion turns to medical records such as progress notes and radiology reports, those items that substantively represent clinical reasoning are predominantly unstructured. The health-care data explosion is overwhelming the ability of individual analysts to process EHR. Thus, improving care based on EHR analysis remains a significant challenge. In order to use EHR to improve patient outcomes and facilitate medical decision-making, the development of systems and tools that bridge heterogeneous IT environments is crucial (Brink et al. 2017).

As part of health-care reform, it is expected that costs of care will diminish and the direct patient benefits will increase when care adheres to evidence-based guidelines. While it is expected that these guidelines will increase in number and complexity, they can be very hard to put into practice (Lacson et al. 2012). Even now, relatively well-known and simple guidelines are difficult to follow, with one study showing radiologists at a major academic center only providing reports that reach 60.8% conformity to Fleischner Society pulmonary nodule guidelines (Eisenberg et al. 2010). It is reasonable to expect that guideline adherence will increasingly affect reimbursement. This may be a major motivating factor to the widespread adoption of structured reporting.

Structured reporting creates opportunities for research, clinical decision support, and quality improvement efforts. For example, uniformity facilitates the radiologists' participation in disease registries. A requirement for Medicare and Medicaid payment for lung cancer screening with low-dose CT includes submitting data to an approved registry for every test performed (cms.gov/Lung Cancer Screening Registries 2015). Currently, the means of recording this data is either through manual entry in a web-based form or manual entry in a spreadsheet template that can be uploaded to the web-based registry (Lung Cancer Screening Registry (LCSR): User Guide 2017). Both of these solutions require a human to extract the information from the report that is generated by the radiologist. A template with pick list and/or coded response options facilitates this current manual extraction of data. Generating the lung cancer screening report directly into a structured database form would eliminate an intermediate translation step between the radiologist and the registry.

It is expected that structured reports will enable the radiologist to provide a more consistent, accurate, and useful report in daily practice as well. Structured reports serve as a checklist for the radiologist. While there are critiques of the role of structured reporting in training, multiple studies are emerging demonstrating that the use of checklist style report templates increases complete reporting and reduces misses for trainees (Lin et al. 2014; Marcovici and Taylor 2014). These checklists are also useful when encountering a disease that is infrequent, as it is difficult to remember all the required elements of a meaningful report. Pancreatic cancer is often cited as a disease where the observations on initial imaging are critical to success but often incomplete (Al-Hawary et al. 2014). A structured template reminds the radiologist to report on all relevant observations, including extent of both venous and arterial vascular involvement as well as nodal location.

It is possible to impose structure on a report after the fact. Machine learning tools like natural language processing (NLP) analyze free-form text using linguistic and statistical methods to convert text into a structured data that is then available for computerized analysis (Cai et al. 2016). NLP performance is maximized when the variety and ambiguity of the text in the radiology reports are minimized (Hassanpour and Langlotz 2016). In constrained settings, the application of NLP to radiology reports has demonstrated benefits to patient care. For example, an interdisciplinary group at Brigham and Women's Hospital used NLP to detect the prevalence of ordering CTPA and the positivity rate of the studies for clinically significant pulmonary embolisms (Raja et al. 2012). After the implementation of a computerized decision support (CDS) algorithm providing real-time guidance to streamline CTPA test ordering, the team compared utilization and positivity rates. The researchers found that the test order rate declined and the positivity rate increased. This represents a means in which the information contained in the radiology reports could be extracted, guidelines could be implemented, and the value of every test ordered is increased, as manifest by a higher test positivity rate.

With multiple radiologists in multiple practice settings, describing disease process lesions using the same terms, radiologists will have the ability to refine the diagnosis and management recommendations. The act of assigning a numeric value to various imaging features and comparing the results to reference standards that include pathology and clinical features provides radiologists the ability to measure and adjust their own clinical care efficacy. By creating the reproducible and reliable evidence and then driving the analysis of the radiologist work product and disease characterization, radiology, as a distinct medical specialty, will be able to claim a direct influence on patient outcomes.

7 Limitations and Concerns

It is difficult to implement structured reporting from both organizational and technical perspectives. While gaining traction, this still significantly changes well-entrenched workflows, may be less efficient, and could result in a more distracted radiologist. The explosive volume of patients that a radiologist is expected to provide care for on a daily basis adds the requirement that reporting increases rather than impedes efficiency. Physician burnout, which is in part driven by a sense that the value a unique physician provides to patient care is diminished, also must be acknowledged (Restauri et al. 2017). A standardized practice may erode the sense of autonomy and intrinsic value of the work for an individual radiologist.

It is essential that radiology use the investments in standardization to promote the role of the radiologist and the direct patient benefits related to the care provided by the radiologist.

Keeping the radiologist role opaque or further masking it behind the anonymity that is imposed by a report that would look the same whether someone with 1 year of training or 15 years of experience interprets the study poses significant risk.

An additional limitation is based on the challenges with maintaining structure through various instances of the digital health system. There are efforts underway to define data structures that will facilitate radiology report information exchange. For example, to address radiology report transmission challenges, the Management of Radiology Report Templates (MRRT) profile has been developed. This specifies a standardized approach for report authoring templates and defines the rules that facilitate the exchange of templates between both vendor-agnostic creation systems and between reporting systems (Kahn et al. 2015; Pinto Dos Santos et al. 2017). An additional effort that is underway is the development of the Common Data Element (CDE) for radiology (Rubin and Kahn 2017). CDEs are "data elements that are collected and stored uniformly across institutions and studies and are defined in a data dictionary" (Winget et al. 2003). The data dictionary specifies the item's name, data type, allowable values, and other attributes. Because of the detail captured by the data dictionary, CDEs will facilitate the collection of contextual information from reports. However, the benefits of information exchange profiles, like MRRT and CDEs, will not be realized until they are requirements of the information systems that create and consume this health information. Until this is the case, building the structured data into reports at the time of report generation is neither an efficiency nor value gain for practicing radiologists.

Conclusion

By decreasing ambiguity, enhancing research opportunities, and facilitating clinical decision support and quality improvement, structured reporting provides many benefits. D'Orsi and Kopans said it well 20 years ago:

> Without standardized terms to describe the important features…there is no means of training or obtaining objective data to improve our specificity. There must be a concise and orderly description of the finding(s) in language understandable to both clinician and radiologist leading to a logical recommendation. Indeed, this format is important for all reports we generate, not only mammography. (D'Orsi and Kopans 1994)

There are legislative efforts underway that encourage radiologists to undertake the process of developing and using structured reports. There are extensive tools available that build structure and enable coded meaning to be imposed on radiology reports. To date, the full realization of the benefits of structured reporting, both to the practicing radiologist and to our patients, is elusive. As our digital systems become more sophisticated, however, these benefits will be achieved. Radiologists should be at the forefront demanding the opportunity to prove the value of our patient interactions, as represented by our radiology reports.

References

Al-Hawary MM, Francis IR, Chari ST, Fishman EK, Hough DM, Lu DS, Macari M, Megibow AJ, Miller FH, Mortele KJ, Merchant NB, Minter RM, Tamm EP, Sahani DV, Simeone DM (2014) Pancreatic ductal adenocarcinoma radiology reporting template: consensus statement of the Society of Abdominal Radiology and the American Pancreatic Association. Radiology 270(1):248–260. https://doi.org/10.1148/radiol.13131184

Bisbal J, Berry D (2011) An analysis framework for electronic health record systems. Interoperation and collaboration in shared healthcare. Methods Inf Med 50(2):180–189. https://doi.org/10.3414/ME09-01-0002

Blumenthal D (2010) Promoting use of health IT: why be a meaningful user? Conn Med 74(5):299–300

Bosmans JM, Weyler JJ, De Schepper AM, Parizel PM (2011) The radiology report as seen by radiologists and referring clinicians: results of the COVER and ROVER surveys. Radiology 259(1):184–195. https://doi.org/10.1148/radiol.10101045

Bosmans JM, Peremans L, Menni M, De Schepper AM, Duyck PO, Parizel PM (2012) Structured reporting: if, why, when, how-and at what expense? Results of a focus group meeting of radiology professionals from eight countries. Insights Imaging 3(3):295–302. https://doi.org/10.1007/s13244-012-0148-1

Brink JA, Arenson RL, Grist TM, Lewin JS, Enzmann D (2017) Bits and bytes: the future of radiology lies in informatics and information technology. Eur Radiol 27(9):3647–3651. https://doi.org/10.1007/s00330-016-4688-5

Cai T, Giannopoulos AA, Yu S, Kelil T, Ripley B, Kumamaru KK, Rybicki FJ, Mitsouras D (2016) Natural language processing technologies in radiology research and clinical applications. Radiographics 36(1):176–191. https://doi.org/10.1148/rg.2016150080

cms.gov/Lung Cancer Screening Registries (2015) U.S. Centers for Medicare & Medicaid Services. https://www.cms.gov/Medicare/Medicare-General-Information/MedicareApprovedFacilitie/Lung-Cancer-Screening-Registries.html. Accessed 1 July 2017

D'Orsi CJ, Kopans DB (1994) The American College of Radiology's mammography lexicon: barking up the only tree. AJR Am J Roentgenol 162(3):595. https://doi.org/10.2214/ajr.162.3.8109503

D'Orsi CJ, Sickles EA, Mendelson EB, Morris EA, Bassett LW, Böhm-Vélez M, Berg WA, Comstock CE, Lee CH (2013) ACR BI-RADS® atlas, breast imaging reporting and data system. In: Radiology ACo (ed). American College of Radiology, Reston

Eisenberg RL, Bankier AA, Boiselle PM (2010) Compliance with Fleischner Society guidelines for management of small lung nodules: a survey of 834 radiologists. Radiology 255(1):218–224. https://doi.org/10.1148/radiol.09091556

Frates MC, Benson CB, Charboneau JW, Cibas ES, Clark OH, Coleman BG, Cronan JJ, Doubilet PM, Evans DB, Goellner JR, Hay ID, Hertzberg BS, Intenzo CM, Jeffrey RB, Langer JE, Larsen PR, Mandel SJ, Middleton WD, Reading CC, Sherman SI, Tessler FN, Society of Radiologists in ultrasound (2005) Management of thyroid nodules detected at US: Society of Radiologists in ultrasound consensus conference statement. Radiology 237(3):794–800. https://doi.org/10.1148/radiol.2373050220

Hassanpour S, Langlotz CP (2016) Information extraction from multi-institutional radiology reports. Artif Intell Med 66:29–39. https://doi.org/10.1016/j.artmed.2015.09.007

Haugen BR, Alexander EK, Bible KC, Doherty GM, Mandel SJ, Nikiforov YE, Pacini F, Randolph GW, Sawka AM, Schlumberger M, Schuff KG, Sherman SI, Sosa JA, Steward DL, Tuttle RM, Wartofsky L (2016) 2015 American Thyroid Association Management Guidelines for Adult Patients with Thyroid Nodules and Differentiated Thyroid Cancer: The American Thyroid Association Guidelines Task Force on Thyroid Nodules and Differentiated Thyroid Cancer. Thyroid 26(1):1–133. https://doi.org/10.1089/thy.2015.0020

Hobby JL, Tom BD, Todd C, Bearcroft PW, Dixon AK (2000) Communication of doubt and certainty in radiological reports. Br J Radiol 73(873):999–1001. https://doi.org/10.1259/bjr.73.873.11064655

Jee K, Kim GH (2013) Potentiality of big data in the medical sector: focus on how to reshape the healthcare system. Healthc Inform Res 19(2):79–85. https://doi.org/10.4258/hir.2013.19.2.79

Jha RC, Mitchell DG, Weinreb JC, Santillan CS, Yeh BM, Francois R, Sirlin CB (2014) LI-RADS categorization of benign and likely benign findings in patients at risk of hepatocellular carcinoma: a pictorial atlas. AJR Am J Roentgenol 203(1):W48–W69. https://doi.org/10.2214/AJR.13.12169

Kabadi SJ, Krishnaraj A (2017) Strategies for improving the value of the radiology report: a retrospective analysis of errors in formally over-read studies. J Am Coll Radiol 14(4):459–466. https://doi.org/10.1016/j.jacr.2016.08.033

Kahn CE Jr, Heilbrun ME, Applegate KE (2013) From guidelines to practice: how reporting templates promote the use of radiology practice guidelines. J Am Coll Radiol 10(4):268–273. https://doi.org/10.1016/j.jacr.2012.09.025

Kahn CE Jr, Genereaux B, Langlotz CP (2015) Conversion of radiology reporting templates to the MRRT standard. J Digit Imaging 28(5):528–536. https://doi.org/10.1007/s10278-015-9787-3

Lacson R, Prevedello LM, Andriole KP, Gill R, Lenoci-Edwards J, Roy C, Gandhi TK, Khorasani R (2012) Factors associated with radiologists' adherence to fleischner society guidelines for management of pulmonary nodules. J Am Coll Radiol 9(7):468–473. https://doi.org/10.1016/j.jacr.2012.03.009

Langlotz CP (2006) RadLex: a new method for indexing online educational materials. Radiographics 26(6):1595–1597. https://doi.org/10.1148/rg.266065168

Langlotz CP (2015) The radiology report a guide to thoughtful communication for radiologists and other medical professionals. CreateSpace Independent Publishing Platform, San Bernardino

Larson DB, Towbin AJ, Pryor RM, Donnelly LF (2013) Improving consistency in radiology reporting through the use of department-wide standardized structured reporting. Radiology 267(1):240–250. https://doi.org/10.1148/radiol.12121502

Lin E, Powell DK, Kagetsu NJ (2014) Efficacy of a checklist-style structured radiology reporting template in reducing resident misses on cervical spine computed tomography examinations. J Digit Imaging 27(5):588–593. https://doi.org/10.1007/s10278-014-9703-2

Lung Cancer Screening Registry (LCSR): User Guide (2017) The American College of Radiology, Reston, VA

Marcovici PA, Taylor GA (2014) Journal club: structured radiology reports are more complete and more effective than unstructured reports. AJR Am J Roentgenol 203(6):1265–1271. https://doi.org/10.2214/AJR.14.12636

Naik SS, Hanbidge A, Wilson SR (2001) Radiology reports: examining radiologist and clinician preferences regarding style and content. AJR Am J Roentgenol 176(3):591–598. https://doi.org/10.2214/ajr.176.3.1760591

Pinto Dos Santos D, Klos G, Kloeckner R, Oberle R, Dueber C, Mildenberger P (2017) Development of an IHE MRRT-compliant open-source web-based reporting platform. Eur Radiol 27(1):424–430. https://doi.org/10.1007/s00330-016-4344-0

Powell DK, Silberzweig JE (2015) State of structured reporting in radiology, a survey. Acad Radiol 22(2):226–233. https://doi.org/10.1016/j.acra.2014.08.014

Pysarenko K, Recht M, Kim D (2017) Structured reporting: a tool to improve reimbursement. J Am Coll Radiol 14(5):662–664. https://doi.org/10.1016/j.jacr.2016.10.016

Radiology Lexicon (RADLEX) (2007) Radiological Society of North America. http://bioportalbioontologyorg/ontologies/RADLEX/. Accessed 1 July 2017

Raja AS, Ip IK, Prevedello LM, Sodickson AD, Farkas C, Zane RD, Hanson R, Goldhaber SZ, Gill RR, Khorasani R (2012) Effect of computerized clinical decision support on the use and yield of CT pulmonary angiography in the emergency department. Radiology 262(2):468–474. https://doi.org/10.1148/radiol.11110951

Reiner BI, Knight N, Siegel EL (2007) Radiology reporting, past, present, and future: the radiologist's perspective. J Am Coll Radiol 4(5):313–319. https://doi.org/10.1016/j.jacr.2007.01.015

Restauri N, Flug JA, McArthur TA (2017) A picture of burnout: case studies and solutions toward improving radiologists' well-being. Curr Probl Diagn Radiol 46(5):365–368. https://doi.org/10.1067/j.cpradiol.2016.12.006

Rosenkrantz AB, Nicola GN, Allen B Jr, Hughes DR, Hirsch JA (2017) MACRA, alternative payment models, and the physician-focused payment model: implications for radiology. J Am Coll Radiol 14(6):744–751. https://doi.org/10.1016/j.jacr.2016.12.001

Rubin DL, Kahn CE Jr (2017) Common data elements in radiology. Radiology 283(3):837–844. https://doi.org/10.1148/radiol.2016161553

Schwartz LH, Panicek DM, Berk AR, Li Y, Hricak H (2011) Improving communication of diagnostic radiology findings through structured reporting. Radiology 260(1):174–181. https://doi.org/10.1148/radiol.11101913

Tessler FN, Middleton WD, Grant EG, Hoang JK, Berland LL, Teefey SA, Cronan JJ, Beland MD, Desser TS, Frates MC, Hammers LW, Hamper UM, Langer JE, Reading CC, Scoutt LM, Stavros AT (2017) ACR thyroid imaging, reporting and data system (TI-RADS): white paper of the ACR TI-RADS committee. J Am Coll Radiol 14(5):587–595. https://doi.org/10.1016/j.jacr.2017.01.046

Wang KC, Patel JB, Vyas B, Toland M, Collins B, Vreeman DJ, Abhyankar S, Siegel EL, Rubin DL, Langlotz CP (2017) Use of radiology procedure codes in health care: the need for standardization and structure. Radiographics 37(4):1099–1110. https://doi.org/10.1148/rg.2017160188

Weinreb JC, Barentsz JO, Choyke PL, Cornud F, Haider MA, Macura KJ, Margolis D, Schnall MD, Tempany CM, Thoeny HC, Verma S (2015) PI-RADS: Prostate Imaging – Reporting and Data System v2

Weiss DL, Langlotz CP (2008) Structured reporting: patient care enhancement or productivity nightmare? Radiology 249(3):739–747. https://doi.org/10.1148/radiol.2493080988

Winget MD, Baron JA, Spitz MR, Brenner DE, Warzel D, Kincaid H, Thornquist M, Feng Z (2003) Development of common data elements: the experience of and recommendations from the early detection research network. Int J Med Inform 70(1):41–48

Clinical Decision Support at the Radiologist Point of Care

Tarik K. Alkasab, Bernardo C. Bizzo, and H. Benjamin Harvey

Contents

T.K. Alkasab, M.D., Ph.D. (✉) • B.C. Bizzo, M.D.
Harvard Medical School, Boston, MA, USA

Department of Radiology, Massachusetts General Hospital, Boston, MA, USA
e-mail: TALKASAB@mgh.harvard.edu

H. Benjamin Harvey, M.D., J.D.
Harvard Medical School, Boston, MA, USA

Department of Radiology, Massachusetts General Hospital, Boston, MA, USA

Institute for Technology Assessment, Massachusetts General Hospital, Boston, MA, USA

1 Introduction

The field of radiology is broad: a single imaging examination can present significant findings that span multiple body systems. For example, an abdominal computed tomography (CT) might show infectious disease of the hepatobiliary system, traumatic injury to the musculoskeletal system, or an obstructive malignancy of the genitourinary tract. In addition to these acute findings, it is not uncommon for a radiologist interpreting an abdominal CT to encounter incidental findings, such as pulmonary nodules, adrenal nodules, renal masses, hepatic hypodensities, pancreatic cystic lesions, or adnexal cysts, among others. This means that radiologists must possess—or have readily available—considerable knowledge of these entities and their management crossing multiple medical specialties to provide accurate and clinically meaningful interpretations.

The challenge of interpreting across a wide range of imaging findings is further complicated by an even wider range of clinical contexts. To provide the necessary flexibility to meet this challenge, radiology has traditionally embraced an open-ended style of reporting. Bordering on conversational, traditional reporting has given radiologists wide berth to marry imaging findings with clinical context to communicate a diagnostic impression. Despite the benefits of this open-ended reporting practice, it also has its drawbacks. Chief among them has been an undesirable

Med Radiol Diagn Imaging (2018)
DOI 10.1007/174_2017_160, © Springer International Publishing AG
Published Online 08 February 2018

variability in reporting between radiologists that can frustrate referring physicians and complicate patient care (Chan et al. 2016; van Riel et al. 2015; Hoang et al. 2014; Elemraid et al. 2014).

2 Addressing the Challenge of Report Variability

To address the issue of report variability, there has been a robust push in recent years toward increased structure and standardization in radiology reporting. Expert panels organized by national bodies such as the American College of Radiology (ACR), the Fleischner Society for Thoracic Radiology, and the Society of Radiologists in Ultrasound have published white papers, best practices, and clinical guidelines to guide radiologist reporting. The most notable example of this is in the field of breast imaging where the ACR developed and promulgated the Breast Imaging Reporting and Data System® (BI-RADS®) for description of breast imaging findings and their clinical management (American College of Radiology (ACR) n.d.-a). Backed by a federal mandate, the BI-RADS® system has achieved ubiquitous use throughout the United States, resulting in a much lower degree of variability in the reporting of breast imaging findings compared to other areas of imaging.

Partially driven by the success of BI-RADS®, other areas of radiology have promulgated similar report standardization efforts across a variety of clinical scenarios. In fact, Centers for Medicare and Medicaid Services (CMS) has mandated the use of standardized lung nodule identification, classification, and reporting system to qualify for reimbursement for lung cancer screening. To meet this requirement many screening programs use the Lung CT Screening Reporting and Data System (Lung-RADS®)—a structured reporting system similar to BI-RADS® (American College of Radiology (ACR) n.d.-b; Centers for Medicare and Medicaid Services 2015).

In addition to achieving language standardization (i.e., ensuring that radiologists use the same words/descriptors to describe an imaging finding), it is equally if not more important to achieve interpretive standardization. Interpretive standardization means ensuring that radiologists seeing the same imaging finding in the same clinical context communicate that same evidence-based interpretation. Expert panels organized by national bodies have addressed the challenge of interpretive variability head on through the development of practice guidelines.

The last decade has seen myriad evidence- and consensus-based guidelines, practice parameters, and technical standards issued to guide imaging interpretation. Much of this guidance for reporting has been structured into algorithms that direct the radiologist to the most likely clinical diagnosis, additional workup if necessary, and standard information to include in the reports. Such guidance is most common for well-recognized imaging findings, such as common incidental lesions. This goal of consistently providing a correct and clinically relevant interpretation is central to radiology's success in value-based payment models and necessary for cost-effective patient care.

Despite the importance and availability of clinical guidelines for interpretation and reporting of imaging findings, in practice, radiologists frequently do not adhere to these guidelines (Lacson et al. 2012).

3 Cracking the Code of Interpretive Variability

Unlike BI-RADS® and Lung-RADS®, use of the clinical guidelines and practice standards by radiologists has been inconsistent at best, with a high degree of report variability persisting across radiology (Lacson et al. 2012; Penn et al. 2015; Eisenberg et al. 2013; Hobbs et al. 2014; Berland et al. 2014; Johnson et al. 2011). This has led some to be skeptical that evidence-based guidelines will inform practice sufficiently to address individual patient needs (Boland et al. 2011). Some advocates of standardized reporting have even suggested extending Clinical Decision Support (CDS) use requirements recently imposed on the image ordering process to the process of image interpretation (Centers for Medicare and Medicaid Services 2017).

Many explanations have been proffered for the ongoing widespread variation in radiologist practice from these guidelines. First, expecting a radiologist to keep up with the ever-growing and changing trove of subspecialty guidelines is increasingly infeasible. The rapid expansion and increasing complexity of radiology guidelines underscore the need for better CDS at the radiologist's point of care. Second, a radiologist may disagree with the national guidelines or favor local guidelines which they believe better address the unique needs of their specific patient population. However, for many radiologists, the most common barrier to consistently applying clinical guidelines is a practical one: in the face of increasing productivity demands, they do not have the time to repeatedly interrupt their workflow to access the relevant clinical guideline. Better workflow integration is essential for removing this practical impediment and achieving more consistent guideline utilization in radiology reporting.

Point-of-care CDS solutions, such as electronic medical record (EMR)-based "best practice alerts," have been shown to improve compliance with guidelines in other areas of medicine (Szlosek and Ferretti 2016; Oluoch et al. 2012). However, these EMR-based systems are less likely to be effective in meaningfully impacting radiologist practice given that the EMR is not as central to the radiologist workflow. A more successful information technology (IT) integration strategy in radiology would be focused on the picture archiving and communication system (PACS) viewer or the voice recognition/reporting software (VRS). The computer-assisted reporting and decision support (CAR/DS) framework aims to accomplish just that (Alkasab et al. 2017).

The CAR/DS solution brings relevant clinical guidelines directly into the radiologist workflow via an easy-to-use, digital format. In the CAR/DS vision, when a radiologist encounters a situation with a relevant imaging finding, instead of issuing an interpretation based on personal preference or experience, a CAR/DS tool incorporated into their PACS viewer or VRS directs the radiologist to conform to recognized best practices. With respect to recommendations for follow-up (FU) imaging, the CAR/DS tool should help less experienced radiologists move toward the recommendation pattern of more experienced radiologists and in so doing substantially reduce variation among radiologists. The usage of such tool comports with the principles of ACR's "Imaging 3.0," a national initiative for increasing radiologists' relevance to the healthcare system.

4 The Open CAR/DS Framework

Moving toward the CAR/DS vision, the ACR has adopted an open format to define clinical guidelines in a standard definition language for the assisted reporting modules. Under the ACR Assist™ initiative, the ACR is in the process of translating its relevant clinical content, including ACR "RADS" and white papers of the Incidental Findings Commission, into this standard definition language. Once accomplished, this ACR clinical content can be readily integrated into Open CAR/DS-enabled PACS viewers and VRS programs to guide radiologists at the point of care. Commercial VRS and PACS are already starting to incorporate these guideline-specific definitions into their products (Alkasab et al. 2017). What's more, other national bodies including the Fleischner Society for Thoracic Radiology and the Society of Radiologists in Ultrasound can use the Open CAR/DS framework to start encoding their clinical practice guidelines into a format which allows vendors to include their content as well.

The Open CAR/DS framework has been designed to separate as much as possible the work of content developers such as the ACR from the development of the image-viewing and report-generating software that will use it. Open CAR/DS includes a freely available, nonproprietary file format that content developers use to specify what data must be collected and how it can be interpreted. It is then up to each PACS or VRS vendor to tailor their tools to implement the specified guideline. The implementing vendors are responsible for storing the

XML modules and offering them to radiologists in appropriate contexts (e.g., appropriate exam type and patient demographics). They must adapt their user interfaces to collect the specified data from radiologists, generate the appropriate text based on responses, and incorporate the text into the report. Finally, Open CAR/DS-compliant systems will store the radiologist responses as structured data and send that data to downstream systems as appropriate.

The Open CAR/DS framework is based around clinical guidelines encoded using the Open CAR/DS schema for describing the data elements, the logic tree, and a report text to be generated. This format is defined using an Extensible Markup Language (XML) schema (Extensible Markup Language (XML) n.d.). A CAR/DS module must define all the potential data elements that serve as the inputs and outputs of the reference radiologic clinical guideline. Likewise, it must define the branching logic rules by which inputs are turned into outputs and specify the appropriate report language for each of these potential outputs. Therefore, at the highest level, a CAR/DS guideline definition contains descriptive metadata, data element definitions, a flowchart-like logic tree, and a set of templates associated with the possible end points.

The metadata section contains general information about a CAR/DS guideline (e.g., text label and description of the guideline, contact information for relevant authors of the document, citations to relevant articles, and may also contain links to other ontologies), information specifying for which examination types and patient demographics the guideline would be relevant, and also provides clues as to how a reporting system might recognize when a user is describing a finding for which the guideline might be applicable.

The data element definitions specify the input values used to drive the clinical decision tree and possibly intermediate or output values associated with an algorithm. These can be collected from the radiologist at reporting time and can be numeric values (e.g., the size of a lesion), integers (e.g., the series or image number a finding is seen on), Boolean values (e.g., the presence or absence of a finding), single-choice values (e.g., categorization of a finding), or multiple-choice values (e.g., presence or absence of findings in multiple locations).

Clinical guidelines are frequently defined as flowchart-like decision trees. For representation in the CAR/DS format, this logic must be formally encoded as a branching structure of binary decision points based on Boolean logic and associated outputs or further decision points. Starting at the first decision point in the branch logic, implementing software finds the contained branches and evaluates the condition of each sequentially. The first branch whose condition evaluates to true is then followed, leading to only one possible true path based on the available choices. If the branch leads to an end point, then that end point is the output of the algorithm.

Each end point of the defined logic tree specifies actions to be taken when user inputs lead to that output, primarily reflected as a set of templates. These templates lay out the text to be inserted in a radiology report by an implementing reporting system. Pieces of text can be defined to insert into the findings section of the report, into the impression section, and into a recommendation section.

To enable development and testing of clinical guidelines encoded into CAR/DS definitions, reference software has been created and is freely available from the ACR. This program loads guideline definition files, enacts the specified user interaction, processes the user-entered data according to the given logic, and generates and presents the defined report text. The software consists of a Web application, where both server-side and client-side components are written using the JavaScript programming language. The reference implementation of the software allows users to test the fidelity of clinical guidelines that they have encoded into a CAR/DS definition and to interact with the encoded CAR/DS guideline to test how different inputs lead to different outputs.

This new CAR/DS framework brings evidence-based guidelines for recommendations and actionable reporting into clinical practice in a structured, vendor-neutral manner. Vendors of VRS, as well as other vendors in the radiology workflow, can implement CAR/DS content to extend the functionality of commercial tools currently in use. Because CAR/DS modules can work as "apps" or "plug-ins" for any vendor's reporting system, it is expected that many professional societies will follow the ACR's lead in making their guidelines available as CAR/DS modules at the radiologist point of care.

5 Radiologist Experience of CAR/DS

The CAR/DS framework makes it easy for radiologists to do the right thing: issue guideline-compliant reports without workflow interruption. From the point of view of a radiologist, a CAR/DS-enabled reporting tool allows real-time reporting guidance based on clinical guidelines integrated into the workflow. By having the tool incorporated into the point of care, radiologists do not have to choose between the time-consuming task of looking up a guideline and trying to use a flowchart to apply to the current clinical situation or the fast, but less reliable cognitive dissonance of improvising to his/her best memory or guess as to what the published guideline instructs. Since clinical guidelines to date primarily focus on incidental lesions, a CAR/DS-enabled reporting system allows a radiologist to focus his/her mental energy on the central clinical question. This is particularly important for generalist radiologists practicing across a broader range of modalities and body regions.

How does CAR/DS-assisted reporting work in everyday practice? Consider an incidentally discovered adrenal nodule on CT as an example. The radiologist is using a CAR/DS-enabled VRS tool which has incorporated an encoded guideline from the ACR based on College's Incidental Findings Commission's white paper for the workup/management of incidentally discovered adrenal nodules. When the radiologist encounters the adrenal nodule, the CAR/DS tool within the VRS aids the radiologist in providing the necessary descriptions of the adrenal nodule by prompting the radiologist to provide the important characteristics of the adrenal nodule including size, presence of macroscopic fat, and stability from prior imaging examinations. Based on the radiologist input, the CAR/DS tool determines the appropriate workup/management and automatically generates and inserts standardized language of the imaging findings and necessary clinical FU into the report (Fig. 1).

Radiologists interact with the CAR/DS framework while reading a study in two ways: either

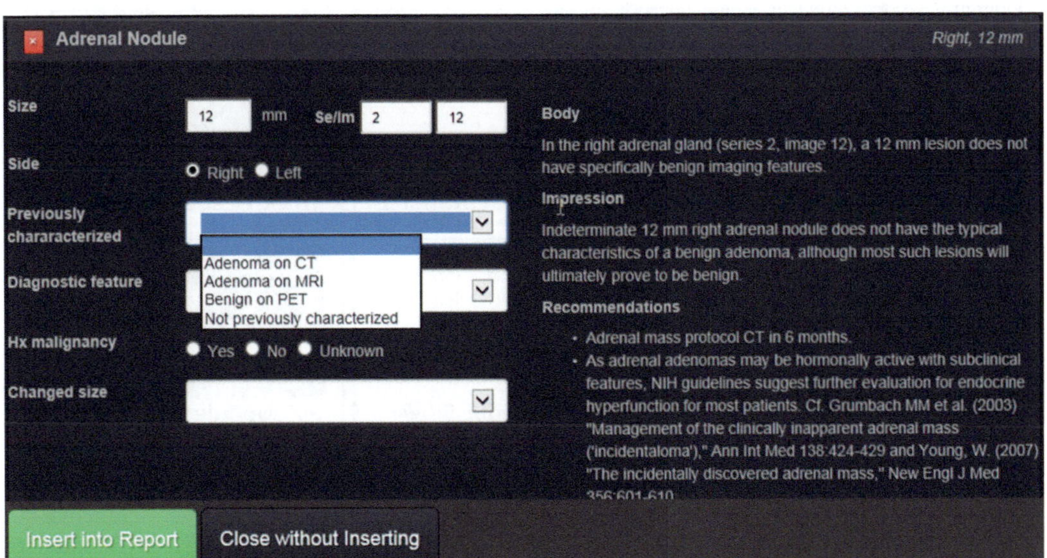

Fig. 1 Web-based reference software CAR/DS incidental adrenal nodule module interface

the reporting system detects specific predetermined voice or text commands corresponding to a given CAR/DS module and offers to launch that tool or the radiologist triggers the CAR/DS tool directly and is given a choice of the available/applicable guideline modules filtered for the type of exam being read and patient age and sex. Either way, the radiologist interacts with a series of relevant questions that can be answered using both the VRS and the mouse and keyboard. In addition to text-based questions, it is also possible to use image-based selection including exemplar images, as well as tables, graphics, and classification/grading figures. These aids allow an easy and practical way to describe and identify more nuanced imaging characteristics (Figs. 2 and 3). As the radiologist answers the required questions (noting that which answers are required may change dynamically based on prior answers), the radiologist sees the proposed text generated based on the provided answers. Upon completion, the generated text is pushed into the correct portions of the radiologist's draft report (findings, impression, and recommendation, as appropriate). The radiologist can reopen the tool, and modify the description of the lesion in question, and the generated report text will be updated.

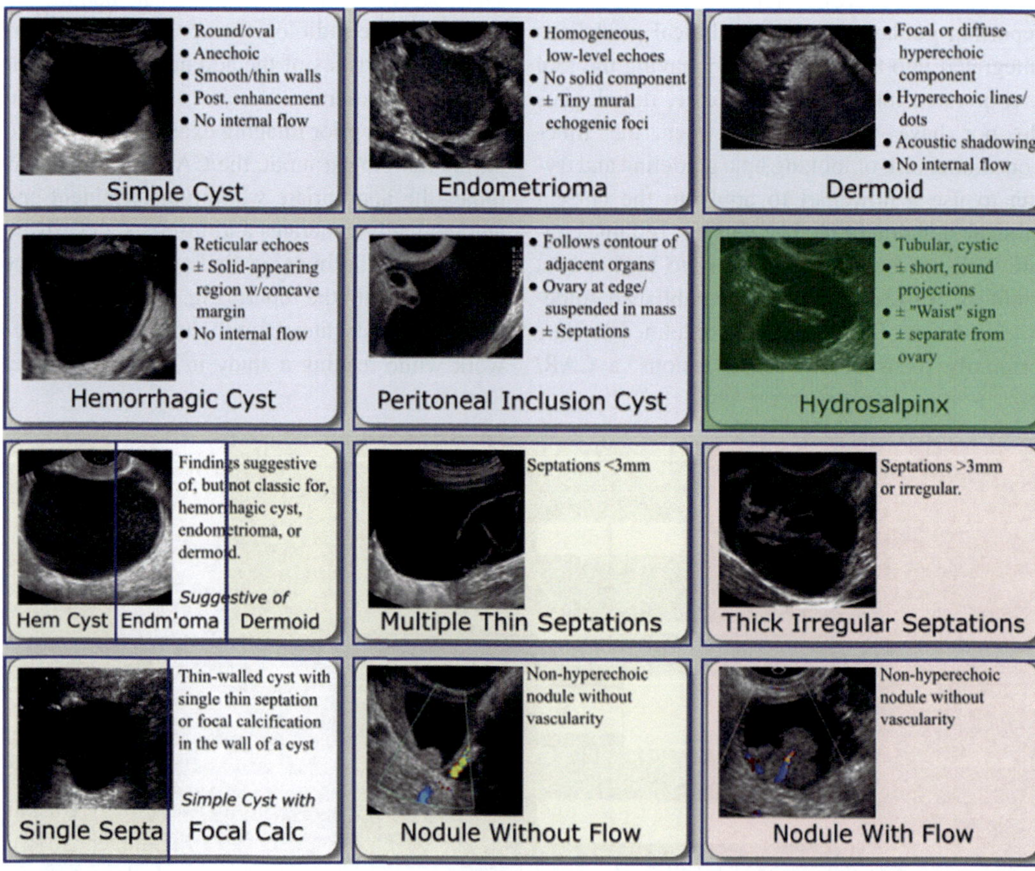

Fig. 2 Clickable schematic image for guidance to report adnexal cyst lesions on ultrasound

		<6 mm	6–8 mm	>8 mm
Solid	Single	Low risk **No routine follow-up**	Low risk **CT at 6–12 months** *(then consider CT at 18–24 mos.)*	**Consider PET/CT or tissue sampling, vs. CT at 3 months**
		Unknown risk **No routine follow-up** *or* **Optical CT at 12 months** *per risk*	Unknown risk **CT at 6–12 months** *(then consider CT at 18–24 mos.) per risk*	
		High risk **Optional CT at 12 months** *Stronger consideration if suspicious nodule morphology and/or upper lobe location*	High risk **CT at 6–12 months** *(then CT at 18–24 months)*	
	Multiple *Most suspicious nodule drives management*	Low risk **No routine follow-up**	Low risk **CT at 3–6 months** *(then consider CT at 18–24 months)*	Low risk **CT at 3–6 months** *(then consider CT at 18–24 months)*
		Unknown risk **No routine follow-up** *or* **Optical CT at 12 months** *per risk*	Unknown risk **CT at 3–6 months** *(then consider CT at 18–24 months) per risk*	Unknown risk **CT at 3–6 months** *(then consider CT at 18–24 months) per risk*
		High risk **Optional CT at 12 months** *Stronger consideration if suspicious nodule morphology and/or upper lobe location*	High risk **CT at 3–6 months** *(then CT at 18–24 mos.)*	High risk **CT at 3–6 months** *(then CT at 18–24 mos.)*

		<6 mm	≥6 mm
Subsolid	Single ground glass	**No routine follow-up**	**CT at 6–12 months** *(then CT every 2 years until 5 years)*
	Single part solid	**No routine follow-up**	**CT at 3–6 months** *(then ann. CT x5 years if unchanged & solid part <6mm)*
	Multiple	**CT at 3–6 months** *(if stable, consider CT at 2 and 4 years)*	**CT at 3–6 months** *(then subsequent management based on the most suspicious nodule)*

Fig. 3 Clickable schematic table for guidance to report incidental pulmonary nodules on CT

6 Benefits from Implementation of CAR/DS

Data have shown significantly improved compliance with guidelines when radiologists use the point-of-care CAR/DS tool for management of incidental pulmonary nodules on abdominal CT (Lu et al. 2016). This suggests that a workstation-integrated, point-of-care CDS tool can improve guideline adherence beyond levels achieved through current, more passive methods of implementation. The impact of using the CAR/DS tool should be reflected in several ways, such as improving the quality and efficiency of radiology reporting; reducing the inter- and intra-radiologist report variability and level of confidence; increasing the report compliance of guideline recommendations for imaging FU, as well as the ordering provider compliance with imaging FU recommendation; and increasing ordering provider satisfaction (Boland et al. 2011; Brink 2014).

Failure to provide guideline-based care has long been recognized as a cause of suboptimal patient care and referring physician dissatisfaction. However, compliance with the guidelines has taken on even greater importance under value-based reimbursement models in which compliance is increasingly being used as a financially tied measure of quality in medicine (Torchiana et al. 2013). As the US healthcare environment continues the transition into value-based payment models, the CAR/DS tool provides an objective metric by which the ACR could measure radiologists' practice quality. To date, these potential financial incentives and penalties have affected radiology indirectly; however, the high frequency of both incidental findings on cross-sectional imaging and recommendations for FU imaging suggest that future radiologist-specific initiatives aimed at these drivers of healthcare costs are likely (Boland et al. 2011).

Use of the Open CAR/DS framework could also offer important protection with respect to malpractice litigation. It is estimated that each year approximately 7% of radiologists will face a lawsuit, and the likelihood of a radiologist being the defendant in at least one lawsuit is 50% by 60 years of age (Jena et al. 2011; Baker et al. 2013). Approximately 35% of claims against radiologists will result in payment to the plaintiff, with the average award being approximately $175,000 (Harvey et al. 2016). Workstation-integrated, point-of-care CDS tool makes it easier to clearly tether one's radiological impression to the prevailing standard of care. If the standard has been met, then there is no liability (American College of Radiology 2005).

The CAR/DS framework also improves the integration of radiology point of care with systems like the EMR that are not usually central to the radiologists' workflow. For example, patient demographic and clinical data, such as a more detailed history of the present illness, current medications, vital signs, laboratory values, genetic tests results, smoking status, and history of malignancy, can be made more easily accessible in the radiologist point-of-care environment and can better shape the radiologist's report. The generated structured data can be embedded into the report and/or communicated to EMR or other systems. For example, the quantitative data from tumor measurements can be inserted into an oncology research registry automatically rather than being copied by hand. CAR/DS can also serve as a cornerstone technology for radiologists playing the role of an "imaging data shepherd." Radiologists can define an essential role in generating and overseeing structured data generated from imaging exams that can be included in the patient's medical record. This can provide higher value reports, and also improve the ability to associate radiology findings and imaging in general with patient outcomes.

The Open CAR/DS framework enables radiologists to generate structured recommendations for FU imaging that automatically incorporate information on the exact exam being recommended, acceptable substitute exams, indication for the FU exam, and timeframe in which that exam should be obtained. This will permit these recommendations to be automatically used by downstream systems. For example, an EMR could offer one-click ordering of the recommended exam. A tracking system could be reliably created to monitor whether the recommended exams have been obtained.

In addition, Open CAR/DS-enabled systems can serve as a channel for incorporating other data science tools such as wearable devices and artificially intelligent (AI) image analysis programs. This would allow the creation of a linkable interface with AI machine learning (AI/ML) algorithms and report generation systems, in which the results of a neural network output could be incorporated into radiology reports using the CAR/DS framework.

All of these improvements contribute to more cost-effective patient care and are fundamental to radiology's success in value-based payment models, as described in the ACR's Imaging 3.0 vision. Large-scale implementation of the CAR/DS tool has the potential to dramatically change the radiologist's practice, by shifting the conventional interpretation task toward a more integrative role, in which report recommendations reliably guide care pathways (Allen and Wald 2013).

7 Future Directions

The Open CAR/DS definition format serves to separate the content of clinical guidelines from the vendor functionality implementing the

CDS tool. From the vendor perspective this means that individual software vendors can decide how best to implement the CAR/DS interaction for their specific use case. This freedom will empower them to adapt the experience for their particular use case and should translate into a growing, evolving ecosystem of CAR/DS functionality, creating a healthy competition to provide the richest CAR/DS implementation. In turn, this should also improve the fluidly of the workflow integration over time. From the guideline creator perspective, this means that anyone (e.g., individual radiologist, radiology group, or professional society) can craft CAR/DS modules and then make available to others, potentially creating a marketplace of CAR/DS modules. From this marketplace practices can choose the best and most trusted tools to make available to their radiologists.

Data to support the value of assisted reporting tools in radiology is still very limited. More robust research assessing for improvements in radiologist practice is expected in the near future. The results of such research will provide objective analyses of the impact of clinical implementation of the CAR/DS tool that would be of value to payers, healthcare IT vendors, policy makers, and practicing radiologists.

Lastly, as a structured reporting system, the CAR/DS will generate large-scale structured clinically relevant data. This means the potential for improved data collection and mining. The CAR/DS framework can be tailored to automatically populate research registries making large-scale outcome studies more feasible and less expensive. On the individual level, the CAR/DS framework will allow for more accurate peer review metrics, including inter- and intra-radiologist report variability, compliance with guidelines' recommendations for imaging FU, and ordering provider compliance with imaging FU recommendations. In an iterative process, the data collection and research fostered by the CAR/DS technology can inform both individual radiologists and societal guidelines, moving radiology practice even more in line with clinical evidence.

References

Alkasab TK, Bizzo BC, Berland LL, Nair S, Pandharipande PV, Harvey HB (2017) Creation of an open framework for point-of-care computer-assisted reporting and decision support tools for radiologists. J Am Coll Radiol 14(9):1184–1189

Allen B, Wald C (2013) Imaging 3.0™ IT reference guide for the practicing radiologist

American College of Radiology (2005) Medical-legal issues in radiology, 3rd edn. ACR, Reston, pp 1–36

American College of Radiology (ACR) (n.d.-a) BI-RADS® atlas [Internet]. https://www.acr.org/Quality-Safety/Resources/BIRADS

American College of Radiology (ACR) (n.d.-b) Lung CT screening reporting and data system (Lung-RADS) [Internet]. [cited 2017 Aug 23]. https://www.acr.org/Quality-Safety/Resources/LungRADS

Baker SR, Whang JS, Luk L, Clarkin KS, Castro A, Patel R (2013) The demography of medical malpractice suits against radiologists. Radiology 266(2):539–547

Berland LL, Silverman SG, Megibow AJ, Mayo-Smith WW, Castro A, Amorosa JK (2014) ACR members' response to JACR white paper on the management of incidental abdominal CT findings. J Am Coll Radiol 11(1):30–35

Boland GWL, Thrall JH, Gazelle GS, Samir A, Rosenthal DI, Dreyer KJ et al (2011) Decision support for radiologist report recommendations. J Am Coll Radiol 8(12):819–823

Brink JA (2014) Clinical decision-making tools for exam selection, reporting and dose tracking. Pediatr Radiol 44(S3):418–421

Centers for Medicare and Medicaid Services (2015) Decision memo for screening for lung cancer with low dose computed tomography (LDCT) (CAG-00439N), pp 1–90. http://www.cms.gov/medicare-coverage-database/details/nca-decision-memo.aspx?NCAId=274

Centers for Medicare and Medicaid Services (2017) Medicare Program; Revisions to Payment Policies Under the Physician Fee Schedule and Other Revisions to Part B for CY 2018; Medicare Shared Savings Program Requirements; and Medicare Diabetes Prevention Program [Internet]. https://www.federalregister.gov/documents/2017/07/21/2017-14639/medicare-program-revisions-to-payment-policies-under-the-physician-fee-schedule-and-other-revisions

Chan TY, England A, Meredith SM, McWilliams RG (2016) Radiologist variability in assessing the position of the cavoatrial junction on chest radiographs. Br J Radiol 89(1065):20150965

Eisenberg RL, Bankier AA, Boiselle PM, Al E (2013) Ways to improve radiologists' adherence to Fleischner Society guidelines for management of pulmonary nodules. J Am Coll Radiol 10(6):439–441

Elemraid MA, Muller M, Spencer DA, Rushton SP, Gorton R, Thomas MF et al (2014) Accuracy of the interpretation of chest radiographs for the diagnosis of paediatric pneumonia. PLoS One 9(8):e106051

Extensible Markup Language (XML) [Internet] (n.d.). [cited 2017 Aug 27]. https://www.w3.org/XML/

Harvey HB, Tomov E, Babayan A, Dwyer K, Boland S, Pandharipande PV et al (2016) Radiology malpractice claims in the United States from 2008 to 2012: characteristics and implications. J Am Coll Radiol 13(2):124–130. [cited 2017 Aug 31] http://linkinghub.elsevier.com/retrieve/pii/S1546144015006869

Hoang JK, Riofrio A, Bashir MR, Kranz PG, Eastwood JD (2014) High variability in radiologists' reporting practices for incidental thyroid nodules detected on CT and MRI. Am J Neuroradiol 35(6):1190–1194

Hobbs HA, Bahl M, Nelson RC, Kranz PG, Esclamado RM, Wnuk NM et al (2014) Journal Club: incidental thyroid nodules detected at imaging: can diagnostic workup be reduced by use of the society of radiologists in ultrasound recommendations and the three-tiered system? Am J Roentgenol 202(1):18–24

Jena AB, Seabury S, Lakdawalla D, Chandra A (2011) Malpractice risk according to physician specialty. N Engl J Med 365(7):629–636

Johnson PT, Horton KM, Megibow AJ, Jeffrey RB, Fishman EK (2011) Common incidental findings on MDCT: survey of radiologist recommendations for patient management. J Am Coll Radiol 8(11):762–767

Lacson R, Prevedello LM, Andriole KP, Gill R, Lenoci-Edwards J, Roy C et al (2012) Factors associated with radiologists' adherence to Fleischner Society guidelines for Management of Pulmonary Nodules. J Am Coll Radiol 9(7):468–473

Lu MT, Rosman DA, Wu CC, Gilman MD, Harvey HB, Gervais DA et al (2016) Radiologist point-of-care clinical decision support and adherence to guidelines for incidental lung nodules. J Am Coll Radiol 13(2):156–162

Oluoch T, Santas X, Kwaro D, Were M, Biondich P, Bailey C et al (2012) The effect of electronic medical record-based clinical decision support on HIV care in resource-constrained settings: a systematic review. Int J Med Inform 81(10):e83–e92

Penn A, Ma M, Chou BB, Tseng JR, Phan P (2015) Inter-reader variability when applying the 2013 Fleischner guidelines for potential solitary subsolid lung nodules. Acta Radiol 56(10):1180–1186

van Riel SJ, Sánchez CI, Bankier AA, Naidich DP, Verschakelen J, Scholten ET, et al (2015) Observer variability for classification of pulmonary nodules on low-dose CT images and its effect on nodule management. Radiology 277(3):863–71

Szlosek DA, Ferretti JM (2016) Using machine learning and natural language processing algorithms to automate the evaluation of clinical decision support in electronic medical record systems. eGEMs 4(3):1222

Torchiana DF, Colton DG, Rao SK, Lenz SK, Meyer GS, Ferris TG (2013) Massachusetts General Physicians Organization's quality incentive program produces encouraging results. Health Aff (Millwood) 32(10):1748–1756

Report Communication Standards

Erik R. Ranschaert and Jan M.L. Bosmans

Contents

E.R. Ranschaert (✉)
Vice-president of EUSOMII, Radiologist,
H. Hartziekenhuis, Gasthuisstraat 1, 2400 Mol, Flanders, Belgium
e-mail: erik.ranschaert@gmail.com

J.M.L. Bosmans
Staff Radiologist, Ghent University Hospital, Ghent, Flanders, Belgium

Visiting Professor, Ghent University, Ghent, Flanders, Belgium

Visiting Lecturer, University of Antwerp, Antwerp, Flanders, Belgium
e-mail: jan.bosmans@ugent.be

Abbreviations

ACR	American College of Radiology
ANCR	Automated critical test result notification system
DICOM	Digital imaging and communications in medicine
EHR	Electronic health record
ESR	European society of radiology
HIS	Hospital information system
NLP	Natural language processing
PACS	Picture archiving and communication system
RIS	Radiology information system
SNOMED-CT	Systematized nomenclature of medicine—clinical terms
SR	Structured reporting

Good communication is essential in medicine, and particularly in radiology. Radiology is a supporting specialty with a mainly consultative function. The service rendered by radiologists can be roughly divided into two distinct but inseparable parts: analyzing the images on the one hand, and reporting the findings on the other. The radiology report

Med Radiol Diagn Imaging (2017)
DOI 10.1007/174_2017_113,
Published Online 01 September 2017

is the core of the communication by the radiologist (Flanders and Lakhani 2012), and in a way our product, the end stage of the workflow.

The report serves several purposes. Its primary role is medical: it usually mentions the clinical information at the time of the examination, the clinical question, the type of study that has been performed, a detailed description of the findings, and finally an impression or a conclusion, i.e., a medical interpretation of the findings, and ideally an answer to the clinical question. But the report is also a medicolegal document: it describes the type of care provided, the question to be answered by the study, the results and limitations of the study, the findings, and the conclusions based on these findings. Moreover, the document justifies reimbursement of the study and may be used for training, education, research, and quality control. Last but not least, it can play a role in the communication with the patient (Flanders and Lakhani 2012).

The interests of both patients and referring physicians are best served if the following conditions are met:

- A thorough preliminary clinical examination of the patient by the referring clinician
- A summary in the examination request of the most relevant clinical information, notably a working diagnosis, relevant symptoms, and open questions

The presence of this information enables the radiologist to interpret the images in the right context, and thus to provide the most accurate and cost-effective diagnostic approach. Access of the radiologist to the electronic health record (EHR) and active consultation of the information by the latter can further facilitate this. The gradual introduction of electronic applications will make it possible to automatically integrate relevant information from the EHR into the request (the so-called integrated and actionable request).

1 The Radiology Report

For many decades, reports and radiological documents were stored and archived in physical form. Results were often delivered late, and a considerable number of radiological documents and reports got lost.

The times when handwritten reports together with the "plates" were delivered to the referring physician by courier, or handed over to the patient, are long gone. Thanks to voice recognition technology and the Internet, great progress has been made in the composition and distribution of the report. Paradoxically, the form and content of the report have changed little since the early years of radiography. In most cases, the radiology report is still a piece of prose, consisting of a description of the findings, followed by a problem-oriented interpretation of those findings.

The introduction of digital solutions such as PACS and RIS, together with voice recognition software, has significantly improved the workflow. Results can now be delivered on time, with or without the intervention of a transcriptionist. The advent of Internet technology has made it possible to immediately communicate critical findings. This, however, is not enough to meet the needs of present-day interdisciplinary medicine.

The report remains the cornerstone of the communication from radiologist to referring physician. However, while the report can now be composed and distributed rapidly, its content still shows a wide variety of style and clarity (Bosmans et al. 2009). The call for a "standardized" type of report is getting stronger. That is not new. Already in 1899, one of the first editors of the American Journal of Roentgenology (AJR), the Detroit, Michigan-based radiologist Preston M. Hickey (1865–1930), expressed the view that there was a need for a more standardized approach to radiological reporting. In the early twentieth century, he introduced the term "interpretation," thus referring to a probability-based process in which specialized knowledge was required to reach a conclusion that could lead to a diagnosis. It was his opinion that reporting was most often so ambiguous that it was impossible to extract a diagnosis out of it, or to correlate radiological findings to the clinical problem (Flanders and Lakhani 2012; Wallis and McCoubrie 2011). He was also very disappointed by the lack of training of residents in describing and characterizing defects. Charles D. Enfield, a contemporary of Hickey, criticized radiologists who did describe findings in detail but omitted a conclusion.

The fundamental purpose of reporting is unchanged from what it was a century ago already. The value of the radiologist resides in his or her ability to recognize and coherently describe relevant findings, but also to express an opinion on the clinical implications. To achieve this, radiological terminology must be clear and unequivocal, and structure consistent. The net result must be that previously open clinical questions get an answer.

To our knowledge, teaching how to report, either in theory or in practice, is rather seldom an essential part of a structured training program for future radiologists (Sistrom et al. 2004). Residents therefore depend on their trainers and fellow trainees to learn the relevant terminology and developing a reporting style. According to this apprenticeship model, the language of the radiology report is handed down from generation to generation. This evokes associations with the storyteller tradition of our ancestors prior to the introduction of writing, a tradition that lives on in some indigenous peoples. During apprenticeship, the apprentice concocts a personal radiological thesaurus from the expressions, standard phrases, and idiosyncrasies passed on by trainers and peers. New technological developments bring along new terms, so this thesaurus continues to evolve. New insights acquired by the apprentice can likewise assert their influence. Simultaneously, language in the broadest sense continues to evolve, a process that speakers are generally little aware of. Taking all this into account, the question remains whether the radiology report ultimately serves the set objective, i.e., to ensure effective communication on the results of the examination (Bosmans 2011).

2 Basic Characteristics of a Radiology Report

While radiology itself from its conception in the dark days of late November 1895 has made progress at a breathtaking rate, how to report the findings has not been of much concern to anybody for almost a century. Grigg (1965) relates that at the beginning of the X-ray era, some considered radiographs as self-explaining. Others used arrows to elucidate pathological findings. Those who took the trouble to describe their findings produced something that looks like a present-day free-text report. The description of an abdominal X-ray quoted by Grigg is an iconic example. Grigg further quotes the US Army X-Ray Manual (1918) and books by the aforementioned Charles D. Enfield (1925); Schinz, Baensch, and Friedl (in German, 1928); Glasscheib (in German, 1936); and Reynburg (in Russian, 1938) as containing passages or chapters on radiology reporting. As to papers in peer-reviewed journals, Grigg states that guidelines were usually presented in editorials, and thus deleted from the annual table of contents (Grigg 1965). Well into the second half of the twentieth century, formulating guidelines for radiology reporting remained a concern for "wise old people," and indeed mostly took the form of an editorial, or even a letter to the editor.

3 Of Wise Men, and the Lack of a Shared Opinion

In the January 1983 edition of the American Journal of Roentgenology (AJR), Paul J. Friedman started his editorial with a sentence that became emblematic: "Communication is the goal of radiologic interpretation and reporting." Friedman stated that the wide variety in style and content of radiology reports is evidence that an optimum format has not yet been found. He reflected on what a good report should look like: concise (no "mindless litany of normal structures"); containing a short description of mild abnormalities which can be attributed to the age of the patient; aimed at answering the clinical question; consisting of a descriptive part in which different observations are neatly organized; and ending on an impression or a conclusion that contains some level of certainty. He mentioned the conviction by some that the impression (the conclusion) should come first, but advocates logical reasoning to come to an impression at the end of the report. In the interest of unequivocal communication, every report that is longer than two sentences should contain an impression (Friedman 1983).

Conrad S. Revak reacted to Friedman's editorial by presenting his own view. Taking into account the brevity of his letter to the editor,

Revak offered the reader a cornucopia of advices to create what he considers a good report: brevity; a narrative style; the use of paragraphs to separate pathology; the present tense; avoid "there is"; respond to questions in the request; avoid rigid word patterns; put the most important findings first; use inductive logic; give an impression if the description contains more than three sentences; discuss complicated cases; mention incidental findings only when relevant; state a degree of certainty; measure what is measurable; avoid radiologic slang; and if something goes wrong, deal with it in a business-like way, avoiding a tale of woe (Revak 1983). Fifteen years later, R.R. Armas will summarize the qualities of a good report as "six c's: clear; correct; containing a confidence level; concise; complete; and consistent (Armas 1998).

In 2000, Harvard's Ferris M. Hall authored an elaborate set of advices. In this "primer for residents and wayward radiologists," Hall points at new developments, such as computer-generated reports and the Breast Imaging Reporting and Data System (BIRADS), which are proof that efficient conveying of information does not require complete sentences in a narrative style. Since Revak's letter, things have clearly evolved! Hall shows himself an adversary of pleonasms ("an aphthous ulcer") an advocate of "there is" (!) and of acronyms ("when usage is well established"); a convincing challenger of expressions nobody understands the meaning of anymore, such as "a wet reading"; and of misconceptions, such as calling a contrast product "a dye." The baseline however is that Hall admits that his own opinions are constantly being challenged by colleagues with differing views (Hall 2000).

In 2008, Francesco Schiavon and Fabio Grigenti bundled the experience of former authors with their own, in the 138 pages of "Radiological Reporting in Clinical Practice." The book offers a solid theoretical basis for some of the principles of radiological reporting. In the introduction, the authors declare that they want to "encourage discussion of reporting within two often distant areas—medical and scientific knowledge, and humanistic and philosophical learning." They rightly state that "people called upon to write a report are not always aware of the technical, logical and conceptual processes governing the operations being carried out." Plato's reflections on how ideas derive from images are never far away in the rest of the book. It is fascinating reading, but residents who are looking for a quick way to improve their reporting skills will have to absorb a considerable amount of philosophy to find practical tips (Schiavon et al. 2008).

Of a totally different order is a more recent book by Curtis P. Langlotz. In "The Radiology Report, a Guide to Thoughtful Communication for Radiologists and Other Medical Professionals" (2015), Langlotz first sketches the history of the report, from the very early days till today's speech recognition, PACS (picture archiving and communication system) and RIS (radiology information system). The highly fashionable trend towards structured reporting gets much attention, and even that appears to be much older than one would suspect, taking into account the plea in favor of standardized roentgen reports, including nomenclature, by the aforementioned Detroit radiologist Preston M. Hickey (Langlotz 2015).

All these laudable attempts to improve the quality of the radiology report only emphasize that there is no universally valid opinion about its structure and content. To this day, both are strongly influenced by the personal preferences and experiences of radiologists. Style and language often depend on the kind of work they perform, on the subspecialty they practice, or on the institution where they have been trained. In addition, culture, traditions, and even limitations of the institution where they work influence reporting style. That is not necessarily negative: referring physicians can get used to the way their fellow radiologists express themselves, resulting in a symbiosis of perfect mutual understanding. On the other hand, radiologists often know how their reports are received and appreciated by referrers, and may do their best to comply with their demands. One may safely assume that most radiology reports are accurate and make a meaningful contribution to diagnostic and therapeutic management of a patient (Flanders and Lakhani 2012; Sherry et al. 2011; European Society of Radiology (ESR) 2011a;

Bosmans et al. 2011a, b). A less positive side is that many radiologists tend to overestimate the quality of their own reports. In the ROVER survey, not less than 40% of the radiologists thought their reports were better than those of their colleagues (Bosmans et al. 2011a).

Theoretically, the effectiveness of radiology reports can be derived from the number of recipients who understand the report. Usual recipients are referring GPs, specialists or residents, other caregivers, and fellow radiologists who consult priors or prepare a multidisciplinary meeting. The number of patients who have access to the report is rising as well (Flanders and Lakhani 2012). While most GPs are highly dependent on the report, many specialists use the report as a reference document when analyzing the images themselves, especially in case of rather simple studies, such as conventional radiographs. The radiologist must also consider that in some cases the recipient will only read the conclusion of the report, although, in the COVER survey, two-thirds of the referring clinicians denied doing so (Bosmans et al. 2011a). Moreover, the digital revolution has considerably widened the gap between referring clinicians and radiologists. Fellow physicians visiting the radiology department to seek additional information have become rare. Due to these evolutions, the radiology report has gained even more importance as a sole means of communication, which must be an additional stimulus to improve its quality.

4 Elements of the Report

The basic components of the radiological report are explained in the Practice Guideline for Communication of the American College of Radiology (ACR) and the Guidelines for Radiological Reporting of the European Society of Radiology (ESR) (Sherry et al. 2011; European Society of Radiology (ESR) 2011a; Kushner et al. 2005). What follows is a concise summary of these guidelines.

Each radiological examination must result in a final (official) written report, regardless of where the examination took place. A typical report consists of a description of the findings and a conclusion/impression or, if necessary, a differential diagnosis. In each report, the following elements should be present:

1. Demographic data of the patient and date and time of the examination
2. Relevant history, clinical information, and questions
3. A description of the procedure and the findings:
   (a) Technique and procedure, including the administration of contrast and/or the use of materials.
   (b) Findings: The author (radiologist) must use the correct anatomical, pathological, and radiological terminology to describe the findings as accurately as possible.
   (c) Potential limitations: the report must mention all factors that hinder proper interpretation, such as artifacts.
   (d) Clinical remarks: the report has to answer as well as possible the clinical question in the examination request.
   (e) Comparative data: the study should be compared with previous similar studies, where available.
4. Impression/Conclusion/Diagnosis
   (a) Unless the report is very short, any report must contain a conclusion in which, if possible, an accurate diagnosis is mentioned.
   (b) Where necessary, a differential diagnosis must be included.
   (c) Advice concerning additional or follow-up examinations shall be given where necessary.

4.1 Demographic Data

Demographic data include the following: identity of the patient (name, date of birth, gender), the patient number in the institution (or the social security number, used to unequivocally identify the patient), the location of the examination, the name of the referring physician, and type, date, and time of the study (Sherry et al. 2011). In most hospitals where such data is exchanged digitally via the HIS, RIS, PACS, and/or the EHR, these elements are automatically added to the report.

4.2 Clinical History, Information, and Questions

This section of the report contains a summary of the condition that necessitates the study ("indications" or "justification"). To make an appropriate analysis of the images and a correct answer to the clinical question possible, it is important that the referring physician briefly states the relevant history of the patient. The importance of repeating concise but relevant clinical information in the report cannot be overestimated, as it offers the recipient an idea of what the radiologist already knew at the time of the examination (Flanders and Lakhani 2012). It allows the referring physician to check if the radiologist has read the clinical question, and, doing so, get more out of the report than when the radiologist did not take the clinical question into account (Wallis and McCoubrie 2011). It is also appropriate to mention in the report the absence of useful clinical information, as this may help the reader to understand any sign of uncertainty or confusion in the report (Wallis and McCoubrie 2011; European Society of Radiology (ESR) 2011a). In a growing number of hospitals, the EHR offers digital imaging requests, which allow easy integration of clinical information. However, studies have shown that even this automated approach can be problematic and does not always correlate with the actual clinical condition of the patient (Flanders and Lakhani 2012; Van Borsel et al. 2016). Another disadvantage of the automatically generated request may be that the radiologist becomes less aware of the need to verify the relevance of the information.

4.3 Technique

In general, it is not necessary to provide a detailed description of the technique used for a simple examination, in contrast to more complex studies, such as radiological interventions, CT, and MR examinations. Both ACR and ESR advise to include a brief description of the examination technique, especially when using a nonstandard approach (e.g., additional MRI sequences). Mentioning contrast administration is recommended, including way of access, type of contrast, and dose. Allergic reactions must be recorded and reported (Sherry et al. 2011; Kushner et al. 2005; European Society of Radiology (ESR) 2011b).

The mention of the technical quality of the study is recommended, especially when it is suboptimal (Wallis and McCoubrie 2011; European Society of Radiology (ESR) 2011b). This is useful to illustrate the limitations of the study, but it should not be used by the radiologist to justify the hedge (Wallis and McCoubrie 2011).

4.4 Comparative Studies

Comparison with previous studies (priors), if available, must be made, including the date of those studies. The unavailability of previous studies should be mentioned as well.

4.5 Findings

This is usually the most extensive part of the report. It consists of a structured, targeted, and comprehensible description of any abnormality. The most relevant findings in the context of the clinical question should be mentioned first. The structure of the report may be either organ oriented or oriented in function of the disease. Consistency in this approach is the basis of the standardized or structured report. A schematic representation of the structure of a report can be found in Table 1.

- The terminology should be as accurate as possible, avoiding loose terms such as "shadowing." Where measurable, data such as physical dimensions, signal intensity, signal change, and/or enhancement of abnormalities should be quantified.
- Specific positive or negative features that will affect interpretation of the abnormalities, such as margin delineation, calcification, or cavitation, should also be described (European Society of Radiology (ESR) 2011b).

Table 1 Components of a structured radiology report

Clinical information and question	• Clinical history and context • Justification of examination: indication, question, medical necessity • Risk factors: allergies (if relevant), renal function
Demographic data	• Identity data (name, sex, date of birth) • Identifier/medical record number • Date, time, and location of image acquisition
Imaging technique	• Type of examination, imaging device • Details about the technique used, imaging parameters • Preparation of patient (if relevant) • Contrast administration (name, dose, route, quantity) • Technical quality of examination
Comparison	• Date and type of previous examinations reviewed, if applicable • Absence of priors should be mentioned
Findings	• Organ- or pathology-oriented structure • Correct and unequivocal descriptive terminology • Precise description of abnormality(ies) with concrete and measurable data • Logical order: most relevant findings first • Accurate morphological description • Correct anatomical description • Correlation with clinical and other relevant data • Relevant negative findings • Relevant incidental findings • Functional information, quantitative data (if available)
Other	• Use of standardized scoring system, if applicable
Conclusion (impression)	• Summary of the most relevant findings • Interpretation of the examination in relation to all other data • Provision of diagnosis if possible, or short differential diagnosis in order of probability • Formulate answer to the question • Recommendation(s) or advice regarding further diagnostics or approach

- The anatomical location of the abnormality should be described as accurately as possible, as well as the relation to the surrounding structures. Including references to relevant images can help the recipient too.
- Negative findings should be mentioned if relevant.
- Incidental findings should be noted and analyzed (see "Incidental findings").

Representing the findings in a structured and standardized way deserves recommendation, especially in case of oncological follow-up studies. Radiologists should adhere as much as possible to standardized scoring systems, such as RECIST for oncological follow-up, BI-RADS for breast imaging, PI-RADS for prostate MRI imaging, C-RADS for colon cancer CT, and LI-RADS for hepatocellular carcinoma. Additional structured approaches may be required in hospitals with specific expertise, e.g., in cancer-related surgery of pancreas or rectum. In close collaboration with referrers, structured checklist-type reports can be developed. A good example of a nationwide accepted type of report is the MRI staging protocol of rectal cancer in the Netherlands, which can be found on The Radiology Assistant website (van Loenhout et al. 2015).

4.6 Conclusion or Impression

The conclusion or impression is the most frequently read part of the report, as it summarizes the most important findings, correlates those to the available clinical information and to additional examination results (e.g., biochemical), and, ideally, answers the clinical question. Where possible, the conclusion will provide a diagnosis, or at least a differential diagnosis, listed in descending order of probability. Arguments that make elements in the differential diagnosis less likely can also be mentioned or explained. The conclusion should contain an answer to the clinical question or a statement explaining why the answer cannot be provided. If no correlation can be found between the clinical condition and the radiological findings, this should also be mentioned (European Society of Radiology (ESR) 2011b). In case of an incidental finding, the conclusion must mention its clinical relevance. Finally, the conclusion may contain recommendations for further studies, either radiological or other. The radiologist, however, must be aware of the value of these supplemental studies for the diagnostic and therapeutic outcome, of the risks involved and of the supplemental cost for patient and healthcare system. Moreover, the advice must be balanced against the risk that the referrer may request additional studies to avoid being held liable if not taking the advice into account (Wallis and McCoubrie 2011). Radiologists who do not have sufficient clinical information are at risk of recommending unnecessary additional studies. It is therefore advisable to specify in the conclusion the logic that justifies those studies.

The phrase "to be correlated with the clinical findings" should be avoided, as it may be considered an attempt by the radiologist to cover up errors or uncertainty. Never must it be used as a substrate for an accurate diagnosis (Wallis and McCoubrie 2011).

Table 2 gives some tips on formulating a good conclusion.

Table 2 Tips for a good conclusion/impression

In short reports no conclusion is necessary
Provide an answer to the clinical question
Try to provide a diagnostic opinion, avoid "hedging" against errors
Restrict the list of differential diagnoses
Adapt the recommendation(s) regarding further examination(s) to its impact on the treatment
Systematically mention that the results were already orally discussed, if applicable, when, and with whom

4.7 Radiation Information

In the European Union, the EURATOM Directive 2013/59, adopted in 2013, will be implemented in 2018. This directive tightens the existing requirements for the registration and reporting of dosimetric data and imposes new legal requirements on all EU member states regarding the information provided to patients about exposure to radiation. From 6 February 2018, the radiological organizations/associations and industry must adapt their regulations, practices, and equipment in accordance with these directives. According to Art. 58.b, information on the patient's exposure radiation during radiological examination has to be included in the report (Anon 2013; European Society of Radiology (ESR) 2015). However, this article does not specify the form in which this information should be provided in the report. Most probably, dosimetric data must be included. This assumption is based upon the recently published ESR summary of Directive 2013/59, which states that "… it contains significant changes regarding … dosimetric information in imaging systems and its transfer to the examination report" (European Society of Radiology (ESR) 2015). This may imply that the data from the dosimetry system will have to be transmitted electronically to the RIS or EHR via an HL-7 link, to include them automatically in the report, which is more or less similar to the way demographics are currently imported in the report. What type of radiation descriptor is to be used (dose area product, dose-length product, organ dose, or other) had not yet been specified at the time this book was prepared. It may be the subject of further interpretation of the directive by individual EU member states, presumably according to the advice by the European Federation of Medical Physics (EFOMP). In the United States, those requirements depend on the individual states.

5 Terminology and Style

The terminology of the report should take into account the expected level of knowledge of the reader. Particular medical abbreviations, for instance, may be perfectly understood by referrers from the same institution, but completely unclear to other recipients. As is the case with esoteric abbreviations in the request form, unnecessary or unusual abbreviations should be avoided in the radiology report as well (Berlin 2013; Bosmans 2013).

It makes little sense to extensively describe findings without any clinical significance. Obsolete and redundant words, such as sentences starting with "There is …" can irritate the recipient. Brevity, as in Revak's time, is still the hallmark of the master (Revak 1983).

The radiologist must always keep in mind which recipients the report is meant for; one size does not fit all. While most surgeons seem to prefer concise, telegram-style reports, other specialists may value grammatically correct sentences. Radiologists provide services; it is necessary that we check whether the services provided meet the expectations of our clients. Particularly the clarity of the report, tailored to the level of knowledge of the recipient, is generally highly valued (Wallis and McCoubrie 2011).

6 The Final Report

The final report is the means by which the results of a study are formally communicated to the referring physician. The report may be delivered either in print or in electronic form. Ideally, the report is incorporated automatically in the RIS or EHR. Other, more direct methods of communication are highly recommended in particular situations. The delay between study and delivery of the report will mainly depend on the level of urgency of the clinical problem.

- All reports must be proofread and signed, electronically or otherwise.
- The final report must be sent to the referring physician. The referring physician shares with the radiologist the responsibility to obtain and read reports of the studies that he or she has requested.
- If possible and useful, at the request of the patient or with his/her consent, a copy of the original report may be sent or made available to other care providers, such as GPs or other specialists.
- If a second reading or opinion diverts from the initial report, an addendum should be added. This addendum should be made known to the author of the initial report, or be added by himself/herself, or at least added with his/her permission.

7 Guidelines and Protocols

Medical diagnoses or decisions regarding therapy increasingly depend on imaging. Even when radiologists make a perfect analysis of the images, patients may not get optimal benefit from the examination if communication about the results is less than perfect. Lack of timely communication between referring physician and radiologist has become one of the five most common causes of malpractice litigation in radiology in the United States (Flanders and Lakhani 2012; European Society of Radiology (ESR) 2011a).

Nowadays, radiological reports are integrated into the RIS or EHR, sent electronically to the referring physician, or, together with the images, saved onto a CD-ROM. Some systems provide delivery monitoring: radiologists automatically receive a notification when the report has not been opened within a reasonable time span. Such systems are still relatively little used. Moreover, they are not entirely watertight, especially with regard to life-threatening situations (Flanders and Lakhani 2012).

Of course, radiologists and referring specialists are not confined to the written exchange of information. Direct communication, either in person, by phone, or by safely encrypted chat, must be encouraged. It helps to select the most appropriate examination, both in terms of medical efficiency and cost-effectiveness, and can help referring physicians to better understand the results and consequences of the examination (Kushner et al. 2005). It is advisable to mention in the report the name of the referrer with whom there has been direct contact, together with the time at which it happened. If the radiologist deems that immediate action must be undertaken, it is his/her duty to contact the referring physician without delay. If the referrer cannot be reached, the radiologist must contact the doctor in charge of the patient at that moment or, if necessary, the emergency department. In all circumstances, including unexpected findings, the radiologist has to make sure that the results have been received and understood by the recipient.

The ESR states that timely communication of urgent incidental findings is the shared responsibility of the institution and the radiologist (Kushner et al. 2005). Hospitals are expected to invest in secure electronic communication systems. Radiologists have to make sure that they have robust protocols to transmit reports in a timely, reliable, and consistent way.

- In those communication protocols, radiologists must specify which means of communication they use, either directly or indirectly. If communication is digital, they must specify how records will be marked as urgent.

- Radiologists are considered to work in accordance with the communication protocols. If there are none such protocols, the radiologist must take initiatives to ensure that the report was communicated effectively, regardless of the means by which this was realized.

For ESR, communication is urgent in case of any finding by which the patient can experience harm if action is not taken urgently. Examples are pulmonary embolism, complicated fractures, and acute hemorrhage. Consequences of nontreatment can be so severe that the radiologist must directly contact the doctor in charge of the patient.

According to the ESR, it is not necessary that the referring physician is contacted directly if the radiologist detects a nonurgent clinically important incidental finding, such as a tumor. In such a case, an electronic marker can be attached to the report, or it can be accompanied by an e-mail message. Incidental findings in general remain a subject for discussion, according to ESR. Urgent communication is necessary when short-term action needs to be undertaken; if not, standard communication protocols can be followed.

In the ACR guidelines, in contrast, it is stated that the radiologist must contact the referring physician in case of urgent or clinically significant incidental findings (Flanders and Lakhani 2012; Sherry et al. 2011). Examples are:

- Findings requiring immediate surgical intervention (e.g., cerebral hemorrhage, cerebral infarction)
- Findings discordant with the previous interpretation of the same study (or with the interim report if available), or when omission of necessary action can have a negative effect on the health of the patient (e.g., a large multiple sclerosis plaque instead of a brain tumor)
- Unexpected findings that can negatively affect the health of the patient (e.g., a renal tumor accidentally discovered on a CT scan of the lumbar spine)

In those circumstances, direct verbal communication is necessary, and this must also be documented.

These ACR guidelines have already caused much debate. Some consider them outdated, as the use of structured reporting is increasing steadily, in conjunction with the secure digital transmission of reports. Others, however, indicate that these new technological developments also steadily augment the expectations of referring clinicians. In addition, parallel to the increasing complexity of imaging studies themselves, communication too becomes more complex, thus increasing the workload and, by consequence, leaving less room for effective communication. And in all cases, radiologists must take care not too frequently being distracted from their primary task. Getting the right physician at the phone at the right time can be a challenge, especially in larger hospitals, where they often work in teams and shifts at the emergency room (ER). The radiologist must try to transmit the information to the person who is most appropriate to take action on short term. A notice to a secretary cannot be accepted as a substitute. Assurance that the message was clearly understood by those in charge is indeed an essential part of the communication process. A difficult question is how the radiologist can be certain that the message has been fully understood, and appropriate action has been undertaken.

In case no suitable person can be reached, the radiologist may consider directly providing the patient with the results, including information on which steps should be undertaken, e.g., referral to ER (Flanders and Lakhani 2012).

8 Closed-Loop Communication

The digitization of radiology, and in particular the use of PACS, has led to the situation that personal communication between radiologists and clinicians has become increasingly rare (Weiss et al. 2014). In patient care, as we already said, it is important that diagnostic information is properly received and understood by the recipient. When communication is synchronous (in person, by phone, or by encrypted chat), that is usually not a problem. The main disadvantage of synchronous communication however is that it can be very time consuming for both the radiologist and the referring physician. Most problems occur in electronic or asynchronous communication. Thanks to speech recognition, radiologists can report their findings almost in real time and send the result to the RIS or EHR. In most of these systems, however, there is no mechanism to ensure that the referring physician has read and understood the report.

Creating a closed-loop communication, providing certainty that results and advice were received and understood is currently one of the most fundamental challenges in radiology management. A system that starts with an electronic request, conduction of the study, creating a report, sending the report to the recipient, and finally confirmation of receipt, all that without the intervention of the radiologist, is currently nonexistent and will perhaps remain utopian (Weiss et al. 2014). To attain a closed-loop communication, it is necessary that all software systems are seamlessly connected, and linked with a data model that allows carrying out the necessary quality controls and benchmarking.

One of the links of the loop is speech recognition. Indispensable as it may be these days, it can be the cause of many errors, due to faulty pronunciation, accent, poor microphone position, background noise, inability of the system to recognize particular words, etc. Speech engines get better all the time, and the brighter cousin of speech recognition, natural language processing (NLP), is coming our way. Some companies already offer this feature as "clinical language understanding" (Weiss et al. 2014). NLP is indeed able to filter meaningful information from dictation, e.g., to produce automatic structured reports. It facilitates text and data search, and thus can be used to automatically correct reports (Weiss et al. 2014). Ideally, NLP would systematically screen reports for critical terms, and warn the radiologist that urgent action needs to be undertaken. After verification by the radiologist, the system could then further automatically activate various communication techniques, such as encrypted messaging services and SMS messages via the internal telephone network. A voice message could be added or linked to the report automatically. Unanswered messages could trigger a call to another person. For less urgent findings (e.g., an incidental lung nodule) an e-mail or nonurgent message might be sent, still with verification that the message has been read (Flanders and Lakhani 2012). If none of the medical recipients can be reached, the assignment could be given to a radiological secretary, to verify manually the timely receipt of the report by the referring clinician, on a regular basis.

Some institutions have developed dedicated software to facilitate critical imaging test result communication. An example of such a system is the Automated Critical Test Result Notification System (ANCR) that was developed at the Brigham and Women's Hospital in Boston. When the radiologist activates the ANCR while reviewing an imaging study in which a critical result was identified, he/she can select an appropriate alert level depending on the emergency of the finding. Consecutively, an alert notification is sent to the referring clinician through a paging and/or e-mail system. The results of a study conducted with this system have shown that the use of ANCR reduces medical errors and improves the quality of patient care (Lacson et al. 2014).

In closed-loop communication, it would also be possible to include follow-up information, such as the advice to carry out additional studies.

9 Structured Reporting

As we have shown earlier, the narrative report has undergone little or no change in the course of 120 years. Since the middle of the 1980s however, numerous surveys have shown that both radiologists and referring physicians prefer structured (preformatted, itemized, tabular ...) reports (Bosmans 2015). Elsewhere in this book, Marta E. Heilbrun elaborates on the subject. Therefore, we only briefly explain why, in most cases, the narrative report should be abandoned in favor of a structured report.

Despite multiple advantages of structuring the radiology report, many radiologists are still reluctant to embrace the idea, which delays its large-scale introduction. One of the reasons for their hesitation is the lack of standardization in reporting. Another reason is the lack of technical support and the scarcity of SR-based applications. In addition, radiologists are afraid that the introduction of SR will necessitate a considerable investment of time, and will hinder and slow down the workflow.

Nonetheless, there is a growing demand and need for SR (European Society of Radiology (ESR) 2011b) for various reasons. Using SR, information is presented in a reproducible, unequivocal way, which contributes to more accurate communication. The radiologist is invited to use a kind of checklist, which facilitates completeness. If the software is good, SR can be time-saving, and thus make workflow more efficient.

SR makes it possible to retrieve data in a (semi-) automated way, by applying techniques such as NLP (natural language processing), and by implementing an underlying standardized coding system, such as RadLex or SNOMED-CT. This is an asset for research, auditing, and education.

At this moment, most models for SR are based on a modular format template, consisting of functional, "itemized" sections. In some centers, starting speech recognition software automatically opens the right template for a particular study. Each section contains a checklist-type summary of the topics that need to be addressed. A large part of this information can be filled in automatically (e.g., demographic data, clinical information, clinical question, technique), which saves valuable time. Theoretically, additional relevant information, such as measurements, comparative metrics, annotations, key images, and multimedia data can also be integrated (semi-) automatically. Copying errors can thus be prevented, which increases the recipients' confidence in the report (European Society of Radiology (ESR) 2011b).

Ideally, structured reports are linked to an underlying coded lexicon or ontology (European Society of Radiology (ESR) 2011b). Not all radiologists are in favor of this approach, as they feel "forced" to adopt a vocabulary which may not be their own. Reports using nonstandardized terminology, however, have been shown to be less understandable (Flanders and Lakhani 2012). Moreover, an underlying ontology makes it easier to automatically translate reports, to extract data for scientific and epidemiological purposes, and to feed "deep learning software" and auto-analysis. To facilitate data exchange and optimize technical support, international standards need to be developed and implemented for SR, similar to the DICOM standards for image exchange (Rylands-Monk 2015). RSNA and ESR support the MRRT ("Management of Radiology Report Templates") standard, which was developed by the IHE Radiology Committee. Adhering to these standards will also facilitate the linking of underlying metadata or encoding(s) of the report to other data, such as those obtained from computer-based morphological image analysis, which is of major importance for the further development of deep learning algorithms. Using advanced techniques such as NLP, it will be possible to develop tools that utilize the data of the reports for other applications, such as clinical decision support (CDS), workflow analysis, and quality management (Weiss et al. 2014).

Increasingly, political decisions in healthcare are based on evidence and cost-benefit analysis. This in turn increases external pressure to implement standardization, such as SR. Although radiology has always embraced new technology, introducing SR will require extraordinary efforts. Financial incentives may be required to motivate the acceptance of new ways of reporting.

10 The Report of the Future

The future radiologist will be a communication specialist. Where today communication is mainly limited to getting requests and providing reports, radiologists will increasingly have to communicate with patients as well. Further integration of structured reporting in the workflow can contribute

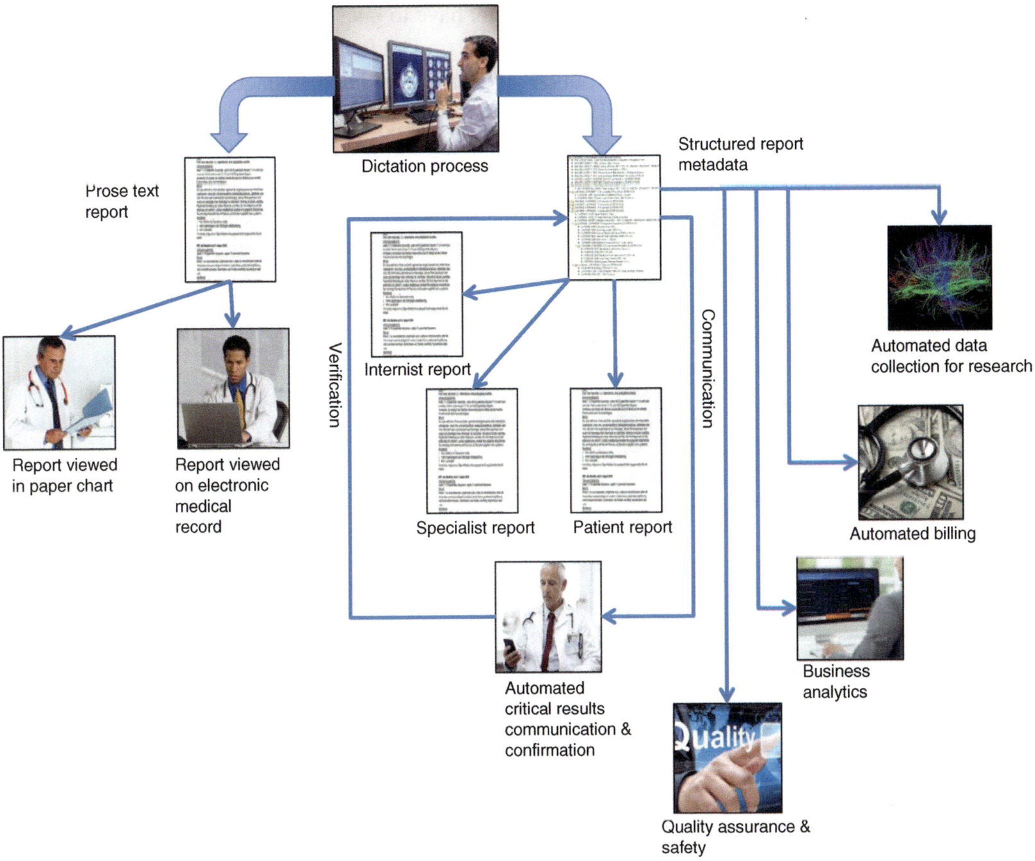

Fig. 1 Comparison of the route of the conventional prose report with the structured report (SR). The conventional report *(left)* is stored in a printed version or electronically in the EHR. The electronic SR *(right)* is rich in metadata and offers the possibility to feed several automated processes, such as the creation of different types of reports, communication of critical findings with verification, automatized collection of data for research, business analytics software, quality management, and invoicing

positively to the transformation of the profession in several ways.

A structured report rich in metadata allows the addition of many other functions (see Fig. 1). The invisible associated metadata and codes can be linked to other databases. This data can then be used for other automated processes, such as the generation of different types of reports, depending on the type of recipient. Using structured report data and associated metadata, a computer would be able to make a prose-rich report. Ambiguous and confusing terminology or structure would be filtered out automatically. The report would also automatically be adjusted to the preferences or the background of the referring clinician (specialist versus general practitioner) or even the patient. Different users, in other words, using a variety of software "glasses" to read the report, would each get exactly the kind and level of information they need, i.e., information pertinent to their needs and expectations. If a standardized lexicon underlies each structured report, relationships can be established more easily with related terminology (synonyms), or even other languages. This would allow the automatic creation of patient-centered reports (using layman's terms) as well as reports with highly specialized content, directed at the specialist. Software to create easy-to-use multimedia structured reports already exists today (Ranschaert 2016). Through incorporation of NLP, metadata are automatically extracted from narrative text dictated by the radiologistwith the purpose of tagging relevant images. All data are assembled into a graphical representation of the patient, with the key images linked to anatomical sites (Fig. 2). Thereport data can also be integrated into a follow-up timeline displaying the evolution of the disease, integrating all therapies and observations. In addition this information can be used for data mining. Media-rich reports will create value for both referencing physicians and patients. From these reports, the referring physicians will not have to guess anymore what the radiologist is referring to. In addition, the need to fully translate reports into lay language could be eliminated, since key findings can be directly annotated and marked on the images so that they are explained for patients in an understandable manner.

Another new development is to provide patients with an online system that adds descrip-

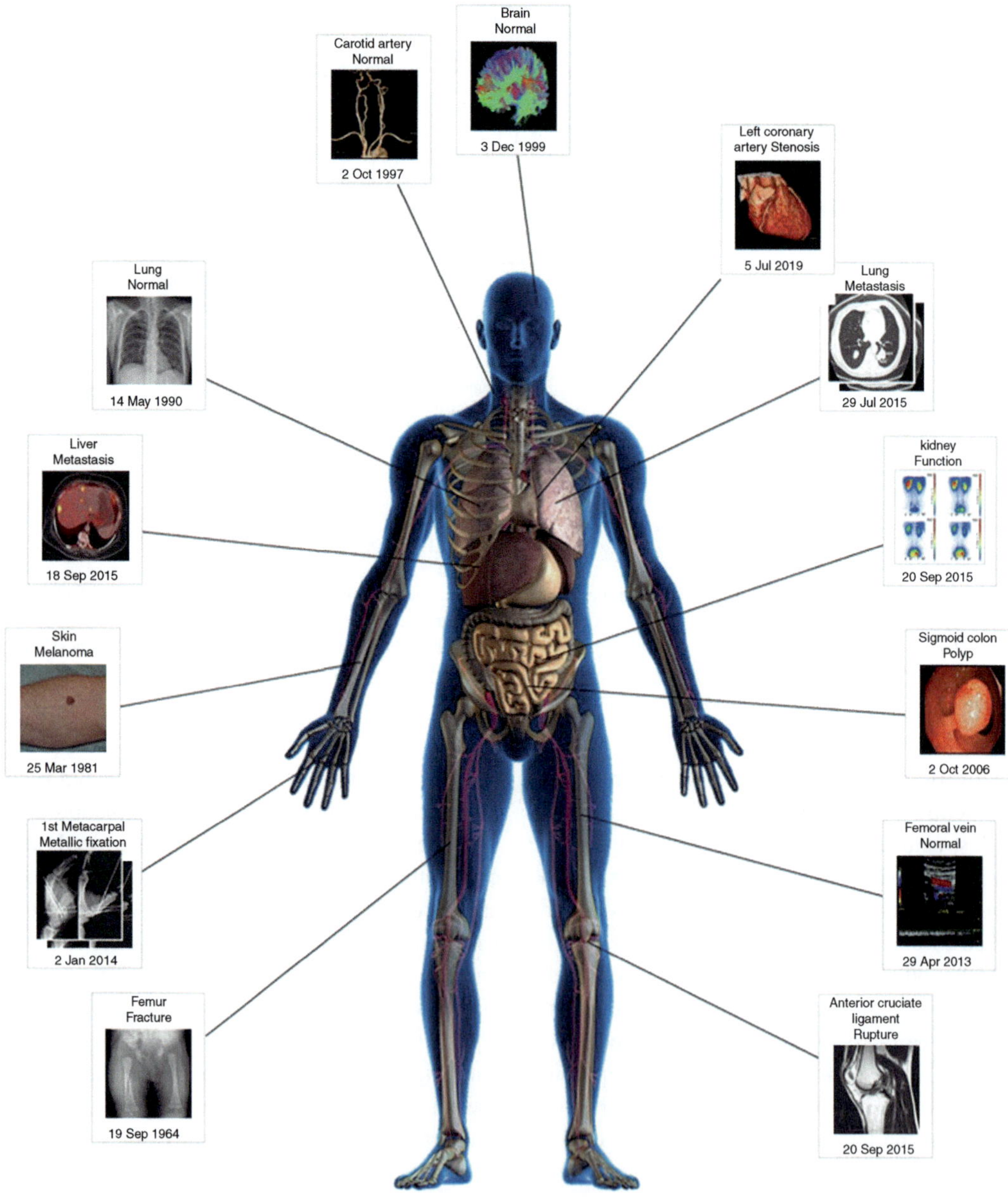

Fig. 2 A software system to create a multimedia structured reporting system presents radiology reports as a graphical presentation of a patient with the key images linked to anatomical sites (with permission of David J. Vining, July 2017)

tions/definitions and illustrations to the medical and technical terms used in the report. A recently published study (Cook et al. 2017) has shown that such a system allows patients to better understand the report. For this purpose, a *Patient-Oriented Radiology Reporter* (PORTER) tool was developed. It uses a Web-based interface for patients to add annotations from a lexicon to the text of the report, as well as anatomical drawings and hyperlinks to additional information. In the study, this PORTER tool was used to clarify reports of knee MRI studies for 7 months. Of the patients who viewed the online report, 77% agreed that the additional annotations helped them to understand the report. To 91% of users, the drawings were very helpful, which proves that anatomical images in multimedia reports can be very useful (Ranschaert 2016; Cook et al. 2017).

New standards need to be developed to ensure that structured reports containing quantitative data, metadata, and multimedia content become easily transportable, exchangeable, and machine readable, so they can be integrated into other applications, such as automatic workflow analysis and invoicing (Fig. 1).

Reports will be used to feed other databases, so clinical decision support software can be improved, and national and international monitoring and/or benchmarking of radiation becomes much easier. Links to imaging biobanks will facilitate deep learning techniques, and thereby contribute to the improvement of automated image analysis. It is however necessary that healthcare organizations and policy makers fundamentally change the way they experience the role of radiology. The seamless sharing of data, with appropriate levels of security and confidentiality, requires new national and international policy guidelines as well as daring strategic investment.

11 Reporting Training for Residents

During training, little attention is paid to reporting skills. The training of radiology residents must lead to well-trained radiologists, who are not only able to interpret radiological examinations but also to communicate efficiently with referring clinicians, patients, and other stakeholders (Cook et al. 2017). Usually, radiology residents learn to report according to the apprenticeship model. That model, however, has many shortcomings (Bosmans 2011). Moreover, the way interim reports are created which need to be reviewed, amended, and validated by a supervisor is prone to errors. In most cases, supervision takes place through oral consultation. The availability and motivation of the supervisor can determine whether the report is reliable or not. In some institutions, residents are expected to actively follow the studies they have made and to check the final report, but this does not always happen consistently. The quality and quantity of the feedback by supervisors can vary widely, and are usually not well documented (Gorniak et al. 2013). At present, it is already possible to evaluate the reporting skills of radiology residents longitudinally and qualitatively in a few digital platforms, but it is not yet a part of their formal evaluation (Gorniak et al. 2013; Surrey et al. 2013). Most tests and evaluation programs focus primarily on the resident's assessment skills, rather than on the ability to create a coherent and proper radiological report (Gorniak et al. 2013).

In view of the increasing importance of good communication in radiology and medicine, we believe that it would be useful to pay more attention to the longitudinal evaluation of the reporting skills of future radiologists. There is certainly space for a formalized test to objectively evaluate their communication skills, including their ability to report. Such implies, of course, that the supervisors themselves are "trained to train," and above all that they acquire excellent communication and reporting skills.

References

Euratom Anon (2013) Council Directive 2013/59 EURATOM of 5 December 2013 laying down basic safety standards for protection against the dangers arising from exposure to ionising radiation, and repealing Directives 89/618/Euratom, 90/641/Euratom, 96/29/Euratom, 97/43/Euratom and 2003/122/Euratom. Available: https://ec.europa.eu/energy/sites/ener/files/documents/CELEX-32013L0059-EN-TXT.pdf. Accessed 8 May 2017

Armas R (1998) Qualities of a good radiology report. Am J Roentgenol 170:1110
Berlin L (2013) TAC: AOITROMJA? (the acronym conundrum: advancing or impeding the readability of medical Journal articles?). Radiology 266(2):383–387
Bosmans J (2011) The radiology report, from prose to structured reporting and back again? Ph.D. thesis, University of Antwerp. Available: http://hdl.handle.net/1854/LU-1900882. Accessed 8 May 2017
Bosmans J (2013) Abbreviations in request forms. Radiology 268(2):610–610
Bosmans J (2015) What are the concrete benefits of structured reporting for the referring physicians? European Congress of Radiology 2015, Vienna (oral presentation)
Bosmans J, Weyler J, Parizel P (2009) Structure and content of radiology reports, a quantitative and qualitative study in eight medical centers. Eur J Radiol 72(2):354–358
Bosmans J, Weyler J, De Schepper A, Parizel P (2011a) The radiology report as seen by radiologists and referring clinicians: results of the COVER and ROVER surveys. Radiology 259(1):184–195
Bosmans J, Peremans L, De Schepper A, Duyck P, Parizel P (2011b) How do referring clinicians want radiologists to report? Suggestions from the COVER survey. Insights Imaging 2(5):577–584
Cook T, Oh S, Kahn C (2017) Patients' use and evaluation of an online system to annotate radiology reports with lay language definitions. Acad Radiol. doi: 10.1016/j.acra.2017.03.005. [Epub ahead of print]
European Society of Radiology (ESR) (2011a) ESR guidelines for the communication of urgent and unexpected findings. Insights Imaging 3(1):1–3
European Society of Radiology (ESR) (2011b) Good practice for radiological reporting. Guidelines from the European Society of Radiology (ESR). Insights Imaging 2(2):93–96
European Society of Radiology (ESR) (2015) Summary of the European directive 2013/59/Euratom: essentials for health professionals in radiology. Insights Imaging 6(4):411–417
Flanders A, Lakhani P (2012) Radiology reporting and communications. Neuroimaging Clin N Am 22(3):477–496
Friedman P (1983) Radiologic reporting: structure. Am J Roentgenol 140:171–172
Gorniak R, Flanders A, Sharpe R (2013) Trainee report dashboard: tool for enhancing feedback to radiology trainees about their reports. Radiographics 33(7):2105–2113
Grigg E (1965) The trail of the invisible light. 1st edn. Charles C Thomas (Ed.). Springfield IL. pp 692–693
Hall F (2000) Language of the radiology report: a primer for residents and wayward radiologists. Am J Roentgenol 175:1239–1242
Kushner D, Lucey L, American College of Radiology (2005) Diagnostic radiology reporting and communication: the ACR guideline. J Am Coll Radiol 2(1):15–21
Lacson R, O'Connor SD, Andriole KP, Prevedello LM, Khorasani R (2014) Automated critical test result notification system: architecture, design, and assessment of provider satisfaction. Am J Roentgenol 203(5):W491–W496. doi:10.2214/AJR.14.13063
Langlotz CP (2015) The radiology report, a guide to thoughtful communication for radiologists and other medical professionals, 1st edn. CreateSpace Independent Publishing Platform, San Bernardino. ISBN 978-1515174080
van Loenhout R, Zijta F, Lahaye M, Beets-Tan R, Smithuis R (2015) Rectal Cancer - MR staging 2.0. Available: http://www.radiologyresident.nl/en/p56195b237699d/rectal-cancer-mr-staging-20.html. Accessed 8 May 2017
Ranschaert E (2016) The impact of information technology on radiology services. Ph.D. thesis, University of Antwerp. Available: https://repository.uantwerpen.be/docman/irua/465bef/134701.pdf. Accessed 8 May 2017
Revak C (1983) Dictation of radiologic reports (letter). Am J Roentgenol 141:210
Rylands-Monk F (2015) Standardization moves streamline Europe's reporting structures. ECR Today newspaper, March 4, 11. Available: http://myesr.org/media/254. Accessed 20 May 2017
Schiavon F, Grigenti F, Van Terheyden N (2008) Radiological reporting in clinical practice, 1st edn. Springer, Milan
Sherry C, Adams M, Berlin L, Fajardo L, Gazelle G (2011) ACR practice guideline for communication of diagnostic imaging findings. Available: http://xray.ufl.edu/files/2008/11/communication-of-diagnostic-imaging-findings.pdf. Accessed 8 May 2017
Sistrom C, Lanier L, Mancuso A (2004) Reporting instruction for radiology residents. Acad Radiol 11(1):76–84
Surrey D, Sharpe R, Gorniak R, Nazarian L, Rao V, Flanders A (2013) QRSE: a novel metric for the evaluation of trainee radiologist reporting skills. J Digit Imaging 26(4):678–682
Van Borsel M, Devolder P, Bosmans J (2016) Software solutions alone cannot guarantee useful radiology requests. Acta Radiol 57(11):1366–1371
Wallis A, McCoubrie P (2011) The radiology report—are we getting the message across? Clin Radiol 66(11):1015–1022
Weiss D, Kim W, Branstetter B, Prevedello L (2014) Radiology reporting: a closed-loop cycle from order entry to results communication. J Am Coll Radiol 11(12):1226–1237

Image Interpretation

Angel Alberich-Bayarri

Contents

A. Alberich-Bayarri, Ph.D.
Biomedical Imaging Research Group (GIBI230), La Fe Health Research Institute, La Fe Polytechnics and University Hospital, Av. Fernando Abril Martorell 106, Tower A, 7th Floor, Valencia 46026, Spain

Quantitative Imaging Biomarkers in Medicine (QUIBIM SL), Valencia, Spain
e-mail: angel@quibim.com

Abstract

Image interpretation is the core process of radiological workflow. Current visualization environments contain a set of tools to help in the annotation of relevant imaging findings. However, there still exist important challenges for interoperability between different platforms when working with annotated images. How the annotations and findings are reported is also evolving, moving from traditional descriptive texts towards item-based structured reports. Finally, thanks to the recent advances in the artificial intelligence science, specifically in machine learning algorithms it has been possible to implement a growing number of computer-aided detection solutions to assist radiologists in the image interpretation process. Image interpretation is under a process of paradigm shift, from traditional image reading through observation and free text reporting of the findings, towards the inclusion of new technologies in the loop such as computer-aided detection and diagnosis (CAD), imaging biomarker extraction, and structured reporting. The advance in interoperability between systems to standardize image annotation formats, together with the growing use of structured reporting and AI-assisted image reading, will shape radiology as one of the most relevant data sciences in the era of precision medicine.

Med Radiol Diagn Imaging (2017)
DOI 10.1007/174_2017_121, © Springer International Publishing AG
Published Online 09 August 2017

1 Introduction

Image interpretation is the core of radiological workflow. The radiologist has to read the images with efficiency and effectiveness and translate them to understandable and meaningful information from the patient health status. The images will be provided by any of the different modalities available nowadays with enough diagnostic quality after a referring physician asked for the examination due to the conditions and symptoms of the patient.

In this process, the radiologist can be abstractly compared to an infinitely complex system with specific inputs, internal processes, and outputs. The inputs consist of all the clinical information available from the patient, together with lab data such as blood test results or genetic information. Previous imaging studies and quantitative information extracted through the image reading process are also considered, among many other inputs. The processing that the radiologists perform to these data does not follow simple rules, but takes into account everything the specialist has learned mainly since the beginning of medical studies and continued through accumulating knowledge and experience in the professional career. Spatial orientation, memory, and even psychological characteristics like self-confidence and attitude can influence how the images are interpreted. All these data and factors are combined together with imaging findings in order to provide an output in the form of a text-based report that has to be as reliable and concise as possible.

The most relevant part of the image interpretation process is the visual analysis of the images themselves. This process is typically performed in the picture archiving and communication system (PACS) visualization environments that contain a set of tools to help in the annotation of relevant imaging findings. These tools allow to indicate alterations, measure lesions, and define regions of interest. Image features and their location within the region examined, either observational or computational, can be attached to an image. As it will be reviewed in this chapter, there still exist important challenges for interoperability between different platforms when working with annotated images, although projects for standardization like the Annotation and Image Markup (AIM) have addressed the problem (Roy et al. 2014; AIM web page https://wiki.nci.nih.gov/display/AIM/Annotation+and+Image+Markup+-+AIM; Mongkolwat et al. 2012).

How image interpretation is well detailed in the radiological report is one of the key issues for understanding the status of the patient. As the end product of radiologist activity, it has an enormous relevance, as it communicates a diagnostic impression from which the care physician makes important therapeutic and prognostic decisions in clinical practice. Its quality and efficacy depend largely on obtaining relevant clinical information from the patient. It also has clear medicolegal implications. There is still a significant lack of training and dedication to the correct elaboration of radiological reports throughout training periods. The radiological report is currently under a paradigm shift process, moving from traditional descriptive texts towards structured reports, an itemized approach to the description of findings. Structured reporting systems can contribute to a greater standardization of processes and improve communication and interpretation of findings obtained from medical imaging. How image interpretation workflow can be integrated with structured reporting is also detailed in this chapter.

Thanks to the advances in artificial intelligence (AI) and image recognition algorithms like convolutional neural networks (CNN) together with high-performance computing (HPC) capabilities such as the graphical processing units (GPU), it has been possible to implement a growing number of computer-aided detection (CAD) solutions to assist radiologists in the image interpretation process. The main goal of CAD software is to increase the detection of disease by reducing the false-negative rate due to observational oversights (Castellino 2005). Although these tools are initially designed as an aid to the specialist, the recent progression of CNN and deep learning (one of the most promising machine learning (ML) technologies especially suited to analyze bidimensional data such as images) has raised some concern among the radiologist community. However, although the technology is showing excellent results for daily life images, the applicability in real clinical scenario for the analysis of radiological images with success within current radiology workflows has still to be demonstrated.

2 Challenges in Image Interpretation

Image interpretation is the most important part of the radiological workflow, in which the images have to be "read" by the radiologist in order to provide the most accurate conclusion on the status of patient organs and tissues. This process is currently surrounded by technology, typically performed in workstations with advanced visualization hardware (monitors) and software (image viewers). Despite image interpretation is technically performed in most centers worldwide in a similar way, agreements on specific standards and criteria for the image interpretation and post-processing are still lacking.

One of the most important issues related to image interpretation is the heterogeneity in characteristics of display devices, mainly due to different luminance and resolutions. In order to minimize heterogeneity across different visualization environments, the grayscale standard display function (GSDF) was introduced in the (digital imaging and communications in medicine) DICOM standard (Fetterly et al. 2008). It consists of the use of a mathematical function that translates from the grayscale signal value to luminance data, ensuring similar contrasts throughout different grayscale ranges in displays. Beyond luminance adaptation, at a single frequency, current regulatory requirements (Ochs et al. 2016) ask for the following tests required nowadays for achieving CE mark and Food and Drug Administration (FDA) 510 k certifications:

- Signal-to-luminance conversion at different spatial frequencies, therefore defining spatial resolution
- Location and count of pixel defects
- Presence of artifacts
- Temporal response of screens
- Maximum and minimum luminance and conformance to the grayscale-to-luminance function
- Others

Regarding image manipulation in software applications, any image visualization or analysis with diagnostic purposes should be performed using uncompressed or lossless compressed DICOM source images (Schulz-Menger et al. 2013) in order to work with real signal intensity from the images.

Apart from visualization, a recurrent task is to create different transformations and annotations to the images. Transformations typically imply zoom modifications, window-level adjustment, image flip, and rotation, while annotations mainly consist of distance measurement, angle measurement, arrow pointing towards a specific finding, and ROI delineation and extraction of mean signal (see Fig. 1). Nevertheless, due to interoperability issues and lack of integration, these new data generated by the radiologist get lost in other viewers. The reason for this is mainly that vendors tend to store the information about the transformations and annotations performed to the image in different places (i.e., different private DICOM tags).

As it can be appreciated, the way proprietary software encodes annotations and markup suffers frequently from problems of incompatibility. Some vendors, however, advancing to the interoperability era, have already set Extensible Markup Language (XML) as the format of election. In this sense, the Annotation and Image Markup (AIM) project was initiated by the National Institutes of Health (NIH) Cancer Biomedical Informatics Grid (caBIG) (Roy et al. 2014; AIM web page https://wiki.nci.nih.gov/display/AIM/Annotation+and+Image+Markup+-+AIM; Mongkolwat et al. 2012) providing a common annotation format that could be used and shared among different PACS vendors. AIM has a double benefit in simplicity and understandability, since it provides a structured and self-defined format using XML for radiological annotations that can be easily parsed. A template builder software is available at NIH National Cancer Institute (NCI) wiki (AIM web page https://wiki.nci.nih.gov/display/AIM/Annotation+and+Image+Markup+-+AIM). In Table 1, the AIM template concepts can be appreciated.

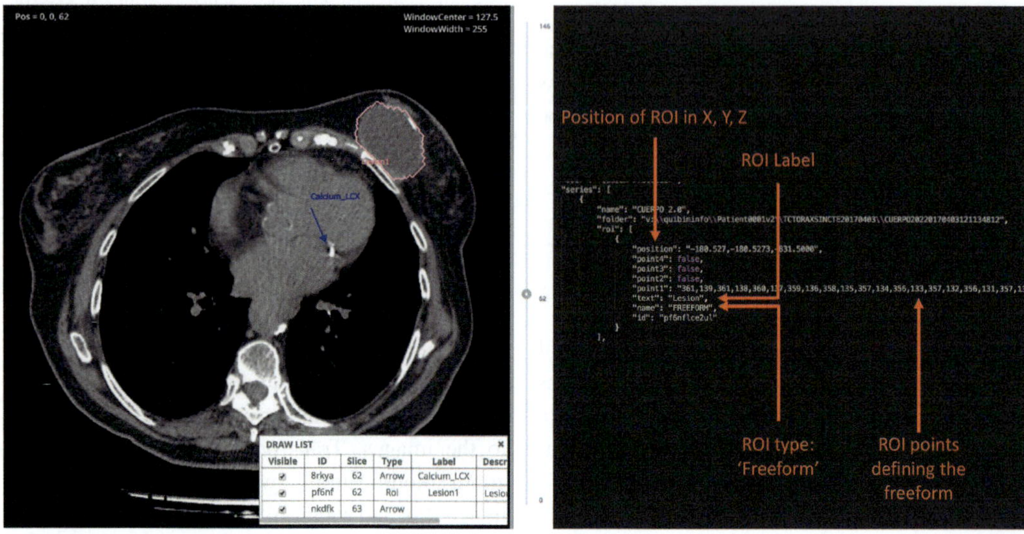

Fig. 1 Lesion delineated in pink color in left breast region. Different image annotations can be observed in the inferior table of the image. On the right, the internal structure of data in a JavaScript Object Notation (JSON) file (similar to XML) in QUIBIM Precision® software platform

Table 1 Annotation and Image Markup (AIM) concepts for the creation of new templates

AIM template builder concept	Annotation concept
Component	Item being annotated; for example, tumor location. A component can be anatomic entity, imaging observation, inference, calculation, and markup or geometric shape
Characteristic	Descriptive element of that item; for example, site of tumor center. Only anatomic entity and imaging observation can have characteristics associated with them
Allowed term	Represents a possible answer choice. It is used to describe the descriptive element of a component or characteristic. For example, frontal lobe is an answer choice for anatomic entity

Adapted from Mongkolwat et al. (2012)

Once the image annotations are already structured in a specific format like the one proposed in AIM, the integration with Health Level 7 (HL7) standard is not a complex process.

3 Integration with Structured Reporting

The wide variety of style in radiologic reporting is evidence that the ideal format for the radiology report has not been found or has not been generally accepted. In fact, it has been demonstrated that referring clinicians and radiologists prefer "itemized," "tabular," or "structured" reports of complex examinations rather than for reports in free text (Bosmans et al. 2011).

Nevertheless, the current radiological workflow is in most cases still consisting of free text and not in a structured and standardized procedure of reading and communicating the findings, despite the efforts of professional societies like the RSNA and ESR in Management of Radiology Report Templates (MRRT). The IHE MRRT profile defines all the procedures for the management of reporting templates (IHE Radiology Technical Committee 2015; IHE Radiology Technical Committee 2012), and also their format and modules. Specifically, it is stated that the templates should be in HTML format and are generated by a "report template creator." Thereafter, the templates are stored and managed by a "report template manager," which then

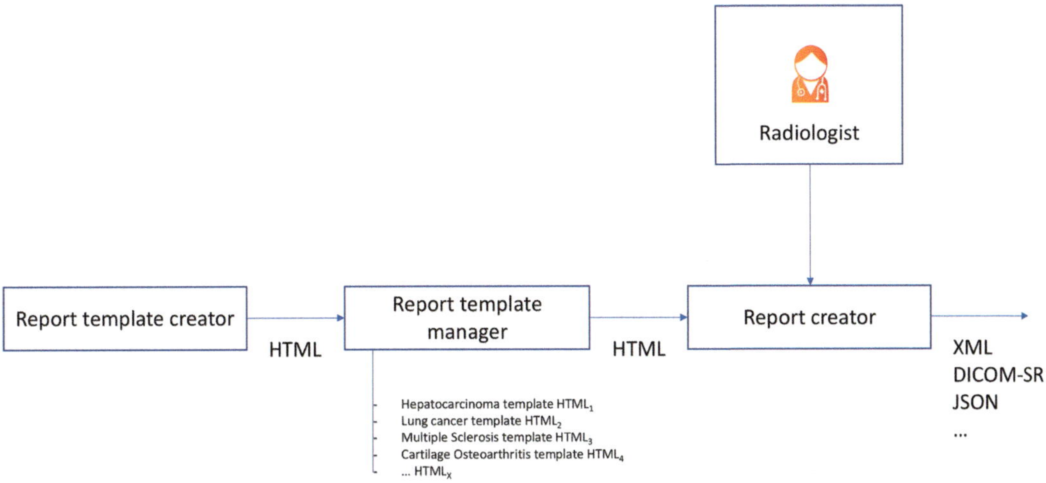

Fig. 2 Different components involved in structured report generation following IHE profile (IHE Radiology Technical Committee 2015)

provides them to a "report creator" where they are made available to a radiologist for reporting (Pinto Dos Santos et al. 2017). See Fig. 2 for this relationship.

Regarding software tools, there is an atomized market of different solutions and open-source tools that can aid to integrate DICOM structured reporting (SR) in clinical routine. These platforms, however, fail to integrate with most PACS and radiology information systems (RIS) in a meaningful way. All these interoperability issues imply a lack of data exploitation capabilities, not only for scientific purposes, but also for a better understanding of the disease. As an example, with an appropriate integration it would be possible to store all the ROIs delineated in hepatocarcinoma cases and automatically handle location, areas, volumes, and shape descriptors. This would not modify workflow, since ROIs or the diameters are today delineated to extract information from lesions. These data, however, are cited in the report but usually are not handled properly in databases of current information systems.

Structured reports, used for appropriate organization of the findings when the radiological reading is performed, have also to be managed, stored, and communicated to referring specialists; therefore they have to follow the description available in supplement 23rd of DICOM standard (Clunie 2000). DICOM Structured Reporting (DSR) defines data structures (patient, episode, images, annotations, derived biomarkers, and short reports) and gives recommendations on storage, consultancy, recovery, analysis, and transference. A structured report is compound by a group of tags related in a treelike hierarchy (Clunie 2000; Pomar-Nadal et al. 2013) organized in XML documents using templates or style sheets.

Besides image annotations, different imaging biomarkers extracted by computational analysis techniques need to be integrated with the structured report (Martí-Bonmatí and Alberich-Bayarri 2017). Most of the imaging biomarker solutions are distributed among workstations and portals offered by big companies like Siemens (Munich, Germany), Philips (Best, The Netherlands), or GE Healthcare (Chicago, IL, USA) and small providers like Cortechs Labs (San Diego, CA, USA), Arterys (San Francisco, CA, USA), Icometrix (Leuven, BE, Belgium), Image Analysis UK (London, UK), Mint Medical (Heidelberg, Germany), Quantib (Rotterdam, The Netherlands), QUIBIM (Valencia, Spain), and Olea Medical (now part of Canon-Toshiba, La Ciotat, France). These quantitative image analysis solutions usually find interoperability issues when trying to transfer information with hospital information systems (HIS) and electronic health records

(EHR); therefore a simple operation like searching in the information systems for the last-year chronic obstructive pulmonary disease (COPD) patients with a percentage of CT-derived emphysema between 5 and 10% is not possible. This kind of data management would allow for a better understanding of the tissue and organ alterations in the disease and their relationship with patient characteristics and associated clinical or lab data.

In order to integrate imaging biomarkers with structured report, a potential solution is to share standardized XML or JSON files containing the imaging biomarkers results with the MRRT software application present in the department. To authors' experience, in order to solve interoperability issues and connect imaging biomarkers together with structured reporting to the PACS and RIS solutions, the architecture of Fig. 3 has been implemented, using QUIBIM Precision® as the imaging biomarker platform, fully developed in-house, and IHE-compliant MRRT web application from Mainz University (Pinto Dos Santos et al. 2017).

4 Artificial Intelligence and Image Interpretation

Data complexity in radiologic examinations is significantly growing with the technology evolution of image acquisition equipment, with a progressive increase in the number of images, and their spatial and temporal resolution, besides other characteristics. Image interpretation workflow is therefore moving from the straight observation and interpretation of these images towards the addition of structural and functional information extracted from them by means of computational analysis. As a consequence, software solutions that assist the radiologist in the image interpretation process in image classification and findings detection as a pre-reading of the studies are a growing need.

The recent AI advances in CNN and HPC already introduced have allowed for the creation of new solutions mainly based on deep learning technology that can be applied mainly in two situations: automated annotations and segmentation.

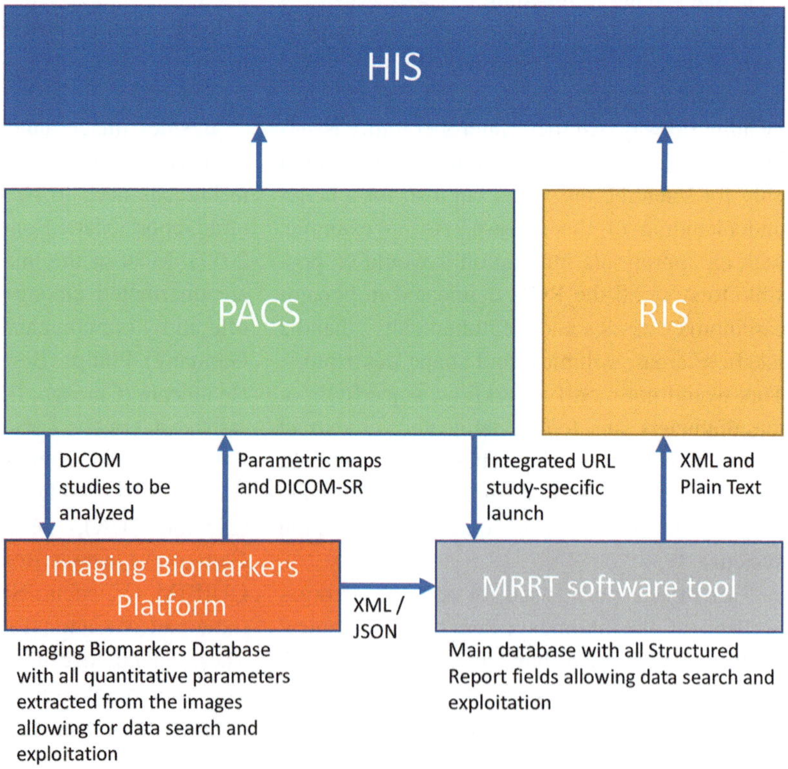

Fig. 3 Architecture of software applications needed to integrate structured reporting with imaging biomarkers in a PACS—RIS environment that initially does not support quantitative imaging data exploitation and structured reporting templates management. An in-house imaging biomarker solution was implemented and the IHE-MRRT software tool was used as the structured reporting platform (Pinto Dos Santos et al. 2017)

The main reason for their application to radiology field is that these technologies have performed with excellent results in daily-life image annotation and region detection. This progress has also been the seed of a growing concern among the radiology community about a potential substitution of radiologists by AI-based algorithms. However, this approach should be carefully considered once we take into account that the amount and complexity of information that has to be processed by radiologist mind are enormous and high, respectively. Radiology is about not only image recognition, but also a high amount of context information. Even more, data managed in the image interpretation process is highly heterogeneous: patient characteristics and habits, clinical status, previous clinical episodes, lab test results, previous examinations, imaging findings, and so on. This should be taken into account in order to avoid reductionist arguments when new human-threating machine learning implementations are currently proposed. To author impression, machine learning capabilities are currently in the top of the hype cycle for emerging technologies (Hype cycle for emerging technologies 2016) and a future normalization is expected where technology will be increasingly adopted in clinical routine as a tool to reduce times in image interpretation and therefore increase productivity. Ethical issues and assignment of responsibilities regarding potential radiologists' mistakes in image interpretations due to a not proper performance of the algorithm remain to be solved.

Algorithms can be classified into different ways but one of the most extended ones is according to the training styles, those unsupervised and supervised. Unsupervised methods are able to clusterize large amounts of data with no previous information. These solutions allow to extract patterns that are not defined by humans and that can potentially provide new disease stratification and phenotypes. In the contrary, supervised methods require a previous dataset annotation by experts in order to train the algorithm. A high percentage of the dataset is frequently dedicated to training the method (typically around 80%) and a part is used for algorithm validation (i.e., 20%). Regarding the algorithm science, the most frequent methods are as follows (Erickson et al. 2017):

- Neural networks: Main machine learning method, consisting of error, search, and update functions. An iterative process is performed in order to adjust the weights of the network that is organized in layers. The error function measures the difference between the generated output and the desired output, the weights of the network are modified, and the error function is measured again in a new iteration. The process will continue until the error is under a specific tolerance. After the adjustment, the network will be ready to be applied in real conditions.
- k-Nearest neighbors: This method looks for classes that contain features similar to the ones found in the input data. Similarity it can be measured by many different ways but one of the most frequently used is the Euclidean distance.
- Support vector machines: This solution consists of modifying the input data in order to ease the separation between groups that were initially not possible to split by linear approaches. For doing so, the widest plane or support vector is calculated.
- Decision trees and forests: This approach is one of the most understandable by humans within the machine learning spectrum, since it is typically based on binary classification rules that are organized together to form a tree of decision points to generate the results. The equilibrium between decision points and accuracy is the main challenge of decision trees. Accuracy of the method can be improved by aggregating multiple trees into forests.
- Naive Bayes algorithm: Following Bayes theorem, this method is based on a calculation of the probability for an output taking into consideration the probabilities of each feature in the input data. One important consideration is that the method does not require dependency among input features, but can work properly with features that have no relationship.

- Deep learning: This technique is the most recently extended among the machine learning field. While standard neural networks contain a few number of layers that can be even interpreted intuitively, deep neural networks consist of concatenating a large number of layers (i.e., tens of them or more). This aggregation is possible due to the improvements in HPC capabilities, specially in the field of GPU. The most suitable algorithm within deep learning for image artificial interpretation is the one based on CNN, which assume that the inputs have a position relationship, like the coordinates of any image matrix. The minimum element of this method is the kernel, a two-dimensional window taking a small part of the image, and the output at the CNN is the convolution of such kernel. The deep neural network will be grouped from basic shape kernels (i.e., corners, edges) to higher level structures (i.e., faces, entire organs). These convolutional layers are combined with activation layers and pooling layers that will reward those convolutions collecting most of the information from the image, that is, the most relevant features describing the image.

Independently of the machine learning algorithm used, care should be taken in designing new image interpretation solutions, since every disease and organ produce specific features at a pixel level that have to be considered together with context information. For this, not only a single machine learning technology may be the solution, but also a combination of them, in order to manage both imaging and one-dimensional data.

Conclusion

In this chapter, the most relevant challenges in the field of image interpretation have been addressed. This topic is the core of the radiological workflow and it is currently under a process of paradigm shift, from traditional image reading through observation and free text reporting of the findings towards the inclusion of new technologies in the loop such as computer-aided detection and diagnosis (CAD), imaging biomarker extraction, and structured reporting. The advance in interoperability between systems to standardize image annotation formats, together with the growing use of structured reporting and AI-assisted image reading, will shape radiology as one of the most relevant data sciences in the era of precision medicine.

References

AIM web page. https://wiki.nci.nih.gov/display/AIM/Annotation+and+Image+Markup+-+AIM. Accessed 1 May 2017

Bosmans JML, Weyler JJ, De Schepper AM, Parizel PM (2011) The radiology report as seen by radiologists and referring clinicians: results of the COVER and ROVER surveys. Radiology 259:184–195

Castellino RA (2005) Computer aided detection (CAD): an overview. Cancer Imaging 5:17–19

Clunie DA (2000) DICOM structured reporting. PixelMed, Bangor, PA

Erickson BJ, Korfiatis P, Akkus Z, Kline TL (2017) Machine learning for medical imaging. Radiographics 37(2):505–515

Fetterly KA, Blume HR, Flynn MJ, Samei E (2008) Introduction to grayscale calibration and related aspects of medical imaging grade liquid crystal displays. J Digit Imaging 21:193–207

Hype cycle for emerging technologies (2016) 19-07-2016. www.gartner.com. Accessed 1 May 2017

IHE Radiology Technical Committee (2012) IHE Radiology (RAD) white paper: management of radiology report templates, pp 1–26

IHE Radiology Technical Committee (2015) IHE radiology technical framework supplement: management of radiology report templates (MRRT), pp 1–50

Martí-Bonmatí L, Alberich-Bayarri A (2017) Development and clinical integration. In: Imaging biomarkers. Springer, New York. isbn: 978-3-319-43502-2

Mongkolwat P, Rubin DL, Kleper V, Chen JJ, Siegel EL (2012) Structured reporting with the caBIG® Annotation and Image Markup (AIM) template builder for AIM Version 4.0; Radiological Society of North America, Chicago, IL November 2012

Ochs R, Chun S, Lam B (2016) Display devices for diagnostic radiology. Draft Guidance for Industry and Food and Drug Administration Staff, pp 1–14

Pinto Dos Santos D, Klos G, Kloeckner R, Oberle R, Dueber C, Mildenberger P (2017) Development of an IHE MRRT-compliant open-source web-based reporting platform. Eur Radiol 27:424–430

Pomar-Nadal A, Pérez Castillo C, Alberich-Bayarri A, García-Martí G, Sanz-Requena R, Marti-Bonmati

L (2013) Integrando el informe de biomarcadores de imagen en el informe radiológico estructurado. Radiología SERAM 55:188–194

Roy S, Brown MS, Shih GL (2014) Visual interpretation with three-dimensional annotations (VITA): three-dimensional image interpretation tool for radiological reporting. J Digit Imaging 27:49–57

Schulz-Menger J, Bluemke DA, Bremerich J et al (2013) Standardized image interpretation and post processing in cardiovascular magnetic resonance: society for cardiovascular magnetic resonance (SCMR) board of trustees task force on standardized post processing. J Cardiovasc Magn Reson 15:35

Transforming from Radiologist Peer Review Audits to Peer Learning and Improvement Approaches

Ronald Eisenberg and Jonathan Kruskal

Contents

Abstract

All radiologists actively practicing in the United States are required to undergo some manner of periodic performance evaluation. This should provide an unbiased, fair, and balanced evaluation of radiologist performance to identify opportunities for additional education, error reduction, and self-improvement. By far the most common method of peer review audit system currently used in radiology is RADPEER, developed almost 15 years ago by the American College of Radiology (ACR), in which originally interpreted images are randomly selected and reviewed by a peer radiologist. However, studies have shown that this time-consuming process has inherent sampling bias, has limited value as an educational tool, and is primarily performed to meet accreditation and hospital credentialing requirements. Moreover, it evaluates the performance of a radiologist in terms of a diagnostic discrepancy score, excluding the myriad of other functions and roles that radiologists play, including teaching, consulting, and communicating abnormal results. Consequently, an increasing number of radiology practices are embracing simple scoring systems that either agree with the prior read or score the interpretation as an "apparent learning case."

Rather than a scoring-based peer review audits of random cases for evaluating radiologist performance, this chapter recommends

R. Eisenberg, M.D., J.D. (✉) • J. Kruskal, M.D., Ph.D.
Department of Radiology, Beth Israel Deaconess Medical Center, Harvard Medical School,
330 Brookline Avenue, Boston, MA 02215, USA
e-mail: rleisenb@bidmc.harvard.edu

Med Radiol Diagn Imaging (2017)
DOI 10.1007/174_2017_114, © Springer International Publishing AG
Published Online 09 August 2017

the adoption of a system based on "peer learning, which consists of peer feedback, learning, and improvement. The goal is not to identify poor-performing physicians, but to improve performance of all members of the group by analyzing the potential contributors to errors through a self-reflection process, as well as peer discussion in a constructive, nonpunitive quality improvement meeting.

Keywords
Learning opportunities • Peer learning • Peer review

The guidelines of the Joint Commission for Accreditation of Healthcare Facilities in the United States (Joint Commission 2007) state that physicians are expected to "demonstrate knowledge of established and evolving biomedical, clinical, and social sciences, and the application of their knowledge to patient care and the education of others." As with other physicians, the initial entry of radiologists into the specialty requires an intense period of residency and fellowship training before they can receive board certification indicating that they are credentialed to practice as radiologists. Periodically thereafter, radiologists must demonstrate that they have retained their medical skill and judgment. For all organizations that are accredited by the Joint Commission, it is mandated that each radiologist be subjected to ongoing professional practice evaluations (OPPE) on an 8-monthly basis, in which radiologist-specific data is collected by the imaging department in six specified categories (Joint Commission 2007; Donnelly and Strife 2005; Donnelly 2007). These include patient care, medical and clinical knowledge, practice-based learning and improvement, interpersonal and communication skills, and system-based practice (Joint Commission 2007; Donnelly and Strife 2005; Donnelly 2007). If the OPPE data raise any question about the performance level of a specific radiologist, this triggers a focused professional practice evaluation (FPPE), in which the performance of the radiologist is further investigated and closely scrutinized to determine whether there has been sufficient deterioration of skills and knowledge over time (or underlying mental or physical illness or substance abuse) that jeopardizes patient care and requires remediation (Steele et al. 2010; Kruskal et al. 2016). Other circumstances that can trigger an FPPE include patient and family complaints, concerns of referring physicians and colleagues, an excessive number of bad outcomes/incident reports ("misses" in diagnostic radiology; complications in interventional radiology), data collected through the peer review process, and malpractice suits (Kruskal et al. 2016; Kruskal and Eisenberg 2016). Measures used to resolve performance issues may include education, proctoring, counseling, practitioner assistance, and suspension or revocation of specific privileges (Larson et al. 2016).

Thus, all radiologists actively practicing in the United States are required to undergo some manner of periodic performance evaluation, and the manner with which this is achieved varies considerably. Of note, no benefit for patients or improved clinical care has ever been shown from participating in scoring audit processes. Hidden within these evaluation processes are ill-defined requirements for peer review, which have been linked to the site accreditation process. The purpose of this chapter is to address the state of peer evaluations of radiologists and to show that scoring audit systems are slowly being replaced by learning and improvement practices.

1 Scored Peer Review Audit Systems

The practice of radiology requires a complex interplay of skills, knowledge, and judgment. Therefore, the most effective way to determine the professional competence of a radiologist is by others in the specialty and clinical colleagues. In most institutions, OPPE includes a peer review audit system based on a template first described by Donnelly (Donnelly 2007). Peer review should provide an unbiased, fair, and balanced evaluation of radiologist performance to identify opportunities for additional education, error reduction, and self-improvement (Mahgerefteh et al. 2009).

In many systems, there are no requirements for providing constructive feedback, or for categorizing the case or type of learning and improvement opportunity. Ideally, the process should be nonpunitive, have minimal effect on work flow, and allow easy participation (Mahgerefteh et al. 2009). The process should also be free of bias both in case selection and case review. Peer review should also be performed by similarly trained colleagues with similar experience and reflect a representative case and modality mix.

By far the most common method of peer review audit system currently used in radiology is RADPEER, developed almost 15 years ago by the American College of Radiology (ACR), in which originally interpreted images are randomly selected and reviewed by a peer radiologist (Borgstede et al. 2004; Jackson et al. 2009). The reviewing radiologist scores the original radiology report on the basis of the RADPEER four-point scoring system, with a score of 1 representing agreement and scores of 2 to 4 representing discrepancies of increasing severity (Jackson et al. 2009; American College of Radiology 2016), with the score of 4 eliminated in May 2016 (American College of Radiology 2016). To evaluate the performance of the radiologist, a disagreement rate is calculated, in which the number of cases scored 3 (or 4) is divided by the number of cases reviewed. In this way, the performance of each radiologist can be compared with the discrepancy rates of other radiologists in the group as well as with national averages (Borgstede et al. 2004; Jackson et al. 2009). In addition, according to those who developed the RADPEER system, any substantial discrepancy detected by the peer reviewer is to be communicated to the initial interpreting radiologist, who is given the opportunity to challenge the finding of the discrepancy and/or its scoring (Larson et al. 2011; Abujudeh et al. 2014). In many institutions, errors scored 3 (or 4) become the subject of regular Quality Assurance conferences. However, in our experience, much more time is typically spent arguing over the score assigned to the discrepancy, rather than focusing on the underlying causes of the error and how to prevent it from recurring.

There has never been a report systematically evaluating the benefits of the RADPEER peer review auditing system or any indication that it has led to widespread performance improvement (Larson et al. 2016). One study reported very low interrater agreement by multiple subspecialists in an academic radiology department, concluding that "a ratings-based peer review system [like Radpeer] is unreliable and subjective for the evaluation of discrepant interpretations" (Bender et al. 2012). Another described substantial selection bias and a strong tendency to underreport the severity of the discrepancy so as to decrease the calculated disagreement rate of fellow radiologists, with 44% agreeing with the statement that scoring-based peer review audit systems are a waste of time (Eisenberg 2014). In a large survey of ACR members, 80% stated that RADPEER was being performed to meet accreditation requirements and 70% indicated that it was being performed to meet hospital credentialing requirements, such as those for OPPE, while 47% believed that their practice patterns had not changed as a result of peer review and only 20% thought it had (Abujudeh et al. 2014). As Donald Berwick succinctly summarized in a recent editorial, the current era of medical practice is one characterized by "excessive measurement, much of which is useless but nonetheless mandated. Intemperate measurement is as unwise and irresponsible as is intemperate health care … The aim should be to measure only what matters, and mainly for learning" (Berwick 2016).

One study demonstrated that peer review audit systems are time-consuming exercises that, in addition to being unpopular among radiologists, have little "bang for the buck" (Eisenberg and Heidinger 2016). Analyzing 6 years' experience of peer review in the chest section of an academic teaching center, of 9441 cases there were only 244 discrepancies scored as 3 or 4 (2.6%). One-third of discrepancies were related to the presence and degree of pulmonary vascular congestion or pleural effusion, or enlargement of the cardiac silhouette, determinations which have a substantial amount of subjective variability in interpretation. For specific diagnoses, it was necessary to peer review 197 cases to detect one level 3 or 4 discrepancy regarding pulmonary vascular congestion, 858 to find a missed pulmonary nodule/mass, and 1574 to detect a rib or other skeletal lesion. It was calculated that radiologists in this four-FTE section spent more than 14 h to detect a discrepant pulmonary nodule/mass and more than 26 h to detect a missed rib or skeletal lesion. Overall, the total time expenditure of these four radiologists in peer review was 157 h (almost 20 full work days).

All currently applied peer review methods assess interpretive disagreement between readers. In the absence of a definitive diagnosis (such as surgery or pathology), it may be impossible to differentiate between an error and a genuine difference of opinion regarding the correct interpretation of an image or an appropriate recommendation for follow-up (Alport and Hillman 2004). Added to this is the inherent high subjectivity, sampling bias, and underreporting of this quantitative measurement, which provides a false impression of accuracy (Larson et al. 2016). Indeed, this has led the Royal College of Radiologists in the United Kingdom to abandon its scoring-based peer review audit program altogether in favor of another approach that focuses on learning and improvement (The Royal College of Radiologists 2014a, b). In the United States, where a form of peer review is currently required, more and more practices are adopting a modification of this change and are embracing simple scoring systems that either agree with the prior read or score the interpretation as an "apparent learning case" (or use some variant term).

In a thoughtful review on this subject, Larson et al. (2016) raised the emotional toll that radiologists may suffer from peer review auditing based a scoring model. Although often considered as nonpunitive, this approach documents medical error in a manner that is "inherently associated with feelings of anxiety, shame, and humiliation." Since all radiologists make errors, the design and implementation of a peer review process have great effect on the painful experience of this realization. As currently constituted in most institutions, the scores of randomly sampled cases in a peer review audit are used to rate the radiologist's overall performance as a professional, rather than focusing on specific areas of practice that might be amenable to improvement. In other words, the performance of a radiologist is evaluated purely in terms of a diagnostic discrepancy score, excluding the myriad of other functions and roles that radiologists play, including teaching, consulting, and communicating abnormal results. A program in which the individual radiologist is judged incompetent on the basis of subjective peer evaluations "engenders feelings of failure, shame, and betrayal, which tend to produce paralysis, disillusionment, and anger, rather than a desire to improve."

If the intention of audit systems is simply to meet regulatory requirements, then such systems are effective. However, if the true intention is to evaluate a radiologist's performance with the goal of providing constructive feedback that leads to learning and improvement, then audit systems have failed miserably. For this reason, much thought is currently going into developing and deploying so-called peer learning systems, of which many are now being used in the clinical setting.

2 Peer Learning and Improvement

In September, 2015, the Institute of Medicine (IOM) issued a widely publicized report, "Improving Diagnosis in Health Care," which focused on the problem of diagnostic errors in medicine (Balogh et al. 2015a). A major recommendation of the report was that "health care organizations should adopt policies and practices that promote a non-punitive culture that values open discussion and feedback on diagnostic performance" (Balogh et al. 2015b). This included the need to "develop and deploy approaches to identify, learn from, and reduce diagnostic errors and near misses in clinical practice," which is not met by current scoring-based peer review audits such as RADPEER and similar systems. Instead, the IOM encouraged the establishment of "work system and culture that supports the diagnostic process and improvements in diagnostic performance," implying implementation of a nonpunitive system that urges open and honest feedback and discussion without public embarrassment and shaming. As another way to improve diagnosis and reduce diagnostic error, the IOM recommended the development of "a reporting environment and medical liability system that facilitates improved diagnosis by learning from diagnostic errors and near misses." Finally, the IOM recognized that the effective practice of medicine is a cooperative effort and encouraged the facilitation of "more effective teamwork in the diagnostic process among health care professionals, patients, and their families." The IOM report strongly recommended team-based care based on shared goals, mutual trust, effective communication, and measureable processes and outcomes. Noting that this approach has been shown to increase safety and quality of care in the face of mounting health care complexity, it recognized that "reframing the diagnostic process as a team-based activity may require changing norms of health care professional roles and responsibilities" that "may take some time and may meet some resistance" (Balogh et al. 2015c).

Based on the IOM report, Larsen et al. (2016) have advocated an alternative to the scoring-based peer review that is based on "peer learning," which consists of peer feedback, learning, and improvement. Rather than having the goal of identifying poor-performing physicians, the aim of peer learning is to improve performance by analyzing the potential contributors to errors through both a self-reflection process and through peer discussion in a constructive, nonpunitive quality improvement meeting.

3 Peer Feedback

Instead of the retrospective reading of a specific percentage of randomly selected cases that characterizes RADPEER and similar peer review auditing systems, which result in disruption of the normal workflow and miss (or fail to report) the majority of cases in which significant or impactful errors have occurred, we have developed an online QA system, in which radiologists and referring physicians voluntarily submit errors detected as part of their normal activities (Kruskal et al. 2016; Eisenberg and Heidinger 2016). Prospective detection of errors, which may come from radiologist review of a prior examination as part of normal clinical activities, consultation with a referring clinician, multidisciplinary conferences, pathology or surgery discrepancy reports, complaints to radiology leadership, and incident reporting systems, is more likely to yield learning and improvement opportunities (Brook et al. 2015).

Rather than being the source of anxiety and shame in an open Quality Assurance conference, feedback should be timely, confidential, and given in a constructive and nonjudgmental manner, always in the spirit of learning and improvement rather than punitive (Alkasab et al. 2014). It can be given either directly by another radiologist who personally observed the discrepancy when reading a subsequent examination or by a designated radiologist in the department to whom errors can be submitted confidentially from a variety of sources and then relayed anonymously to the original radiologist (Larson et al. 2016). In either case, the feedback ideally should summarize the discrepancy and any adverse effect it may have had upon the patient. When appropriate, it should provide suggestions as to how to avoid the mistake in the future.

4 Peer Learning and Improvement

Although direct feedback to the one who has made an error is valuable, the intent of peer learning is to improve the performance of all radiologists through group conferences (Halsted 2004), or even a wider audience through secure dissemination of appropriately edited teaching cases. If scoring systems are going to persist, and we strongly advocate that they do not, then one approach is to cast a wider net for relevant case capture by changing the current scoring system for peer review audits to "Agree" or "Apparent Learning Opportunity" (rather than score discrepancies). This shifts the focus away from unhelpful and often time-consuming debates about how to score a case and its impact, rather than thinking about what lessons the case provides for reflection and improvement. Some institutions have added a third category of "Great Call/Pickup," which is defined as a difficult case in which a radiologist made the correct call or interpretation that could reasonably be missed by another radiologist (Larson et al. 2016). It is important that efforts be made to shift the focus to positive constructive feedback rather than highlighting negative aspects of interpretive errors. Some authors have recommended categorizing cases identified as learning opportunities into issues that relate to the radiologist or to system and process contributors. In our own practice we use the system shown in Fig. 1 when analyzing possible contributors to an error.

A Guide for Analysis of Contributors

Radiologist contributors

- Near miss, or caught in time
- Perceptual
    - Observational
    - Satisfaction of search
- Cognition/interpretive
    - Overcall
    - Undercall
    - Misclassification
    - Knowledge gap
- Report-related
    - Content
    - Recommendations
    - Communication

System contributors

- Indication or Information provided
- Imaging technique or protocol
- Patient factors & comorbidities
- Teaching & supervision related
- Work environment
- PACS factors
- Other process related factors

Fig. 1 A guide for analysis of radiologist and system contributors to errors. This checklist facilitates analysis of cases and identification of different categories of contributors. Part of the peer learning process is to teach participants that human errors are only a small component of the many additional contributors that lead to the occurrence of errors and near misses

We have also developed a template for learning case submission, based in part on similar systems that have been developed by the Royal College of Radiologists (The Royal College of Radiologists 2014a, b). This template (Fig. 2) shows how information is submitted and includes the initial interpretation, the final interpretation, and possible contributing factors that are identified using the guide on the left. Additional data include potential improvement opportunities and lessons learned from review of the case. We have found that such a system also allows near-miss cases to be identified and can be used to collect procedure-related cases. Our own radiologists prefer to submit a few cases into a system such as this, rather than spending the time and effort that go into agreeing with the vast majority of reviews of original interpretations with traditional retrospective audit systems.

We have developed and implemented a so-called Contributor-Impact Chart (Fig. 3), which facilitates the root-cause analytical process when thinking about an error. This novel approach considers the major contributors to an adverse event or a diagnostic error and allows the case reviewer to think about ways in which different contributors might have led to an error occurring. Such a process also allows for analysis of the factors contributing to learning cases and is used for prioritizing the order in which improvement activities should be addressed.

The format of a peer learning conference depends on the size and degree of subspecialization of the radiology practice at a particular institution, ranging from a general monthly session in small imaging departments to independent conferences for each subspecialty area in larger institutions. In academic and teaching programs, the monthly learning conferences should include trainees, both for the educational

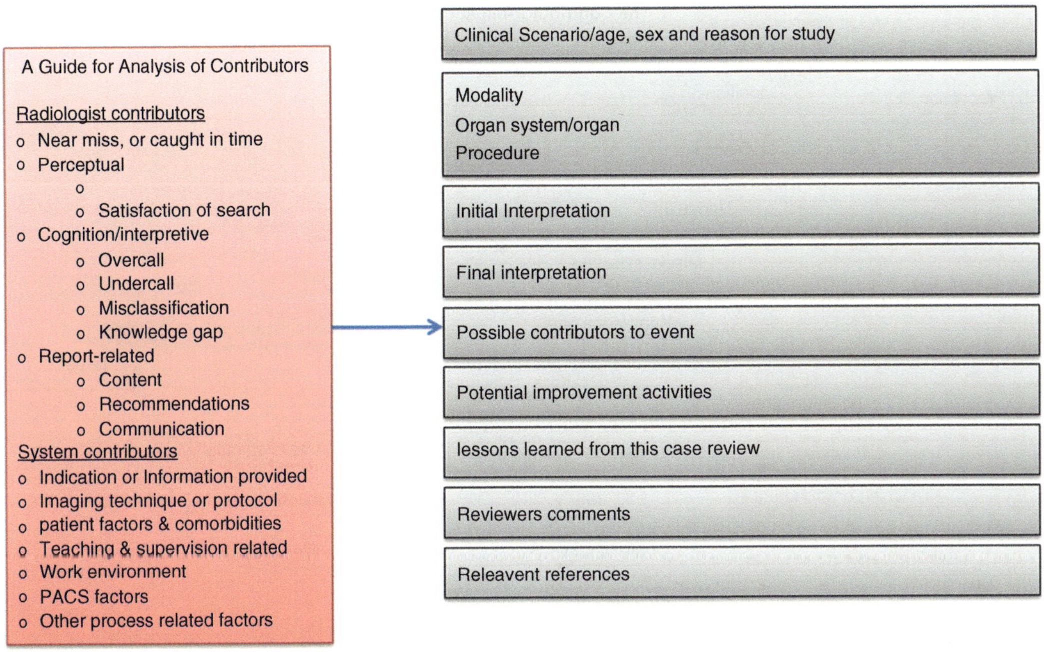

Fig. 2 Template for learning case submission. Case submission template (in *grey* on the *right* of image) illustrating how the contributor list links into completing the different boxes. This template was designed to allow analysis of cases, along with relevant demographics, study type, organ system, and the actual change in interpretation that was made. Note also the opportunity to share potential improvement activities (such as lectures or reading materials, protocol or policy changes, or even remedial training). The box for lessons learned from review of a case is especially important to share. Since we mentor the process, a review also can provide additional feedback and suggestions

opportunities they offer and as an early introduction to the modern culture of peer learning in which they all will need to participate. In the United States, national education regulatory groups require that trainees are taught about and participate in root-cause analyses, and such conferences go a long way towards meeting this requirement. Some have advocated videotaping these conferences, which enables radiologists who could not attend in person to review the learning principles discussed from a secure site at a later date (Larson et al. 2016).

An emerging concept gaining support is to host cloud-based repositories of edited and authored learning cases. Similar to the American College of Radiology's "Case-in-Point" system, learning cases can be submitted, reviewed, accepted, and published into such a learning repository, and then downloaded to enrich the Quality Improvement meeting experience of smaller practices. Such repositories could also be searched to select specific case examples for learning and improvement purposes, as well as for remedial training and even trainee examinations.

Those participating in these conferences should constantly be reminded that their purpose is solely educational, to learn and improve rather than to find fault. The conferences should emphasize potential pitfalls and mimics that might lead to the errors being discussed and strategies for preventing them. When appropriate, there could be more formal educational presentations and reviews of relevant literature. Note that difficult cases categorized as "great calls" should be included in these conferences. Since by definition many radiologists would have missed the finding, the cases provide valuable opportunities for learning (Larson et al. 2016).

Peer learning conferences must always be conducted in a constructive and cooperative manner, with disparaging comments strictly forbidden. The initial interpreting radiologist must be strictly

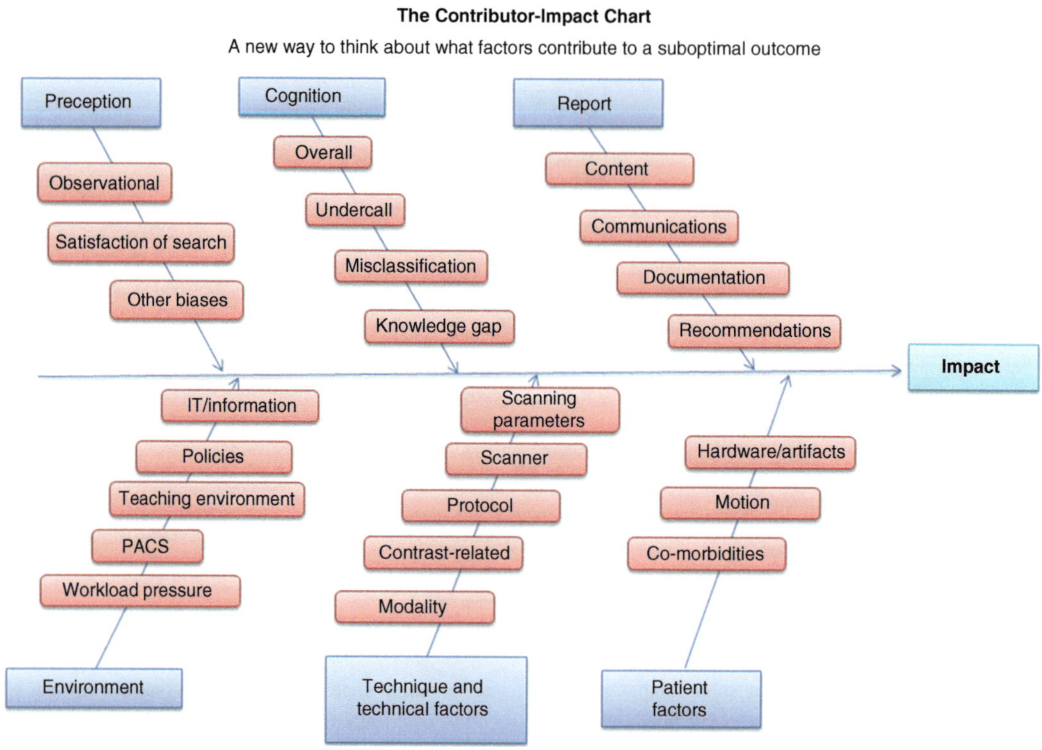

Fig. 3 Contributor-impact chart. This modification of the Ishikawa or cause-and-effect chart was developed to facilitate self-reflection and analysis of cases. Unlike a simple checklist, this chart was created to help identify potential improvement activities and their associated lessons that can be learned from analysis of a case

anonymous; the identity of the person who made the error is immaterial, since every error offers an opportunity for everyone to improve. Perceptual errors are generally the most common and can be reviewed quickly because their major teaching value is for participants to share tips on how to avoid missing them in the future. Interpretive errors often are the subject of more extensive discussions, which may be enhanced by someone presenting a brief review of the topic that includes a differential diagnosis and how to distinguish among various diagnostic possibilities. A radiologist making an interpretative error may benefit from a review of the topic, which can be provided in person by a supportive colleague or by the recommendation of an appropriate videotape or journal article (Larson et al. 2016).

Larson et al. (2016) coined the term "virtuous cycle" to refer to a self-reinforcing process related to the enhanced interpersonal professional relationships generated by the peer learning approach to errors. Unlike the competitive environment engendered by a scoring-based peer review program, when a deficiency in knowledge or skill is discovered in a radiologist working within a group practicing peer learning, colleagues of the individual share knowledge and provide support to help the individual improve (Larson et al. 2016).

5 The Future

As forward-looking radiology departments increasingly adopt the concept of peer learning, the age of scoring-based peer review audits of random cases for evaluating radiologist performance hopefully will come to a merciful end. There is no justification for continuing to record, calculate, or report overall radiologist discrepancy rates as part of an OPPE that triggers an FPPE to determine whether there has been sufficient deterioration of skills and knowledge over time that jeopardizes patient care and requires remediation (Larson et al. 2016). Focused auditing of sample cases should be limited to assessing specific performance elements, such as report errors or adherence to standard reporting templates, to identify those radiologists who need to improve in these areas. This can all be effectively achieved by creating systems that allow the giving of constructive feedback. "Focused auditing of specific examination types, disease states, or modalities also can be of value in helping a radiology practice improve specific aspects of performance." As Larson et al. (2016) note, "The critical difference between this approach and one of peer scoring is that in this case, the topic targeted for improvement is determined prospectively and constitutes a limited, focused, and actionable aspect of performance, rather than a general assessment of radiologist competence."

We have introduced a system for providing direct anonymous constructive feedback about report contents. Figure 4 shows the drop-down menu that allows a reviewing radiologist to provide specific constructive feedback to the original interpreting radiologist. The intent here is to share feedback (including positive feedback!) for the radiologist to consider adopting. Peer feedback systems must accept that not all will agree with the reviews and should allow for independent practice changes to be made or not. Of note, providing effective and helpful feedback about report content is simply addressing one of many roles that being a radiologist embraces, but our reports are an extremely important product of what we do.

Indeed, there is much opposition to including actual peer review data in the OPPE process. Such a process should evaluate the many contributions that radiologists make to patient care. Under the domain of practice-based learning, participation in any effective peer review process should be more than acceptable, and for OPPE purposes, the tendency is to shift away from actual data analysis and to encourage case review and submission instead. Participation in a review process is sufficient for OPPE purposes. We strongly suggest that contributing a few helpful learning cases is far more constructive than contributing a large number of category 1 "agrees."

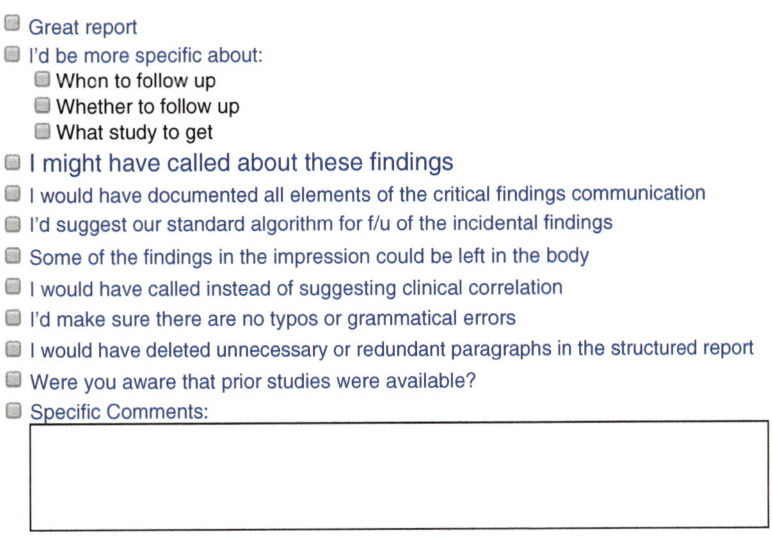

Fig. 4 Drop-down menu for providing constructive feedback on radiologist reports. One very important product that a radiologist produces is the report, and reports offer many opportunities for providing constructive feedback. In the peer learning domain, being able to provide constructive feedback to a radiologist regarding report content, grammar, and recommendations, and the effectiveness of result communications is very helpful, providing data that are not typically collected from traditional peer review audits

Unfortunately, current ACR modality certification requirements make it difficult to transition from scoring-based audits to peer learning by specifically calling for metrics based on a practice's peer review program (Lucey 2014). Therefore, it is critical that all regulatory and certifying bodies accept active participation in a peer learning program as an alternative to fulfill current scoring-based peer review requirements.

Peer learning based on discrepancies encountered during regular clinical activities also detects a much higher rate of clinically significant errors, especially those with high learning potential, which are only rarely discovered through a random audit process. Consequently, the focus of learning and improvement should be on cases that have the greatest learning potential, including examples of both suboptimal and outstanding performance (Brook et al. 2015; Halsted 2004; Larson and Nance 2011).

Eliminating the scoring-based audit model excludes the use of peer review data to evaluate physician competence. As noted above, this is not necessarily a problem, since peer review data have been shown to be biased, unreliable, and not easily actionable (Abujudeh et al. 2014; Eisenberg 2014). Moreover, interpretive skill is merely one element of physician competence. Other important aspects include professional behavior, continuous improvement efforts, and adherence to professional guidelines (Donnelly and Strife 2005; Donnelly 2007; Steele et al. 2010), which often are easier to measure and enforce. For example, instead of using traditional peer review data, compliance with the OPPE requirement can be achieved by documenting active participation in the peer learning program, as well as radiologist performance in the six core competencies of the (American Board of Medical Specialties 2017). Instead of measuring discrepancy rates, it is possible to assess participation at conferences, case submissions, and improvement initiatives completed (Larson et al. 2016).

Lack of competency in professional practice can be based in part on complaints from referring clinicians, anonymous trainee evaluations, and sentinel events (Kruskal and Eisenberg 2016). Although not mathematically precise, these sources can provide evidence of important practice deficits, which is the primary goal of competence assessment. "This approach shifts responsibility for determining competency from the radiologists' community of peers to radiology practice leaders, presumably following a predefined process" (Larson et al. 2016). This improves radiologist esprit de corps, allowing the professional community to focus purely on learning rather than being forced to determine the competence of peers. With practitioners and practice leaders held accountable for fulfilling their specific professional roles according to their best judgment, a continuous learning approach is far superior in maintaining a high level of quality than any existing scoring-based peer review program (Larson et al. 2016).

As an increasing number of radiology departments develop peer learning systems, opportunities for improvement could be shared among various institutions throughout the country. It would be possible to assemble a national repository of de-identified cases, which could be accessed by small practices to enrich their peer learning experience. Analysis of these cases could be used to inform decisions about educational materials and testing for trainees and for CME purposes. Similarly, lessons learning from case analysis could be used to structure educational conferences at many levels. Interactive modules could be developed in which questions are sent electronically to radiologists on a periodic basis (e.g., the daily "Case-in-Point" produced by the ACR), which would permit immediate feedback, case discussion, and readings or videos for further learning opportunities.

Transforming from peer review to peer learning must achieve initial acceptance by practicing radiologists. They must be assured that submitted cases of discrepancy will not be used for any potentially punitive purpose, such as OPPE or FPPE, but only as learning opportunities for all radiologists in the department. Referring clinicians must be urged to contribute imaging studies in which errors may have been made, not for the purpose of blaming their radiology colleagues but rather to further their learning experiences.

Those interested in reading an excellent overview of a prototype for a group learning program can consult *Standards for Learning from*

Discrepancies Meetings, a publication of the Royal College of Radiologists (The Royal College of Radiologists 2014b).

References

Abujudeh H, Pyatt RS Jr, Bruno MA et al (2014) RADPEER peer review: relevance, use, concerns, challenges, and direction forward. J Am Coll Radiol 11(9):899–904

Alkasab TK, Harvey HB, Gowda V, Thrall JH, Rosenthal DI, Gazelle GS (2014) Consensus- oriented group peer review: a new process to review radiologist work output. J Am Coll Radiol 11(2):131–138

Alport HR, Hillman BJ (2004) Quality and variability in diagnostic radiology. J Am Coll Radiol 1:127–132

American Board of Medical Specialties Web site. http://www.abms.org/board-certification/a-trusted-credential/based-on-core-competencies/. Accessed July 5, 2017.

American College of Radiology Web site. http://www.acr.org. Accessed May 12, 2016.

Balogh EP, Miller BT, Ball JR, eds. Board on Health Care Services, Institute of Medicine. Improving diagnosis in health care. Washington, DC: The National Academy of Sciences, The National Academies Press, 2015a.

Balogh EP, Miller BT, Ball JR, eds. Board on Health Care Services, Institute of Medicine. Organizational characteristics, the physical environment, and the diagnostic process: Improving learning, culture, and the work system. In:Improving diagnosis in health care. Washington, DC: The National Academy of Sciences, The National Academies Press, 2015b; 263–306.

Balogh EP, Miller BT, Ball JR, Board on Health Care Services, Institute of Medicine. Diagnostic team members and tasks: Improving patient engagement and health care professional education and training diagnoses. In: Improving diagnosis in health care Washington, DC: The National Academy of Sciences, The National Academies Press, 2015c; 145–216.

Bender LC, Linnau KF, Meier EN, Anzai Y, Gunn ML (2012) Interrater agreement in the evaluation of discrepant imaging findings with the RADPEER system. AJR Am J Roentgenol 199(6):1320–1327

Berwick DM (2016) Era 3 for medicine and health care. JAMA 315:1329–1330

Borgstede JP, Lewis RS, Bhargavan M, Sunshine JH (2004) RADPEER quality assurance program: a multifacility study of interpretive disagreement rates. J Am Coll Radiol 1(1):59–65

Brook OR, Romero J, Brook A, Kruskal JB, Yam CS, Levine D (2015) The complementary nature of peer review and quality assistance data collection. Radiology 274:221–229

Donnelly LF (2007) Performance-based assessment of radiology practitioners: promoting improvement in accordance with the 2007 joint commission standards. J Am Coll Radiol 4(10):699–703

Donnelly LF, Strife JL (2005) Performance-based assessment of radiology faculty: a practical plan to promote improvement and meet JCAHO standards. AJR Am J Roentgenol 184(5):1398–1401

Eisenberg RL (2014) Survey of faculty perceptions regarding a peer review system. J Am Coll Radiol 11:397–401

Eisenberg RL, Heidinger B (2016) Peer review: a better way. Acad Radiol 23:1071–1072

Halsted MJ (2004) Radiology peer review as an opportunity to reduce errors and improve patient care. J Am Coll Radiol 1(12):984–987

Jackson VP, Cushing T, Abujudeh HH et al (2009) RADPEER scoring white paper. J Am Coll Radiol 6(1):21–25

Joint Commission (2007) Comprehensive accreditation manual for hospitals: The official handbook. Oakbrook Terrace, Ill. Joint Commission

Kruskal J, Eisenberg R (2016) Focused professional performance evaluation of a radiologist—a centers for medicare and medicaid services and joint commission requirement. Curr Probl Diagn Radiol 45(2):87–93

Kruskal JB, Eisenberg RL, Brook O, Siewert B (2016) Transitioning from peer review to peer learning for abdominal radiologists. Abdom Radiol (NY) 41(3):416–428

Larson DB, Nance JJ (2011) Rethinking peer review: what aviation can teach radiology about performance improvement. Radiology 259(3):626–632

Larson PA, Pyatt RS Jr, Grimes CK, Abudujeh HH, Chin KW, Roth CJ (2011) Getting the most out of RADPEER. J Am Coll Radiol 8(8):543–548

Larson DB, Donnelly LF, Podberesky DJ, Merrow AC, Sharpe RE, Kruskal JB (2016) Peer feedback, learning, and improvement: answering the call, of the Institute of Medicine Report on diagnostic error. Radiology 27:161254. doi:10.1148/radiol.2016161254. [Epub ahead of print]

Lucey L. The American College of Radiology Accreditation Overview. https://www2.rsna.org/re/QIBA_Annual_Meeting_2014/Index_files/Presentations/11-LUCEY-ACR.pdf. Published May 21, 2014. Accessed Apr 23, 2016

Mahgerefteh S, Kruskal JB, Yam CS, Blachar A, Sosna J (2009) Peer review in diagnostic radiology: current state and a vision for the future. Radiographics 29:1221–1231

Steele JR, Hovsepian DM, Schomer DF (2010) The joint commission practice performance evaluation: a primer for radiologists. J Am Coll Radiol 7(6):425–430

The Royal College of Radiologists. Quality assurance in radiology reporting: peer feedback. http://www.rcr.ac.uk/quality-assurance-radiology-reporting-peer-feedback. Published 2014a. Accessed Apr 23, 2016

The Royal College of Radiologists. Standards for learning from discrepancies meetings. http://www.rcr.ac.uk/publication/standards-learning-discrepancies-meetings. Published 2014b. Accessed Apr 23, 2016

Part VI

Technology's Value During a Time of Health Spending Cuts

IT Innovation and Big Data

Peter Mildenberger

Contents

P. Mildenberger
Department of Radiology, University Medical Center Mainz, Mainz, Germany
e-mail: peter.mildenberger@gmail.com

1 Introduction

Radiology and IT have had an established "symbiosis" for many years. Fundamental requirements and opportunities in the usage of IT in radiology have been described and developed more than 30 years ago (Arenson and London 1979; Arenson 1984).

New developments in IT have been implemented in radiology over the last decades for several different tasks, e.g., PACS (Picture Archiving and Communicating System), teleradiology, image processing, and many others. Therefore, radiology has a leading role, in promoting IT in healthcare overall. In addition, the increase in data generation and knowledge drives new methods like deep learning and machine learning.

IT innovation in radiology could be divided into four pillars:

- Basic IT infrastructure, as RIS, PACS, teleradiology
- New tools improving the basic infrastructure, as order entry solutions, decision support, structured reporting, etc.
- Cross-enterprise communication and patient involvement
- "Disruptive" new developments, as deep learning, artificial intelligence, Big Data, etc.

Over the last decades, these continuous improvements in IT have been essential for quality and workflow improvements in radiology.

Med Radiol Diagn Imaging (2017)
DOI 10.1007/174_2017_144, © Springer International Publishing AG
Published Online 18 August 2017

The next step with introduction of "Big Data," deep learning, or artificial intelligence will change radiology even as much as RIS and PACS did 20 years ago. There is little discussion whether radiology will survive, but the question is "Will radiologists survive?" (Chockley and Emanuel 2016; Jha 2016; Jha and Topol 2016). In many radiology departments, dedicated IT experts have been or are still part of the team and proving special expertise to the IT developments. This might change over time, and rethinking radiology informatics could be relevant (Kohli et al. 2015a, b).

2 Basic IT Infrastructure

Radiology information systems (RIS) have been probably the first IT systems in clinical routine use. RIS solutions have been widely implemented during the 80s and 90s of the last century. The basic functions have been described by Arenson more than 30 years ago as registration, scheduling, patient tracking, film library management, consultation reporting, billing, keeping a teaching file, and providing an imaging system interface (Arenson 1984). Over time, new functionalities have been integrated in RIS solutions, like physician-based order entry, report communication with EMR, worklist provision for imaging modalities, and strong interfacing with PACS. The utilization of RIS solutions has to be feasible in multi-site and multi-user environments. There is an ongoing discussion about the future of RIS as an independent IT system; some vendors do already provide RIS functionality within their EMR solutions, and others argue for an integration of dedicated functions (e.g., reporting) into the PACS and let the EMR provide all other functions.

PACS has been invented in parallel with digitization of imaging systems, which started in the 70s of the last century. Pioneers in Europe have been the University Hospital in Graz (1988) and Donauspital SMZO in Vienna (1992) (Hruby 2003). The introduction of a new standard for "Digital Imaging and Communication in Medicine (DICOM)" in 1993 has been a key factor in the wide adoption and introduction of PACS, because of the new possibilities for interfacing different vendors within the same environment (Mildenberger et al. 1999, 2002). Since then, many different evolutions have taken place, e.g.:

- Integration of high-end image processing (MPR, 3-D, segmentation, image fusion, volumetric measurement, etc.)
- Integration of imaging beyond radiology ("enterprise-wide imaging solution")
- Separation of archiving in dedicated systems ("vendor-neutral archives"), sometimes within the same enterprise, sometimes in cloud-based independent systems
- Support of multi-site enterprises
- Integration within regional or national eHealth systems for seamless image exchange.

Teleradiology has been one of the first telemedicine applications ever, and is probably the most used today. Several societies have published statements on appropriate use of teleradiology, because there are different aspects beyond the technical issues (2002; Radiologists 2012; Ranschaert et al. 2015). A lot of discussion took place about the legal aspects, radiologist's responsibility beyond reporting, or even more on services from abroad using the night shift or offering "low-cost reporting" (Boland 1998, 2008; McLean 2009; Pattynama 2010).

While the first teleradiology systems have been dedicated proprietary solutions, the full integration within PACS is reality today. Such an integration could be established with different technical solutions, like "DICOM-eMail" (a national standard in Germany), web-based systems, or integration with IHE-based "cross-enterprise communication - solutions" (XDS-I) (Weisser et al. 2006; IHE 2017a, b).

3 New Tools Improving the Basic Infrastructure in Radiology Informatics

As RIS and PACS are standard solutions today, there is a continuous demand for further improvements in IT tools supporting radiology. It is expected that radiologists with a better understanding of IT are more efficient in their work and having the appropriate IT tools is a prerequisite to drive performance or use of strategic business and analytics. In the USA, the American College of Radiology has developed the Imaging 3.0™ initiative to empower radiologists in IT, and create and demonstrate value for their patients (Kohli et al. 2015a, b). Typical tools, which have been adopted in radiology today, are speech recognition, advanced visualization, image access from remote, and supportive data for workflow management including information on the referrer and on the patient with access to the EMR.

A key tool to improve efficiency and quality is providing order entry with clinical decision support (CDS). Such tools could help to identify the most appropriate examination based on clinical data. These decision support solutions are based on guidelines, e.g., ACR Appropriateness Guidelines or European Imaging Referral Guidelines. They could be used as a separate tool or with full integration into an order entry solution. In the USA, ACR is providing the ACR Select, and in Europe there is iGUIDE by ESR. CDS is seen as helpful to cope with unnecessary imaging or imaging without reliable indications. It has been demonstrated that especially high-cost procedures could be used more efficiently. In healthcare system with pre-approval for such high-cost procedures, CDS can be used for the approval process and therefore for relevant workflow improvements by reducing the time for approval by 90% and more.

The most relevant reasons to use CDS are the improvement of quality by reducing the number of low-utility examinations and therefore reducing radiation exposure and costs. Rosenthat et al. could demonstrate a decline of such low-utility examinations from 6 to 2% by using CDS already 10 years ago (Rosenthal et al. 2006). Typical examinations with lower evidence are MRI for lumbar pain, head MRI, sinus CT, and CT for pulmonary embolism. It is supposed that CDS could help to reduce the imaging utilization growth (Blackmore et al. 2011; Raja et al. 2014; Moriarity et al. 2015; Yan et al. 2017). CDS is the best way to support standardized clinical practice while allowing some flexibility to adopt local requirements (Allen 2014). Providing the actual recommendations within an electronic ordering system, these criteria could be used also by the referring physicians, who would not use dedicated resources otherwise. CDS could be more relevant in the future with payment based on value instead of volume (Allen 2014). Of course, wide adoption of CDS relies on several requirements. There should be consensus-based criteria for appropriateness, which have to be interdisciplinarily discussed and updated on a regular basis. Actually, a relevant part of indications (over 60%) is not covered by such guidelines (Jensen and Durand 2017). This could lead to relevant differences in the use of CDS-based order entry systems, especially in cases with limited or incomplete clinical information (Schneider et al. 2015). Using CDS usually requests structured information, while conventional ordering is done in a free-text, more unstructured form. This could be a barrier in the acceptance of CDS, if design and integration don't support workflow expectations accordingly. So far, it is not clear if natural language processing (NLP) would help to improve the usability and acceptance (Moriarity et al. 2015, 2017).

However, decision support is not intended to be used for ordering imaging examinations only, but also to support radiologists in reporting and the management of recommendations for follow-up studies or handling of incidental findings. This is also linked with the Imaging 3.0®—Initiative of ACR. Several applications are already available, e.g., for liver imaging, lung nodule follow-up, management of incidental findings, prostate imaging, and others (McGinty et al. 2014; Nielsen and Clark 2016). More advanced solutions are provided using a naive Bayesian decision support tool for mammographic lesions, which is based on the BI-RADS lexicon (Benndorf et al. 2015).

Radiology reporting is evenly discussed on different levels. Usually, radiology reports are in natural language with varying levels of structure and certainty. It is not unusual that wording is vague, probably misleading, or reports don't acknowledge prior examinations accordingly.

Key elements for radiology reports include consistent format, awareness of clinical context, clarity, evidence-based recommendations, or readability also for patients (Boland et al. 2011; Ware et al. 2017; Wildman-Tobriner 2017).

For many years, the term "structured reporting" (SR) has been seen as a key for improvement in radiology reporting. There are several reports showing that SR-formatted reports would be preferred by referring physicians and radiologists. There is an expectation of reduced variability in terms and wording used and a more easy access to information. Also, SR could be linked with coding of information, which could support clinical research and computer-based analyses. Several groups and scientific societies have been active in the field of SR; esp. RSNA's reporting initiative and the joined RSNA-ESR Template Library Advisory Panel (TLAP) have contributed to this field. IHE has provided the technical frame with a dedicated profile for the "Management of Radiology Report Templates". First solutions providing tools to handle such templates within a reporting process are available today (Pinto Dos Santos et al. 2017). Such reporting tools could also be used to integrate radiation dose information, which is automatically collected and fed into the reporting template (Lee et al. 2016).

Another aspect to improve the quality of reports is including images into radiology reports as "image-rich radiology reports" (IRRR). This could be done in different ways, e.g., as embedded images or as hyperlinks with online access. Based on a survey, it is expected that such IRRR could improve the communication and workflow efficiency (Patel et al. 2017).

Different tools, especially the introduction of voice recognition (VR) and enterprise-wide online access, have reduced the turnaround time. Less focus has been set on the quality of reports, and it has been demonstrated that the use of VR could increase the number of mistakes and errors in reports (Chung et al. 2016). Therefore, there is a need to identify errors in reports and potentially clinical significant implications. Systematic peer review could be established by tools like ACR's RADPEER™ (Maloney et al. 2012; Moriarity et al. 2016). Peer review could also be used for structured education and feedback ("peer learning") (Butler and Forghani 2013; Larson et al. 2017). Another approach for quality improvement is a regular comparison of preliminary and final reports in the teaching of residents. There are many organizational issues, which is why there are many barriers for such a comparison, as high study volume, rotation, and remote finalization of reports. An automated system could enable such a comparison on a more consistent way (Kalaria and Filice 2016).

Natural language processing (NLP) is another new trend introduced in radiological IT at the moment (Cai et al. 2016; Pons et al. 2016). Even though there is a growing interest in structured reporting templates, in reality most of the reports are still in unstructured form without standardized terminology. Therefore, it is a challenge to analyze radiological reports with conventional IT tools. NLP could enable "mining" of large datasets of such unstructured reports. The goal is to transform the free-form reports into some kind of structured information, which could be analyzed with database queries or used for business analytics. NLP is based on a set of theories and technologies, including linguistics. First, NLP has to identify individual terms and their modifiers based on pattern matching and linguistic analyses. Further steps are based on rules and machine learning for determination of specific characteristics and relationships in the report (e.g., specific findings). NLP has the potential to identify terms in their different ways of wording respective synonyms or even misspelled terms. So far, domains for NLP have been large-scale testing for CDS, quality assurance and performance monitoring, and appropriate use of imaging as well as screening for patient's eligibility for clinical studies (Cai et al. 2016).

While CDS is used to check the appropriateness of imaging requests to reduce unnecessary imaging, there is also a growing interest to monitor radiation exposure and analyze such numbers. It is expected that with the transition of the EU Euratom Directive 2013/59 into national law, more requirements for systematic registration and analyses will be established. DICOM has developed the concept of radiation dose structured reporting, which allows the documentation of radiation data in a DICOM object that can be handled and stored like other objects. This is a relevant difference from the former practice using DICOM MPPS (Modality Performed Procedure Step), which is just a message form requiring systems able to handle such messages. The adoption of MPPS for systematic dose evaluation has been limited over the years. Now, IHE has developed a profile on radiation exposure monitoring describing three different new roles in this workflow. These are the *Report Dose Information* based on objects from acquisition modalities, the *Dose Register* for building individual or cross-enterprise databases, and the *Dose Info Consumer* for analyzing results. Several use cases can be supported by this approach, as population dose and dose indicators, dose reference levels, site benchmarking, and clinical trials (IHE). Meanwhile, several open-source-based and commercial tools for dose management and dose tracking are available. This can help with auditing patient safety, e.g., in controlling the correctness of imaging protocols or problems following scanner modifications or software updates. Alert levels could help to optimize the analyses and allow efficient online or near-online recognition of critical events. This automation by such dose tracking software enables a more representative overview on dose levels compared with manual, sample-based methods as used before (which are still in use in several countries for establishing official recommendations). Radiation dose tracking and evaluation are part of an outcome-based approach. Several campaigns in the USA, Africa, and Europe support radiation awareness. ACR has established a dose registry for CT studies. The main metrics are of course $CTDI_{vol}$ and DLP. Some solutions could also register size-specific data for further individual estimations (Parakh et al. 2016; Weisenthal et al. 2016).

The development of new tools supporting radiology is going on. Especially the IHE Radiology Domain is working on different new profiles (see also wiki.net.ihe). Some examples for these activities are as follows:

"Cross-Enterprise Remote Reporting for Imaging Workflow Definition", which is relevant for access to the different clinical information types besides imaging such as patient summaries and laboratory results in a distributed interpretation workload of radiologists.

"Standardized Operational Log of Events" (SOLE) for an easy way to collect and compile events coming from different systems, generating an event repository, supporting business intelligence tools or tools related to performance measurement.

"Enterprise Scanner Protocol Management" will allow the central management of scanning protocols and distribution to the different modalities within an enterprise. This is especially relevant for CT and MRI scanners and would improve the standardization of study descriptions. Based on that, the possibilities for the observation of radiation dose exposure and other quality issues could be improved.

"Critical Finding Follow-up Workflow" will improve the tools to mark unexpected, but noncritical, observations requiring a follow-up study (e.g., smaller lung nodules). There is no doubt that radiologist should care about the communication of such additional findings to the referring physician and about appropriate actionable measures. As part of this development, there is also a new concept for "Report Distribution" as part of the developing cycle 2016–2017 in progress.

4 Cross-Enterprise Communication and Patient Involvement

New technical developments have a great potential to change the kind of communication and cooperation between healthcare professionals and also the interaction with patients itself. This parallels with other challenges in radiology, as improved customer service, the call for "patients first", or shortage of radiologists or technicians (Becker et al. 2016; European Society of and American College of 2016). Developing a patient-centered radiology process model is one example for taking these challenges into account and provides metrics for measuring patient experiences (Swan et al. 2017).

Enabling cross-enterprise and cross-sectorial communication and involvement of citizens or patients is a political goal in many countries. It is expected that better communication and information flow could simplify diagnostic and therapeutic processes, leading to improved care provision. Also, the access to healthcare, optimization of quality, and cost reduction are in the focus of such concepts. In Europe, the European Commission has founded many projects promoting eHealth including interoperability, e.g., epSOS or eStandards. As part of this propagation, an eHealth European Interoperability Framework has been developed, which addresses different topics like governance, legal interoperability, organizational interoperability, and semantic interoperability. Sharing radiological workflow and imaging result distribution is included in the list of high-level use cases (European Commission 2013). At present, several countries in Europe already have national eHealth strategies which are implemented or in implementation (e.g., Austria, Denmark, Luxemburg, Switzerland). Most of such national or regional eHealth plans incorporate the IHE concepts for cross-enterprise communication (IHE XDS profiles family).

However, improved information exchange with other care providers has an impact on radiological workflow. This includes the access to electronic health records (EHR) or even the handling of media with imaging studies from abroad. EHR deployment interfaces with the role of RIS. The structures for managing the IT systems become more complex and require a more sophisticated team approach (Sachs and Long 2016).

The implementation of diagnostic imaging repositories (DIRs) allows seamless patient data sharing between separate organizations. There is an increasing interest in the outcome of such networks. Some metrics have been proposed for such an analysis, e.g., the number of access to foreign studies, the impact of CD imports, and reduction of reimaging of patients. In a Canadian study referring to the Toronto region, it could be demonstrated that about 40% of in-house patients have priors in the DIR, a marked reduction of CD imports could be achieved, and an estimated rate of about 15% of patients could be prevented from repeated imaging (Nagels et al. 2017).

5 Artificial Intelligence and Big Data

Decision making is one of the core tasks in radiology with finding the best diagnosis and differential diagnosis in a given imaging study. There is a long tradition of analyzing the "Reasoning Foundations of Medical Diagnosis" — R. Ledley and L. Lusted, pioneers in this field, already described basic principles of logic, probability, and value theory in 1959. Also, they discussed the potential of computers in supporting diagnostic procedures (Ledley and Lusted 1959). More than 50 years later, these visionary ideas could become a reality and people are asking: Will computers replace radiologists? (Jha 2016).

There is no doubt that progression in computer science has made huge contributions to imaging technologies and also that image processing with 3D visualization, segmentation, and volumetric analyses is established in radiology today. But such tools have a supportive intention in improving decision making of diagnosis. They are based on definite algorithms. The process of image analysis is reproducible for humans and results are predictable.

New developments based on "artificial intelligence" (AI) are completely different, because the approach is disruptive from former image processing technologies and the goal and potential are to find the best diagnosis, even without understanding the way and why the computer system gets the specific result. Therefore, it is not surprising that visionary computer scientists are convinced that computers will be able to take over the decision making in image interpretation. This might be one reason why several companies are active in this domain. For example IBM with the Watson Health Imaging program has acquired a PACS company, Google is in cooperation with a National Health Service Trust in the UK, and several other new players (e.g., Enlitic) are very active (Jha 2016).

It might be more realistic to see AI as a supportive approach in radiology to improve the quality and precision of diagnosis instead of a "black-and-white" discussion on replacing radiologists. There are many new challenges in radiology with an increasing number of images per study; the requirement for volumetric analysis, e.g., in oncology or liver surgery; the differential diagnosis of less common findings; and the increasing workload itself. AI-based tools could help to separate normal findings from pathologies, finding lung nodules, detecting fractures or lung embolism, and many others. On the other hand, there are different obstacles for AI to overcome. For example for the training of AI tools, many thousands or even million cases have to be analyzed. One relevant challenge is that for the training of AI tools, qualified radiology reports are required. But it is known that extraction of validated and/or coded information out of conventional free-text reports is not an easy task. Besides this, also consistency in radiological diagnosis will be another challenge.

Several terms are in use to describe such computer-based tools. Besides AI, there is "machine learning" (ML), "deep learning," "data mining," or "Big Data," which are sometimes mixed or have some overlap. AI and machine learning might be understood as higher ranking concepts, which are using different specific tools (Erickson et al. 2017b; Wikipedia 2017a). For example, deep learning is part of machine learning using specific artificial neural networks with a wide range of different architectures as deep neural networks, deep belief networks, or recurrent neural networks (Erickson et al. 2017a; Wikipedia 2017c). Typical fields of application are computer vision, speech recognition, natural language processing, machine translation, etc.

Machine learning could be used in pattern recognition in medical images and rendering medical diagnosis. In machine learning, different techniques are in use, such as linear models for classification and regression, artificial neural networks, kernel-based tools, probabilistic models, cluster analysis, dimensionality reduction, reinforcement learning, multiple instance learning, graph matching, or structured prediction. Conventional applications of machine learning in the past have been image segmentation, image registration, computer-aided detection and diagnosis, functional analysis, content-based image retrieval, and text analysis of radiology reports by NLP (Wang and Summers 2012; Erickson et al. 2017b; Wikipedia 2017d).

Usually, several methods of machine learning can be combined. Especially deep learning methods could perform better when combined with pre- or postprocessing by conventional algorithms. There are open-source tools available for use in different platforms. Also, there are pre-trained neural networks available, which were originally not intended for radiological images, but could be adopted and already perform well (e.g., AlexNet, GoogleNet). Training of such systems could be done in a non-supervised or in a supervised form. Supervised learning requires labeled information for training of the system and could be done on smaller datasets in a more efficient and faster way. However, there often is a drawback in the labeling of data, because radiology reports are not available with codes. Probably, structured reporting could improve this approach in the future.

Advantages of these machine learning tools could be reducing workload and improving accuracy, e.g., segmentation of anatomical structures or pathologies. Examples for this are CAD in breast imaging or detection and identification of lung nodules or colonic polyps. Most times, such tools might focus on sensitivity, which means that there could be a lot of false-positive findings that have to be sorted out by a radiologist. Barriers in the adoption of these methods are, e.g., in the transition of use in small datasets to large datasets, which could have different features, and in the potential complexity based on many variables (Wang and Summers 2012).

There are some promising results with the use of a deep learning approach. Lakhani and Sundaram published a study on automated classification of pulmonary tuberculosis by using deep convolutional neural networks. They used the AlexNet and the GoogleNet in different settings including preprocessing techniques. It could be shown that the best performing classifier could reach an AUC of 0,99 (Lakhani 2017).

Kline et al. have tested a deep neural network for fully automated segmentation of polycystic kidneys to measure the total kidney volume. Based on a set of 2000 cases, they found that fully automated segmentation works at a level comparable to interobserver variability and could be used as a replacement for conventional segmentation (Kline et al. 2017).

Brain imaging is another field in the application of machine learning, in which a lot of classical algorithms have been established for segmentation of normal and abnormal tissue (Akkus et al. 2017). In the past, the limiting factor in the use of tools like this was the missing ability to generalize. Also, normal variations are difficult to handle by conventional image segmentation. This explains the relevant interest in deep learning tools for analyzing brain imaging. Different datasets are available and have been provided for competitions for several years; these include brain tumors, stroke detection, traumatic injuries, etc. Erickson and his coworkers stated in their review that there is a significant potential for deep learning techniques. Even though deep learning tools have been established only recently, it seems like they will one day outperform conventional image processing techniques (Akkus et al. 2017).

Predicting the future might be difficult, Obermeyer and Emanuel stated in their position paper in late 2016, saying that conventional expert systems, which adopt general rules to new patients, will be overcome and machine learning tools will succeed, because these are learning rules from data. They expect that ML will replace much of the work of radiologists and anatomical pathologists (Obermeyer and Emanuel 2016).

While others do have a different view on radiology, there is a challenge to find the optimal approach for translating artificial intelligence into clinical care. In case there will be a functional deep learning system for analyzing dedicated images, this could outperform radiologists in regard of processing time and costs, and also error rate. This will impact practice and clinical training, and also payment systems in the future (Beam and Kohane 2016). This might change or improve the role of radiologists as information specialists handling the different kinds of information advise on further test and guide clinicians (Jha and Topol 2016).

Another topic in general is "Big Data", which will have some impact on radiology, too. Big Data is used for datasets so large or complex that traditional data processing algorithms are not appropriate anymore. Big Data challenges different fields from data capturing and data storage to privacy issues. Volume, variety, and velocity are key elements in handling "big" data, which requires new tools including machine learning and high-performance computing with massive parallel computing. Different aspects in healthcare could benefit from this approach using large datasets, e.g., in genomics, electronic health records, and also medical imaging (Brink et al. 2017; Brink 2017; Wikipedia 2017b).

For the development of tools especially in imaging data science, huge datasets will be required. Such datasets should be organized by different sites to avoid selection of site-specific issues based on protocols, patient selection, or demographics. Such datasets, as already available for some regions including brain, lung, or liver, could be evaluated with different algorithms and programs to validate their capabilities. The advantage of these tools could be the correlation of different health information coming from radiology, pathology, lab results, etc. Tools based on such algorithms could be used for decision support, online guidance in standardized reporting, improved quantification, and quality in reporting in general. Hurdles could be limited quality of data itself with inconsistent information, and of course security and privacy aspects. Privacy aspects are relevant for the use of data in research, because the recombination of different information even out of pseudonymized or anonymized date could identify distinct persons (Brink 2017; Brink et al. 2017; Kruskal et al. 2017). In the UK, Google Deep Mind has developed an app based on millions of regular NHS datasets.

This approach has been found to break UK privacy laws (BBC 2017). Professional organizations are acting on these issues. ACR (American College of Radiology) has started the ACR Center for Imaging Data Science, which will go beyond diagnostic performance of machine learning algorithms. Issues like data ownership, access rights, liabilities, education, and creation of datasets will be addressed as well (Brink 2017). In Europe, similar questions will be in the focus of an ongoing EU project called MEDIRAD, which is coordinated by the European Institute for Biomedical Imaging Research (EIBIR 2017) and in which ESR will be the leading organization.

Data mining and business analytics are other items coming on stage now in radiology, too. Data mining is about knowledge detection in databases, which is relevant in the field of radiology for imaging data and associated metadata as technical parameters of imaging procedures, reports, information in the EHR, etc. Several techniques are used in data mining, e.g., grouping of similar data objects, heuristic search algorithms, neural networks, or decision trees. Data mining could be used to establish references or standards from a trusted cohort or to identify reference images for a given finding. The combination of data mining and radiomics could improve the detection of features that could not be identified by visual analysis alone. As Gillies et al. stated, “Radiomics: Images are More than Pictures, They are Data” (Gillies et al. 2016), radiomics is about the extraction of statistical features out of images. Subsequent analysis could feed decision support, especially in combination with other data sources, or could be used to monitor therapeutic concepts.

Besides imaging data, there is a growing demand and pressure to care about economics in radiology. Radiology is faced with high fixed costs for providing up-to-date imaging quality and 24h service for emergency cases. Therefore, there is a need to know about the resources, imaging capacity, turnaround times, quality indicators, etc. Business analytics (BA) can help to analyze such data and provide results for decision making, resource allocation, and more. The quality of such analyses relies on the metrics used and the consistency of primary data. The Society of Imaging Informatics (SIIM) has developed a workflow lexicon for harmonization of terms and leveraging workflow management tools (Erickson et al. 2013). Also, BA and BI are often used in radiology to improve quality and safety or patient outcome. An example for this is radiation dose monitoring with benchmarking on different levels, e.g., study or institutional. As part of the discussion on value-based radiology, such data is more relevant than before. Different levels of BI can be found with the differentiation in descriptive, predictive, or even prescriptive analytics (Cook and Nagy 2014).

Conclusion

There is no doubt on the relevance of IT in radiology. Actual developments will have different effects on radiology. Better solutions for IT tools and for business analytics will improve the efficiency, workflow, quality, and safety in radiology. Otherwise, artificial intelligence, machine learning, Big Data will probably have a more disruptive effect. Radiologists should be interested in these techniques and try to understand the underlying concepts. Also, they should realize the opportunities for better results in image interpretation, providing new findings and conclusions based on such analysis, which could not be given before. Finally, all these improvements should ensure better care and a better outcome for patients and population health.

References

ACR (2002) ACR standard for teleradiology. 13–21. http://imaging.stryker.com/images/ACR_Standards-Teleradiology.pdf

Akkus Z, Galimzianova A, Hoogi A, Rubin DL, Erickson BJ (2017) Deep learning for brain MRI segmentation: state of the art and future directions. J Digit Imaging:1–11

Allen B Jr (2014) Five reasons radiologists should embrace clinical decision support for diagnostic imaging. J Am Coll Radiol 11(6):533–534

Arenson RL (1984) Automation of the radiology management function. Radiology 153:65
Arenson RL, London JW (1979) Comprehensive analysis of a radiology operations management computer system. Radiology 133:355
BBC (2017) Google DeepMind NHS app test broke UK privacy law. http://www.bbc.co.uk/news/technology-40483202. Accessed 31 July 2017.
Beam AL, Kohane IS (2016) Translating artificial intelligence into clinical care. JAMA 316(22):2368–2369
Becker E, Fishman EK, Horton KM, Raman SP (2016) Leading in the world of business and medicine: putting the needs of customers, employees, and patients first. J Am Coll Radiol 13(5):576–578
Benndorf M, Kotter E, Langer M, Herda C, Wu Y, Burnside ES (2015) Development of an online, publicly accessible naive Bayesian decision support tool for mammographic mass lesions based on the American College of Radiology (ACR) BI-RADS lexicon. Eur Radiol 25(6):1768–1775
Blackmore CC, Mecklenburg RS, Kaplan GS (2011) Effectiveness of clinical decision support in controlling inappropriate imaging. J Am Coll Radiol 8(1):19–25
Boland GW (1998) Teleradiology: another revolution in radiology? Clin Radiol 53(8):547–553
Boland GW (2008) Teleradiology coming of age: winners and losers. AJR Am J Roentgenol 190(5):1161–1162
Boland GW, Thrall JH, Gazelle GS, Samir A, Rosenthal DI, Dreyer KJ, Alkasab TK (2011) Decision support for radiologist report recommendations. J Am Coll Radiol 8(12):819–823
Brink JA (2017) Big data management, access, and protection. J Am Coll Radiol 14(5):579–580
Brink JA, Arenson RL, Grist TM, Lewin JS, Enzmann D (2017) Bits and bytes: the future of radiology lies in informatics and information technology. Eur Radiol:1–5
Butler GJ, Forghani R (2013) The next level of radiology peer review: Enterprise-wide education and improvement. J Am Coll Radiol 10(5):349–353
Cai T, Giannopoulos AA, Yu S, Kelil T, Ripley B, Kumamaru KK, Rybicki FJ, Mitsouras D (2016) Natural language processing technologies in radiology research and clinical applications. Radiographics 36(1):176–191
Chockley K, Emanuel E (2016) The end of radiology? Three threats to the future practice of radiology. J Am Coll Radiol 13(12 Pt A):1415–1420
Chung JH, MacMahon H, Montner SM, Liu L, Paushter DM, Chang PJ, Katzman GL (2016) The effect of an electronic peer-review auditing system on faculty-dictated radiology report error rates. J Am Coll Radiol 13(10):1215–1218
European Commission E (2013) eHealth European interoperability framework: overall executive summary. https://doi.org/10.2759/10138 ISBN 978-92-79-30389-0
Cook TS, Nagy P (2014) Business intelligence for the radiologist: making your data work for you. J Am Coll Radiol 11(12 Pt B):1238–1240
EIBIR (2017) MEDIRAD Project. http://www.eibir.org/news-2/horizon-2020-news/medirad-project-kicks-off-today-in-barcelona-under-eibir-coordination/. Accessed 31 July 2017.
Erickson BJ, Meenan C, Langer S (2013) Standards for business analytics and departmental workflow. J Digit Imaging 26(1):53–57
Erickson BJ, Korfiatis P, Akkus Z, Kline T, Philbrick K (2017a) Toolkits and libraries for deep learning. J Digit Imaging:1–6
Erickson BJ, Korfiatis P, Akkus Z, Kline TL (2017b) Machine learning for medical imaging. Radiographics 37(2):505–515
European Society of, R. and R. American College of (2016) European Society of Radiology (ESR) and American College of Radiology (ACR) report of the 2015 global summit on radiological quality and safety. Insights Imaging 7(4):481–484
Gillies RJ, Kinahan PE, Hricak H (2016) Radiomics: images are more than pictures, they are data. Radiology 278(2):563–577
Hruby, W. (2003). "Digitale Radiologie und Teleradiologie: Zukunftsvision oder moderne Radiologie?"
IHE (2017a) Cross-enterprise document sharing. http://wiki.ihe.net/index.php/Cross-Enterprise_Document_Sharing. Accessed 2 Aug 2017.
IHE (2017b) IHE radiology: technical framework supplement – radiation exposure monitoring (REM). http://www.ihe.net/Technical_Framework/upload/IHE_RAD_Suppl_REM_Rev2-1_TI_2010-11-16.pdf. Accessed 31 July 2017.
Jensen JD, Durand DJ (2017) Partnering with your health system to select and implement clinical decision support for imaging. J Am Coll Radiol 14(2):262–268
Jha S (2016) Will computers replace radiologists? Medscape. http://www.medscape.com/viewarticle/863127. Accessed 12 May 2016.
Jha S, Topol EJ (2016) Adapting to artificial intelligence: radiologists and pathologists as information specialists. JAMA 316(22):2353–2354
Kalaria AD, Filice RW (2016) Comparison-bot: an automated preliminary-final report comparison system. J Digit Imaging 29(3):325–330
Kline TL, Korfiatis P, Edwards ME, Blais JD, Czerwiec FS, Harris PC, King BF, Torres VE, Erickson BJ (2017) Performance of an artificial multi-observer deep neural network for fully automated segmentation of polycystic kidneys. J Digit Imaging 30(4):442–448
Kohli M, Dreyer KJ, Geis JR (2015a) The imaging 3.0 informatics scorecard. J Am Coll Radiol 12(4):396–402
Kohli M, Dreyer KJ, Geis JR (2015b) Rethinking radiology informatics. AJR Am J Roentgenol 204(4):716–720
Kruskal JB, Berkowitz S, Geis JR, Kim W, Nagy P, Dreyer K (2017) Big data and machine learning—

strategies for driving this bus: a summary of the 2016 intersociety summer conference. J Am Coll Radiol 14(6):811–817
Lakhani P (2017) Deep convolutional neural networks for endotracheal tube position and X-ray image classification: challenges and opportunities. J Digit Imaging:1–9
Larson DB, Donnelly LF, Podberesky DJ, Merrow AC, Sharpe RE Jr, Kruskal JB (2017) Peer feedback, learning, and improvement: answering the call of the Institute of Medicine Report on diagnostic error. Radiology 283(1):231–241
Ledley R, Lusted L (1959) Reasoning foundations of medical diagnosis. Science 130(3366):9–21
Lee M-C, Chuang K-S, Hsu T-C, Lee C-D (2016) Enhancement of structured reporting – an integration reporting module with radiation dose collection supporting. J Med Syst 40(11):250
Maloney E, Lomasney LM, Schomer L (2012) Application of the RADPEER scoring language to interpretation discrepancies between diagnostic radiology residents and faculty radiologists. J Am Coll Radiol 9(4):264–269
McGinty GB, Allen B Jr, Geis JR, Wald C (2014) IT infrastructure in the era of imaging 3.0. J Am Coll Radiol 11(12 Pt B):1197–1204
McLean TR (2009) Will India set the price for teleradiology? Int J Med Robot 5(2):178–183
Mildenberger P, Heussel C, Walther S, Thelen M (1999) Three years experience with DICOM in a multivendor PACS. Eur Radiol (Suppl 1.-European Congress of Radiology ECR):99–229
Mildenberger P, Eichelberg M, Martin E (2002) Introduction to the DICOM standard. Eur Radiol 12(4):920–927
Moriarity AK, Klochko C, O'Brien M, Halabi S (2015) The effect of clinical decision support for advanced inpatient imaging. J Am Coll Radiol 12(4):358–363
Moriarity AK, Hawkins CM, Geis JR, Dreyer KJ, Kamer AP, Khandheria P, Morey J, Whitfill J, Wiggins RH, Itri JN (2016) Meaningful peer review in radiology: a review of current practices and potential future directions. J Am Coll Radiol 13(12):1519–1524
Moriarity AK, Green A, Klochko C, O'Brien M, Halabi S (2017) Evaluating the effect of unstructured clinical information on clinical decision support appropriateness ratings. J Am Coll Radiol 14(6):737–743
Nagels J, Macdonald D, Coz C (2017) Measuring the benefits of a regional imaging environment. J Digit Imaging:1–6
Nielsen JP, Clark TJ (2016) Radiologist-Centered decision support applications. J Am Coll Radiol 13(9):1083–1087
Obermeyer Z, Emanuel E (2016) Predicting the future – big data, machine learning, and clinical medicine. N Engl J Med 375(13):1212–1216
Parakh A, Kortesniemi M, Schindera ST (2016) CT radiation dose management: a comprehensive optimization process for improving patient safety. Radiology 280(3):663–673
Patel BN, Lopez JM, Jiang BG, Roth CJ, Nelson RC (2017) Image-rich radiology reports: a value-based model to improve clinical workflow. J Am Coll Radiol 14(1):57–64
Pattynama PM (2010) Legal aspects of cross-border teleradiology. Eur J Radiol 73(1):26–30
Pinto Dos Santos D, Klos G, Kloeckner R, Oberle R, Dueber C, Mildenberger P (2017) Development of an IHE MRRT-compliant open-source web-based reporting platform. Eur Radiol 27(1):424–430
Pons E, Braun LMM, Hunink MGM, Kors JA (2016) Natural language processing in radiology: a systematic review. Radiology 279(2):329–343
Radiologists T. R. C. o (2012) The regulation of teleradiology: A position statement by the Royal College of Radiologists. https://www.rcr.ac.uk/docs/newsroom/pdf/Telerad_PS_May2012.pdf. Accessed 4 June 2013.
Raja AS, Gupta A, Ip IK, Mills AM, Khorasani R (2014) The use of decision support to measure documented adherence to a national imaging quality measure. Acad Radiol 21(3):378–383
Ranschaert ER, Boland GW, Duerinckx AJ, Barneveld Binkhuysen FH (2015) Comparison of European (ESR) and American (ACR) white papers on teleradiology: patient primacy is paramount. J Am Coll Radiol 12(2):174–182
Rosenthal DI, Weilburg JB, Schultz T, Miller JC, Nixon V, Dreyer KJ, Thrall JH (2006) Radiology order entry with decision support: initial clinical experience. J Am Coll Radiol 3(10):799–806
Sachs PB, Long G (2016) Process for managing and optimizing radiology work flow in the electronic heath record environment. J Digit Imaging 29(1):43–46
Schneider E, Zelenka S, Grooff P, Alexa D, Bullen J, Obuchowski NA (2015) Radiology order decision support: examination-indication appropriateness assessed using 2 electronic systems. J Am Coll Radiol 12(4):349–357
Swan JS, Furtado VF, Keller LA, Lotti JB, Saltalamacchia CA, Lennes IT, Salazar GM (2017) Pilot study of a patient-Centered radiology process model. J Am Coll Radiol 14(2):274–281
Wang S, Summers RM (2012) Machine learning and radiology. Med Image Anal 16(5):933–951
Ware JB, Jha S, Hoang JK, Baker S, Wruble J (2017) Effective radiology reporting. J Am Coll Radiol 14(6):838–839
Weisenthal SJ, Folio L, Kovacs W, Seff A, Derderian V, Summers RM, Yao J (2016) Open-source radiation exposure extraction engine (RE3) with patient-specific outlier detection. J Digit Imaging 29(4):406–419
Weisser G, Walz M, Ruggiero S, Kämmerer M, Schröter A, Runa A, Mildenberger P, Engelmann U (2006)

Standardization of teleradiology using Dicom e-mail: recommendations of the German radiology society. Eur Radiol 16(3):753–758

Wikipedia (2017a) Artificial intelligence. https://en.wikipedia.org/wiki/Artificial_intelligence. Accessed 31 July 2017.

Wikipedia (2017b) Big data. https://en.wikipedia.org/wiki/Big_data. Accessed 31 July 2017.

Wikipedia (2017c) Deep learning. https://en.wikipedia.org/wiki/Deep_learning. Accessed 31 July 2017.

Wikipedia (2017d) Machine learning. https://en.wikipedia.org/wiki/Machine_learning. Accessed 31 July 2017.

Wildman-Tobriner B (2017) Mean what you say and say what you mean. J Am Coll Radiol 14(7):862

Yan Z, Ip IK, Raja AS, Gupta A, Kosowsky JM, Khorasani R (2017) Yield of CT pulmonary angiography in the emergency department when providers override evidence-based clinical decision support. Radiology 282(3):717–725

Healthcare Technology Assessment of Medical Imaging Technology

Jaap Deinum, Gabriela Restovic, Peter Makai, Gert Jan van der Wilt, and Laura Sampietro-Colom

Contents

Abstract

This chapter provides a view of how due to the health systems and technologies development in the last century a series of functions have been developed to achieve an optimal health for the entire population with available resources. Considering the particularities of the imaging technology area, the authors describe in what manner the value of these technologies should be defined, what are the approaches proposed for assessing this value, both by academia and by several institutions and finally by looking specifically at the SPARTACUS case an approach to compare two diagnostic modalities in terms of their impact on patient outcome is described. The author's description of the SPARTACUS project is particularly informative. The results of this project made the authors concluding that, although RCT are not commonly used in the context of evaluating diagnostic tests, its use allows for the assessment of a wider scope of outcomes that are arguably relevant from an HTA perspective.

1 Health Technology Assessment

The beginning of this century is being characterized by an exponential development of disruptive (e.g., Hepatitis C drugs) and innovative (e.g., hybrid technologies such as PET-MRI or MRI for prostate cancer) health technologies

J. Deinum, M.D. • P. Makai, Ph.D.
G.J. van der Wilt, Ph.D.
Department for Health Evidence, Health Technology Assessment Group, Radboud Institute for Health Sciences, Radboud University Medical Center, Nijmegen, The Netherlands

G. Restovic, M.Sc.
L. Sampietro-Colom, M.D., Ph.D. (✉)
Health Technology Assessment Unit, Research and Innovation Directorate, Hospital Clínic, University of Barcelona, Barcelona, Spain
e-mail: LSAMPIET@clinic.ub.es

Med Radiol Diagn Imaging (2017)
DOI 10.1007/174_2017_86, © Springer International Publishing AG
Published Online 23 June 2017

which are accessing the healthcare market. Additionally other technologies are emerging, and expecting, to quickly also access the market (e.g., molecular diagnostics). These new technologies usually are costly, either in their acquisition, installation, operation, or maintenance. This trend is paralleled with the growth and aging of populations which will imply an increased demand for medical imaging services, obviously associated to higher costs. These expected raising costs are a concern for finite healthcare budgets of health systems. Policy decision-makers, healthcare managers, and clinicians have to be wise on how to allocate these scarce economic resources. They need to base their decisions in comprehensive, objective, health system tailored information. Questions faced by decision-makers when deciding on one innovative and new health technology (HT) include: is this new HT necessary for my country/hospital? Is the new HT justified sufficiently by the overall benefits achieved in terms of safety, health outcomes, and costs in my country/hospital? Which patients can benefit the most from this new HT in my country/hospital? Among the big number of choices of HT, which are the most appropriate for a specific health problem in my country/hospital?

Healthcare Technology Assessment (HTA) aims to explore in what way and under what conditions the use of specific healthcare technologies can help to create value for patients and society at large (Banta and Luce 1993). Such value may derive from the fact that healthcare technologies can help to restore functioning, alleviate suffering or pain, or avert death in an affordable and sustainable way. Value may also derive from fostering moral values such as bolstering patients' autonomy and promoting equity. HTA provides with the information decision-makers need to base their decisions. HTA is a tool used more and more around the world by health system decision-makers in their process of deliberating and deciding which innovative and emerging technologies deserve allocation of resources. The International Network of Agencies for Health Technology Assessment (INAHTA) define HTA as "the systematic evaluation of the properties and effects of a health technology, addressing the direct and indirect effects of this technology, as well as its indirect and unintended consequences, and aimed mainly at informing decision making regarding health technologies" (INAHTA 2017). HT is defined as "an intervention that may be used to improve health, to prevent, diagnose or treat acute or chronic disease, or for rehabilitation". Therefore, HTs include pharmaceuticals, devices, procedures, and organizational systems used in healthcare (INAHTA 2017). The goal of HTA is provide input into decision-making in policy and practice (Health Technology Assessment 2009), it is not research for research or for the sake of knowledge, it has to be aimed to advice and influence decision-making.

HTA takes a broad view of the HT; it takes into account a comprehensive set of aspects that can impact in the healthcare system when the HT accesses the market. The aim of HTA is to determine the "added value" that the HT brings into the system, especially considering its benefits and financial costs, what is it known as cost-effectiveness analysis (i.e., looking at the incremental cost-effectiveness ratio, ICER). Besides to consider costs and effectiveness (i.e., the effects of HT in real life), HTA include in their analysis, insofar as possible, information on organizational impact (i.e., how the technology is going to impact the current provision of care), patient impact (i.e., how the HT is going to impact the quality of life of the patient and in its relations with his/her environment), and ethical, legal, and social consequences of using the HT. Moreover, sometimes it gives guidance on where and how the HT should be implemented in clinical practice (Goodman 2014). To notice that the comprehensive amount of information that HTA embraces make it different from the evidence requirements asked by regulatory agencies when granting the market access for a HT, which are mainly based in looking at the safety (i.e., HT is not going to incur in an unacceptable risk for patients) and efficacy (i.e., benefits from the HT in "ideal"/"controlled" conditions of practice). Figure 1 depicts the differences in informational requirements from regulatory agencies and HTA agencies; it also

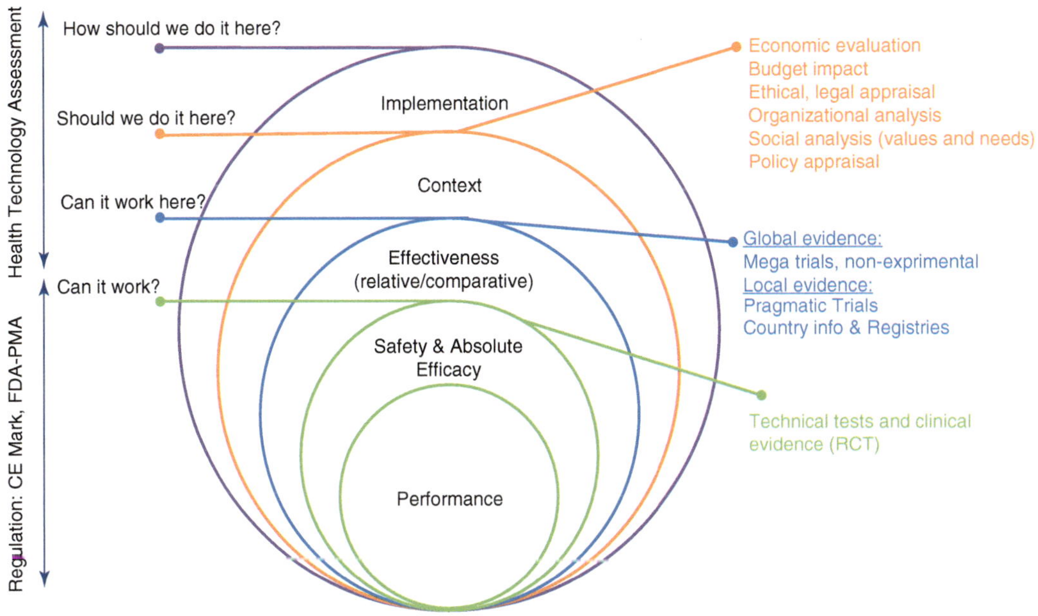

Fig. 1 The path for the assessment of health technologies

shows the sources where information is obtained. Although ideally an HTA report would have to include all the steps and information shown in Fig. 1, the real world make that this happens in few occasions. This is so because decision-makers not always asked for all these information, moreover since the main feature of HTA is that considers the context where the decision should be taken (Sampietro-Colom 2012; Kidholm et al. 2015), different healthcare context ask for different types of information or conducts the assessment process differently. For example, in France, the organization in charge for assessing HTs (i.e., HAS) look first at the effectiveness of the HT; if the available data is not good enough, they do not look at the cost aspects. For the contrary, in the United Kingdom, the organization in charge of doing the assessments (i.e., NICE) performs directly a cost-effectiveness analysis comparing the effects and the cost of the new HT with the current standard of care (Oortwijn 2017).

Given the wide scope of HTA, it needs to be a systematic interdisciplinary process based on scientific evidence and other type of information (Health Technology Assessment 2009). HTA aims to achieve this by producing, critically appraising, and synthesizing relevant evidence. Such evidence may derive from various sources, e.g., randomized controlled trials (RCTs) and clinical registries, and entail the use of both, qualitative and quantitative research methods (Bailar and Mosteller 1992).

In their process to elaborate the HTA report, a wide range of professionals such as clinicians, nurses, economists, social scientists, ethicists, public health and health services researchers and, more and more, patients and their relatives are included. The most frequent activity and product of HTA has traditionally been the systematic review of published evidence regarding the HT, and cost-effectiveness analysis also based on published data (Goodman 2014). Nevertheless, more and more HTA is being introduced in prospective clinical studies, which collect information in all the aspects required to inform a decision in a specific context (Zboromyrska et al. 2016).

As mentioned before, HTA is aimed to advice and influence decision-making. HTA since its origins, in the 80s decade, was devoted to inform coverage and reimbursement decisions. Nevertheless,

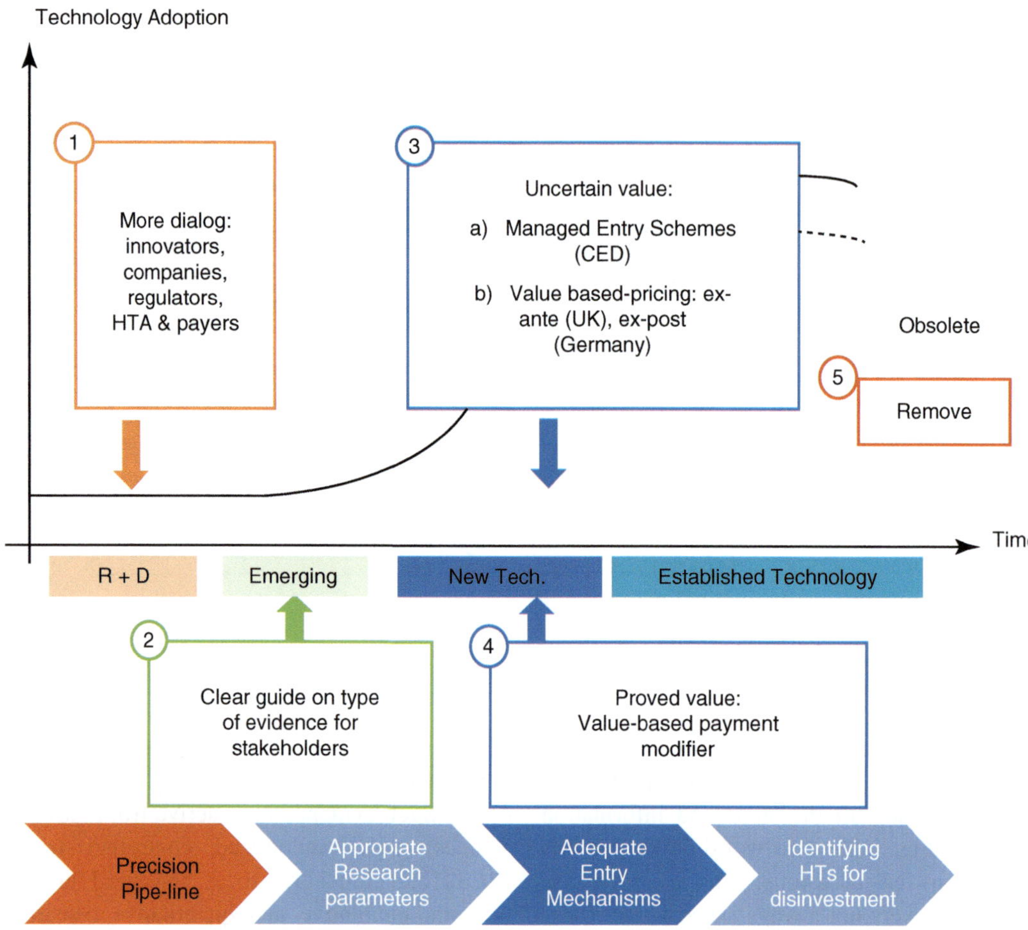

Fig. 2 Use of HTA in the life cycle of health technologies and in the decisions across development

currently HTA is used along the life cycle of the HT to either inform early decisions about whether to pursue development of a HT in the stage of R&D, to later decisions on disinvestment of HT (Facey et al. 2015; Henshall et al. 2012). Figure 2 shows the uses of HTA along the lifecycle of a HT and across the several decisions that should be made in their development.

The use of HTA around the world is continuously expanding. Nowadays, the International Network of Agencies for Health Technology Assessment (INHTA) includes 47 public HTA organizations from all the continents. These are mainly governmental agencies. Besides there are a growing trend to establish hospital-based HTA units (HB-HTA) around the world (Sampietro-Colom and Martin 2016). Moreover, the use of HTA when deciding the added value of HT is being strongly promoted by the European Union and the World Health Organization (WHO). The former has formally established an HTA Network that is aimed to fulfil the Directive 2011/24/EU which enforces to use HTA before introducing innovative technologies in Europe (Health Technology Assessment Network 2017). Additionally, the 67th world health assembly approved a resolution in May 2014 urging member States "to consider establishing national systems of health intervention and technology assessment, encouraging the systematic utilization of independent health intervention and technology assessment in support of universal health coverage to inform policy decisions, including priority-setting, selection, procurement supply system management and use of health interventions and/or technologies, as well as the formulation of sustainable financing benefit packages, medicines, benefits management including pharmaceutical formularies, clinical practice guidelines and protocols for public health programmes" (WHA67.23 2014). Finally, HTA is also being grounded in the USA through the enforcement of comparative-effectiveness research (Riaz et al. 2011).

The current paradigm of evidence-based policy and clinical decision-making requires that the potential value of any specific healthcare technology be defined and operationalized through an HTA. In addition, it requires an understanding of the factors that jointly determine a healthcare technology's actual value in a specific context. Both of these—how should value be defined and what factors seem to determine a healthcare technology's actual value in a specific context—are highly relevant to the HTA of imaging technologies.

2 HTA and Diagnostic Imaging

2.1 Recognizing the Challenges

New diagnostic imaging technologies, as any HT in the era of evidence-based decision-making, need to prove what added value brings to what it is already in place. Nevertheless, worth to mention that to assess diagnostic imaging technologies is more complex than assessing treatments. Metrics for assessing the effectiveness of treatments usually include surrogate outcomes (e.g., bone mass levels) and end-point outcomes (e.g., clinical morbidity, functional status, quality of life, and mortality) and usually a direct relationship between the treatment and the result can be established. For diagnostic imaging technologies there is not such a direct relationship between their use and final patient outcomes; its final impact in patient outcomes depends on the effect of the clinical intervention selected from the information provided by the diagnostic image (Fryback and Thornbury 1991). Therefore, one challenge for assessing diagnostic imaging technologies is the need to evaluate the technology in the context of its effect on the pathway of care, which makes the assessment more complex. Moreover, it is not always obvious where in the care pathway the diagnostic technology is best placed, which require evaluating different strategies. Additionally, since diagnostic tests are frequently done in conjunction with other tests or measurements, it is the composite of the results from the series of tests that is used in decision-making and, therefore, what should be assessed. Another challenge deals with the fact that diagnostic technologies, especially those based on electronics, often change rapidly as new methods, upgrades, and capabilities are added. This situation poses difficulties when looking for the right comparator for the assessment (i.e., risk of outdated comparisons). Comparisons are also challenged by machine and inter-reader variability, and operator learning curves which impact on diagnostic performance and, finally, in outcomes (Gazelle et al. 2011).

2.2 Assessing the Value of Medical Imaging Technology

Although challenges for assessing diagnostic imaging technologies exist as mentioned above, frameworks for assessing their value have been in place for long time. The most used framework dates from 1991 (Fryback and Thornbury 1991) and includes six progressive levels of efficacy assessment: level (1) technical efficacy (e.g., imaging resolution); level (2) diagnostic accuracy efficacy (e.g., test sensitivity/specificity); level (3) diagnostic thinking efficacy (e.g., pre- and post-test changes in subjective determined outcome); level (4) therapeutic efficacy (e.g., effects of diagnostic on choice of therapy); level (5) patient outcome efficacy (e.g., value of test information including measures of morbidity, quality of life, and mortality); level (6) societal efficacy (e.g., cost-effectiveness analysis from societal point of view). This framework was mainly addressed to be guidance for making decisions on the type or characteristics of the research needed for assessing the value of a specific technology.

Building on this framework, the Working Group on Comparative Effectiveness Research for Imaging has recently developed taxonomy for classifying diagnostic imaging technologies according to the extent of outcomes data needed for determining their added value (Gazelle et al. 2011). The taxonomy is based in three pillars, which are: (1) size of the at-risk population (i.e., number of people affected by the technology); (2) anticipated clinical impact (i.e., expected net health benefits compared with the standard of care); and (3) potential economic impact (i.e., unit cost downstream healthcare cost, and relative cost of the technology compared with standard of care). Each of these three pillars has three levels of impact: small, medium, large. The combination of the pillars and their levels determines the characteristics and robustness of data and outcomes requirements to prove the added value of the technology. For example, the higher the population at risk and the smaller the anticipated clinical impact the higher level and robustness of outcome data required. The data and outcomes considered in this taxonomy relates to the six levels of efficacy assessment mentioned above. To mention, that the type of outcomes considered relevant can differ substantially depending on the type of decision-maker looking at the value of the technology. Regulators, politicians, healthcare managers, clinicians, and patients can all have different requirements for the type of data and outcomes they consider relevant. This is very important to take into account when designing original research studies as well as when synthesizing the available evidence for testing the added value of a technology. Involvement of all relevant stakeholders is highly advisable to look at the most appropriate outcomes to include in the assessment.

Traditionally, the value of imaging technology has been defined in terms of its capacity to accurately distinguish between persons who do, and persons who do not have a particular condition of interest. Key parameters to express such diagnostic performance are sensitivity, specificity, positive and negative predictive value, and likelihood ratio. Such measures determine to what extent prior probability of disease is affected as the result of diagnostic test information.

Increasingly, however, such diagnostic test parameters are considered surrogate endpoints, and patient outcome is considered the key parameter of interest (Schünemann et al. 2008). In other words, the value of a diagnostic test cannot be inferred from its capacity to establish or exclude disease, but from patient outcome: how does using the diagnostic test improve the prognosis of patients? Clearly, this requires a different study design to produce the requisite data. Classical diagnostic test research requires a systematic comparison of results of an index test with results of a reference test (gold standard). Data are analyzed through cross-tabulation, yielding parameters such as sensitivity and specificity and positive and negative predictive values. When patient outcome is used as a criterion for a diagnostic test's value, an RCT is required, randomly allocating eligible patients to two or more different diagnostic trajectories, followed by clinical management on the basis of these trajectories. Patients are then followed up for sufficiently long periods of time to allow to decide whether the different diagnostic trajectories translate into clinically meaningful and statistically significant differences between the groups of patients. Recent examples of such RCTs include the studies of computed tomographic angiography in patients with clinically suspected coronary disease (Douglas et al. 2015; Newby et al. 2015; see Table 1 for a summary of these trials).

An advantage of this approach is that it also allows for assessment of other endpoints, such as cost-effectiveness of a novel diagnostic test as compared to current diagnostic practice. Another advantage is that there is no need for a gold standard. A possible drawback of this approach is that it represents the combined assessment of a diagnostic test and subsequent clinical management. Theoretically, it is possible that a novel diagnostic test outperforms currently available diagnostic tests, but that this fails to translate into improved clinical outcome because there are insufficient therapeutic opportunities to take advantage of such difference.

Table 1 Examples of recently published findings of RCTs of diagnostic technologies

Reference	Patient population	Comparison	Primary endpoint	Follow-up	Results	Conclusion
Douglas et al. (2015)	Patients with clinical symptoms suggestive of coronary artery disease (mostly chest pain and dyspnea on exertion); $n = 10{,}003$	Coronary computed tomographic angiography (CTA) vs. functional testing (FT); (exercise electrocardiography, nuclear stress testing, or stress echocardiography)	Composite endpoint consisting of death, myocardial infarction, hospitalization for unstable angina, or major procedural complication	Median of 2 years	Occurrence of primary end-point event of 3.3% (CTA) vs. 3.0% (FT); HR = 1.04 (95% CI 0.83–1.29; $p = 0.75$)	In symptomatic patients with suspected CAD who required noninvasive testing, a strategy of initial CTA, as compared with FT, did not improve clinical outcomes over a median follow-up of 2 years
Newby et al. (2015)	Patients with suspected angina from coronary heart disease; $n = 4146$	Standard care plus CTCA vs. standard care alone	Certainty of the diagnosis, change of planned investigations and treatments, 6-week symptom severity, admittance to hospital for chest pain, fatal and non-fatal myocardial infarction	1.7 years	Certainty of CAD increased (RR 2.56; 95% CI 2.33–2.79, $p < 0.0001$); change in planned investigations (15% vs. 1%, $p < 0.0001$) and treatments (23% vs. 5%, $p < 0.0001$); no difference in 6-week symptom severity or in admittance to hospital for chest pain; 38% reduction in fatal and non-fatal myocardial infarction (HR 0·62, 95% CI 0·38–1·01; $p = 0{\cdot}0527$)	In patients with suspected angina due to coronary heart disease, CTCA clarifies the diagnosis, enables targeting of interventions, and might reduce the future risk of myocardial infarction

CTCA computed tomographic coronary angiography, *CTA* computed tomographic angiography, *FT* functional test, *CI* confidence interval, *HR* hazard ratio, *CAD* coronary artery disease, *RR* relative risk

Thus, such trials aim to optimize the entire patient-pathway instead of determining the best possible diagnostic strategy. In that sense, RCTs testing combinations of different diagnostic strategies and successive treatment may be considered truly pragmatic trials: they aim to establish whether different diagnostic strategies result in better outcomes that matter to patients, not in evidence of different diagnostic test performance (Ford and Norrie 2016).

Besides the frameworks proposed by academia, the European Network of Agencies for Health Technology Assessment (EUnetHTA) has also developed the HTA Core Model for Diagnostic Technologies (2008). This Core Model is proposed to standardize the assessment of diagnostic technologies and it is addressed mainly to scientists performing HTA. Nevertheless, this framework could also be a guidance to take into account when designing clinical trials for imaging technologies in order to include all relevant data that will be asked when the HT will want to access the market. This Core Models uses ten main domains of assessment including: (1) current use of technology (implementation level); (2) description and technical characteristics of technology; (3) safety; (4) accuracy; (5) effectiveness; (6) cost (economic evaluation); (7) ethical aspects; (8) organizational aspects; (9) social aspects; (10) legal aspects. For each domain, there are a variable set of topics to consider (e.g., for clinical effectiveness the topic could be life expectancy, or for societal aspects could be ability to work). Moreover, for each topic, there are different issues to take into account or explore (e.g., for the domain on clinical effectiveness and the topic mortality, two issues could be the effect of the intervention on the mortality caused by the target disease and the effect of the intervention on the mortality due to other causes than the target disease).

Public organizations performing HTA (e.g., Governmental agencies, hospitals, universities) have been assessing diagnostic imaging technologies for long time. A research performed under the Euro-Bioimaging Project which include 33 organizations performing HTA from 17 European countries showed their experience in assessing diagnostic images technologies as well as the type of contribution these organizations could provide in a network assessing this type of technologies (Fig. 3). Therefore, considering the existence of available frameworks for assessing diagnostic imaging technologies and the experience and willingness of collaboration from orga-

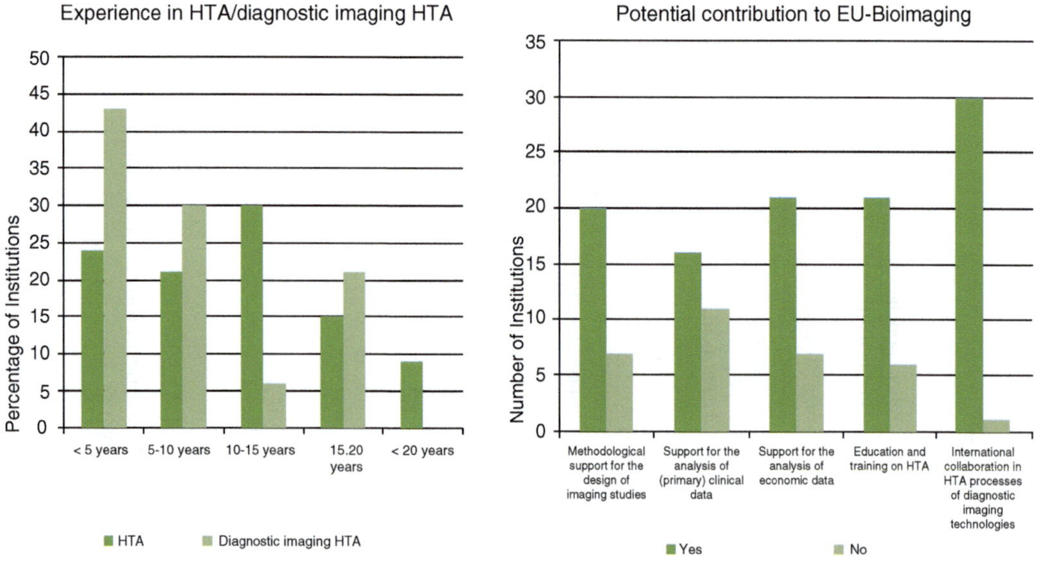

Fig. 3 EU experience in HTA on diagnostic imaging technologies

nizations performing HTA, the assessment of the added value of innovations in the field of diagnostic imaging should become a systematic procedure before their access to the healthcare arena.

2.3 Considering Determinants of Value of Medical Imaging Technology in Daily Practice

It is widely recognized that results from RCTs need not translate into similar results in daily practice. Patients may be selected more carefully, users may be more experienced, or more appropriate action may be taken in case of adverse events in the context of an RCT as compared to daily practice. This definitely also seems to hold with respect to imaging technology. Although the value of specific imaging technologies itself need not be challenged, the overall "community value" is seriously challenged because of suspected wide and systematic over-utilization (Hendee et al. 2010). Average annual growth rates of use of CT of 10.2% (1998–2005) and of 4.2% (2005–2008) among HMO enrolees in the USA have been reported; for MRI, these figures were 14.5% and 6.5%, respectively. Concurrently, associated radiation exposure has increased during this period (Smith-Bindman et al. 2012). An estimated 20–50% of imaging is deemed unnecessary, and imaging is by far the most common service on the list of unnecessary tests and procedures of the Choosing Wisely campaign. In response, professional organizations have started to put more focus on the development of criteria for the appropriate use of imaging technologies (e.g., Carr et al. 2013), which, of course, requires a relevant and reliable evidence base, in conjunction with some form of monitoring (Durand et al. 2015). In the remainder of this chapter, we will present a more detailed example of an RCT of an imaging technology (the SPARTACUS trial, comparing CT scan versus Adrenal Vein Sampling in patients with hypertension due to primary aldosteronism). This will serve as a basis for a discussion of the strengths and weaknesses of such approach, resulting in concrete recommendations for deciding when an RCT might be appropriate to assess the value of medical imaging technology.

3 Case Study: Imaging Versus Functional Testing in Patients with Primary Aldosteronism: The SPARTACUS Trial

The SPARTACUS trial was conducted to assess whether imaging (computed tomography, CT) or functional testing (Adrenal Vein sampling, AVS) is the preferred mode of distinguishing between bilateral adrenal hyperplasia and unilateral aldosterone-producing adenoma in patients with primary aldosteronism (PA) (Dekkers et al. 2016). Increasingly, PA is being recognized as an important cause of hypertension and its squeals (Abad-Cardiel et al. 2013). PA may originate from bilateral adrenal hyperplasia (BAH) or from unilateral adenoma-producing adenoma (APA). Clinically, it is important to distinguish between the two subtypes of PA, since patients with BAH are treated with mineralocorticoid receptor antagonists and patients with APA are offered adrenalectomy. Conventionally, imaging (CT) is used to differentiate between the two subtypes. The limitations of this particular use of CT have been widely recognized (e.g., Patel et al. 2007). On the one hand, the resolution of CT may be insufficient to detect small nodules. On the other hand, it may lead to the detection of non-productive nodules. AVS involves a percutaneous femoral vein approach, taking blood samples from the inferior vena cava and both adrenal veins, allowing for the measurement of aldosterone and cortisol levels at each of these sites (Daunt 2005). Although AVS is less readily available, technically more demanding, more invasive, and more costly than CT, it might still be the preferred option if it would more accurately discriminate between BAH and APA. The SPARTACUS trial was designed to address this issue. In the absence of a gold standard, we chose to conduct an RCT. This allowed us to compare the two diagnostic modalities in terms of their impact on patient outcome (achieving target blood pressure: <135/85 mmHg according to daytime ambulatory blood pressure monitoring). The hypothesis was that if the two diagnostic modalities (imaging (CT) and functional test (AVS)) would differ in their capacity to accurately distinguish between APA and BAH, this would translate into a difference in optimal treatment (adrenalectomy for patients with APA and mineralocorticoid receptor antagonists for patients with BAH), which, in turn, would translate into differences in proportion of patients reaching target blood pressure. However, since the effect of suboptimal treatment of PA may be masked by more intensive antihypertensive medication, the primary endpoint of the study was intensity of antihypertensive medication needed, expressed in daily defined doses (ddd). The trial was designed to achieve a 80% statistical power to detect a difference of 0.8 in ddd between the two groups. All patients were followed up for a period of 1 year. The RCT design also allowed us to assess whether the two diagnostic modalities resulted in differences in quality of life and costs. The trial was an investigator-driven study, conducted at five university-based hospitals in Europe.

At 1 year follow-up, no differences were found between the two groups in terms of median intensity of antihypertensive medication (ddd of 3 in both groups, $p = 0.52$), median number of antihypertensive drugs (2 in both groups, $p = 0.87$), proportion of patients achieving target blood pressure (43% and 45% in the CT group and AVS group, respectively, $p = 0.82$), or median 24 h ambulatory blood pressure (systolic: 127 (IQR: 120–138) vs. 128 (IQR: 121–135) mmHg; diastolic: 80 (IQR: 75–86) vs. 81 (IQR: 76–85) mmHg, in the CT and AVS group, respectively). No difference was found in terms of median quality adjusted life years either (1.29 (IQR: 1.23–1.35) and 1.24 (IQR: 1.18 1.30) in the AVS and CT group, respectively; $p = 0.26$). Median total costs were higher in the AVS group (€6746; IQR 5965–7527) as compared to the CT group (€4228; IQR 3604–4852), $p < 0.001$. Costs included costs of drugs, surgery, AVS, CT, ambulatory visits, and costs associated with complications. These figures translate into a low probability that AVS should be considered a cost-effective alternative to CT in the diagnostic workup of patients with PA, with a probability of 0.02, 0.24, and 0.35 at cost-effectiveness thresholds of €20,000, €50,000, and €80,000 per QALY, respectively.

Although on theoretical grounds AVS might be expected to be superior to CT in distinguishing between patients with BAH and patients with APA, the results of our trial suggest that this may not actually be the case. Although the design of our trial does not allow to draw conclusions regarding the diagnostic performance of the two modalities (accuracy of identifying the two subtypes of PA), the results do suggest that even if there were such a difference, this does not translate into clinically meaningful and statistically significant differences in patient outcomes (blood pressure control, quality of life). Also, from a societal perspective, using AVS instead of CT in the diagnostic workup of patients with PA is unlikely to constitute an efficient use of resources. An RCT, then, although not commonly used in the context of evaluating diagnostic tests, allows for the assessment of a wider scope of outcomes that are arguably relevant from an HTA perspective. A drawback might be, however, the higher costs that are associated with conducting an RCT as compared to conventional diagnostic test research. It would be important, then, to assess upfront whether conducting a specific RCT might be worthwhile. In the following, we will briefly outline a modelling procedure that could be used for such purpose.

4 Value of Information Analysis

Resource scarcity does not only hold for healthcare interventions, it also holds for research into the safety and clinical and cost-effectiveness of those interventions. Spending wisely is not only a mandate for healthcare, it is also a mandate for healthcare research. It would be helpful to assess upfront, then, whether a specific RCT might constitute a worthwhile use of resources. A potentially fruitful approach to this question might be value of information analysis (Keisler et al. 2014). Basically, in this approach, conducting research is a matter of reducing uncertainty. In addition, it is acknowledged that uncertainty can incur certain costs. The approach offers a framework for integrating costs and anticipated benefits (resulting from reducing uncertainty) of conducting a specific study. In the case of AVS and CT in the diagnostic workup of patients with PA, this could work out as follows. At the time, prior to the conduct of the SPARTACUS trial, there was genuine uncertainty regarding the benefits of AVS as compared to CT in the diagnostic workup of patients with PA. Theoretically, AVS could be superior to CT, but there was hardly any evidence to substantiate such claim. In such a situation ("equipoise"), it is defensible to subject half of the patients to AVS, and half of the patients to CT. In the absence of evidence of the comparative value of AVS versus CT, this could mean that there is a 50% probability that patients are subjected to AVS, while it has no added benefit to patients. Likewise, there is a 50% probability that patients are *not* subjected to AVS, while it would confer a benefit to patients. In the former case, a more invasive and (arguably) more expensive diagnostic test is being used, in the absence of an added benefit. In the latter case, costs are incurred because patients are treated suboptimally, resulting in unnecessary persistence of poorly controlled blood pressure and associated cardiovascular events. Conducting a study should result in either reducing or increasing the likelihood that AVS is beneficial to patients. Assuming that clinical practice will be adjusted accordingly (i.e., AVS is offered less, or more, frequently to patients with PA), this would result in a reduction of those costs. This represents the "value of information" in this context. This value can be compared with the costs associated with conducting the trial. Those costs need not be prohibitive, if we may assume that, as long as the evidence has not been produced, it is reasonable that half of the patients would get the experimental procedure, and half of them would not. The incremental costs of conducting a trial would, then, consist of developing a research protocol, obtaining approval from the relevant review boards, developing patient information, setting up an infrastructure for screening, informing and randomly allocating patients, collecting, analyzing, interpreting, and reporting the data. A realistic estimate of such costs would, in case of the SPARTACUS trial (five centers, two European countries, 200 patients, 3 year follow-up) be approximately €650 K. Such costs should be compared with the costs associated with reducing the then existing uncertainty. These can be estimated through modelling, which would, of course, require several assumptions from experts. Scenario analysis could be used to calculate best and worst case scenarios. Important assumptions underlying the value of information approach are the following: (1) the study will, in fact, reduce uncertainty. This assumption critically hinges on the methodological quality of the trial and features such as inclusion of an appropriate trial population, accurate measurement of relevant endpoints, maintenance of randomization throughout a sufficiently long follow-up period (i.e., limited loss to follow-up, limited missing values, limited cross over or contamination, etc.). (2) How the data from a novel trial compare to currently available evidence. (3) Adjustment of clinical practice in accordance with trial results. If the trial results would suggest that AVS has, in fact, added value as compared to CT, capacity for conducting AVS would have to be augmented. If, as was the case, the results of the trial suggested that AVS does not have such added value, the community needs to accept this and revise guidelines and practice accordingly. As already mentioned in the introduction of this chapter, this may prove a considerable challenge (Durand et al. 2015). A further challenge is posed by the rapid pace of technological development: by the time the results of a trial have become available, the technology may have changed in such a way as to make these data of limited relevance (the "moving target problem") (Sorenson et al. 2008). Arguably, these aspects need to be taken into account, alongside the formal value of information analysis.

Conclusion

The HTA of diagnostic imaging poses several challenges. A key problem in recent years has been the indiscriminate use of diagnostic services, rather than the value of those services per se. This has renewed interest in the development of guidelines and in the monitoring of the compliance with those guidelines. Clearly, this requires the availability of evidence that is both, robust and relevant to daily clinical practice. Following recent methodological guidelines (e.g., Schünemann et al. 2008), we have argued that conventional diagnostic test research, resulting in information of diagnostic test characteristics (sensitivity, specificity, etc.) is insufficient to produce such evidence. Instead, RCTs comparing different diagnostic strategies in terms of their impact on clinical outcomes, quality of life, and costs appear to be more useful and capable of producing information that is needed for a comprehensive HTA of medical imaging technologies. A drawback of such studies may be that they are time-consuming and costly. We suggest that a value of information approach may be helpful in deciding whether a particular RCT seems a worthwhile use of R&D resources.

References

Abad-Cardiel M, Alvarez-Álvarez B, Luque-Fernandez L, Fernández C, Fernández-Cruz A, Martell-Claros N (2013) Hypertension caused by primary hyperaldosteronism: increased heart damage and cardiovascular risk. Rev Esp Cardiol (Engl Ed) 66:47–52

Bailar JC III, Mosteller F (1992) Medical technology assessment. In: Medical uses of statistics. NEJM Books, Boston, pp 393–411

Banta DH, Luce BR (1993) Health care technology and its assessment. Oxford University Press, New York, pp 23–57

Carr JJ, Hendel RC, White RD, Patel MR, Wolk MJ, Bettmann MA, Douglas P, Rybicki FJ, Kramer CM, Woodard PK, Shaw LJ, Yucel EK (2013) Appropriate utilization of cardiovascular imaging: a methodology for the development of joint criteria for the appropriate utilization of cardiovascular imaging by the American College of Cardiology Foundation and American College of Radiology. J Am Coll Cardiol 61:2199–2206

Daunt N (2005) Adrenal vein sampling: how to make it quick, easy, and successful. Radiographics 25:S143–S158

Dekkers T, Prejbisz A, Kool LJ, Groenewoud HJ, Velema M, Spiering W, Kołodziejczyk-Kruk S, Arntz M, Kądziela J, Langenhuijsen JF, Kerstens MN, van den Meiracker AH, van den Born BJ, Sweep FC, Hermus AR, Januszewicz A, Ligthart-Naber AF, Makai P, van der Wilt GJ, Lenders JW, Deinum J, SPARTACUS Investigators (2016) Adrenal vein sampling versus CT scan to determine treatment in primary aldosteronism: an outcome-based randomised diagnostic trial. Lancet Diabetes Endocrinol 4:739–746

Douglas PS, Hoffmann U, Patel MR et al., PROMISE Study Investigators (2015) Outcomes of anatomic versus functional testing for coronary artery disease. N Engl J Med 372:1291–1300

Durand DJ, Lewin JS, Berkowitz SA (2015) Medical-imaging stewardship in the accountable care era. New Engl J Med 373:1691–1693

Facey K, Henshall C, Sampietro-Colom L, Thomas S (2015) Improving the effectiveness and efficiency of evidence production for health technology assessment. Int J Technol Assess Health Care 31(4):201–206

Ford I, Norrie J (2016) Pragmatic trials. New Engl J Med 375:454–463

Fryback DG, Thornbury JR (1991) The efficacy of diagnostic imaging. Med Decis Mak 11(2):88–94

Gazelle SG, Kessler L, Lee DW, McGinn T, Menzin J, Neumann P et al (2011) A framework for assessing the value of diagnostic imaging in the era of comparative effectiveness research. Radiology 261(3):692–698

Goodman CS (2014) HTA 101: introduction to health technology assessment. Bethesda, MD: National Library of Medicine (US). https://www.nlm.nih.gov/nichsr/hta101/HTA_101_FINAL_7-23-14.pdf. Accessed 21 Feb 2017

Health Technology Assessment (2009) Int J Technol Assess Health Care 25(Suppl. 1):10

Health Technology Assessment Network (2017). https://ec.europa.eu/health/technology_assessment/policy/network_en. Accessed 3 Mar 2017

Hendee WR, Becker GJ, Borgstede JP et al (2010) Addressing overutilization in medical imaging. Radiology 257:240–245

Henshall C, Schuller T, Mardhani-Bayne L (2012) Using health technology assessment to support optimal use of technologies in current practice: the challenge of "disinvestment". Int J Technol Assess Health Care 28(3):203–210

HTA Core Model for Diagnostic Technologies (2008). http://www.eunethta.eu/outputs/hta-core-model-diagnostic-technologies-10r. Accessed 3 Mar 2017

INAHTA (2017). www.inahta.org. Accessed 21 Feb 2017

Keisler JM, Collier ZA, Chu E, Sinatra N, Linkov I (2014) Value of information analyses: the state of application. Environ Syst Decis 34:3–23

Kidholm K, Olhom AM, Birk-Olsen M, Cicchetti A, Fure B, Halmesmaki E et al (2015) Hospital managers' need for information in decision-making- an interview study in nine European countries. Health Policy 119:1424–1432

Newby D et al., SCOT-Heart Investigators (2015) CT coronary angiography in patients with suspected angina due to coronary heart disease (SCOT-HEART): an open-label, parallel group, multicentre trial. Lancet; 385:2383 2391.

Oortwijn W. (2017) HTA and value: assessing value, making value-based decisions, and sustaining innovation. HTAi Policy Forum background paper. Edmonton: Health Technology Assessment International (HTAi)

Patel SM, Lingam RK, Beaconsfield TI, Tran TL, Brown B (2007) Role of radiology in the management of primary aldosteronism. Radiographics 27:1145–1157

Riaz A, Hanger M, Carino T (2011) Comparative effectiveness research in the United States: a catalyst for innovation. Am Health Drug Benefits 4(2):68–72

Sampietro-Colom L (2012) Consider context and stakeholders. Int J Technol Assess Health Care 28(2):166–167

Sampietro-Colom L, Martin J (eds) (2016) Hospital-based health technology assessment: the next Frontier for health technology assessment. Springer-Verlag, London. 978-3-319-39203-5

Schünemann HJ, Oxman AD, Brozek J, Glasziou P, Jaeschke R, Vist GE, Williams JW Jr, Kunz R, Craig J, Montori VM, Bossuyt P, Guyatt GH (2008) Grading quality of evidence and strength of recommendations for diagnostic tests and strategies. BMJ 17:1106–1110

Smith-Bindman R, Miglioretti DL, Johnson E, Lee C, Feigelson HS, Flynn M, Greenlee RT, Kruger RL, Hornbrook MC, Roblin D, Solberg LI, Vanneman N, Weinmann S, Williams AE (2012) Use of diagnostic imaging studies and associated radiation exposure for patients enrolled in large integrated health care systems, 1996–2010. JAMA 307:2400–2409

Sorenson C, Drummond M, Kanavos P (2008) Ensuring value for money in health care. The role of health technology assessment in the European Union. European Observatory. Observatory Studies Series No. 11. World Health Organization, on behalf of the European Observatory on Health and Systems Policies. www.curo.who.int/pubrequest

WHA67.23 (2014) Health intervention and technology assessment in support of universal health coverage. WHA Resolution; Sixty-seventh World Health Assembly http://apps.who.int/medicinedocs/en/d/Js21463en/. Accessed 3 Mar 2017

Zboromyrska Y, de la Calle C, Soto M, Sampietro-Colom L, Soriano A, Alvarez-Martínez M et al (2016) Rapid diagnosis of staphylococcal catheter-related bacteraemia in direct blood samples by real-time PCR. PLoS One 11(8):e0161684

Index

Med Radiol Diagn Imaging (2018)
DOI 10.1007/978-3-319-42578-8, © Springer International Publishing AG, part of Springer Nature

F

G

H

I

S

GPSR Compliance

The European Union's (EU) General Product Safety Regulation (GPSR) is a set of rules that requires consumer products to be safe and our obligations to ensure this.

If you have any concerns about our products, you can contact us on ProductSafety@springernature.com

In case Publisher is established outside the EU, the EU authorized representative is:

Springer Nature Customer Service Center GmbH
Europaplatz 3
69115 Heidelberg, Germany

Batch number: 10684391

Printed by Printforce, the Netherlands